Cerebrovascular Disease and Dementia

Cerebrovascular Disease and Dementia

Pathology, Neuropsychiatry and Management

Edmond Chiu MBBS DPM FRANZCP AM
Associate Professor in Psychiatry of Old Age, University of Melbourne and Director, Aged Psychiatry Education and Research, St George's Health Service, Melbourne, Australia

Lars Gustafson MD PhD
Department of Psychogeriatrics, University Hospital Lund, Lund, Sweden

David Ames BA MD FRCPsych FRANZCP
Academic Unit for Psychiatry of Old Age, North West Hospital Psychogeriatric Service, Melbourne, Australia

Marshal F Folstein MD
Department of Psychiatry, New England Medical Center, Boston, USA

MARTIN DUNITZ

© Martin Dunitz Ltd 2000

First published in the United Kingdom in 2000 by

Martin Dunitz Ltd
The Livery House
7–9 Pratt Street
London NW1 0AE

Reprinted 2000

All rights reserved. No part of this publication may be reproduced, stored in a retrieval system, or transmitted, in any form or by any means, electronic, mechanical, photocopying, recording, or otherwise, without the prior permission of the publisher or in accordance with the provisions of the Copyright Act 1988 or under the terms of any licence permitting limited copying issued by the Copyright Licensing Agency, 90 Tottenham Court Road, London W1P 0LP.

A CIP record for this book is available from the British Library.

ISBN 1-85317-759-8

Distributed in the United States by:
Blackwell Science Inc.
Commerce Place, 350 Main Street
Malden MA 02148, USA
Tel: 1-800-215-1000

Distributed in Canada by:
Login Brothers Book Company
324 Saltaux Crescent
Winnipeg, Manitoba R3J 3T2
Canada
Tel: 1-204-224-4068

Distributed in Brazil by:
Ernesto Reichmann Distribuidora de Livros, Ltda
Rua Coronel Marques 335, Tatuape 03440-000
Sao Paulo,
Brazil

Composition by Wearset, Boldon, Tyne and Wear.
Printed and bound in Great Britain by Biddles Ltd. Guildford and King's Lynn.

Contents

	Contributors	vii
	Introduction Edmond Chiu	1
1	Historical overview Lars Gustafson	3

Epidemiology

2	Epidemiology of vascular dementia in Europe Ingmar Skoog and Olafur Aevarsson	15
3	Epidemiology of vascular dementia in North America Robin Eastwood	25
4	Epidemiology of vascular dementia in Japan Akira Homma and Kazuo Hasegawa	33
5	Epidemiology of vascular dementia in China Yucun Shen and Xin Yu	47
6	Epidemiology: meta-analysis Anthony F Jorm	55
7	The epidemiology of vascular dementia: an overview and commentary Anthony F Jorm	63

The pathology of cerebrovascular disease – with reference to dementias

8	The neuropathology of vascular dementia Arne Brun	69
9	White matter pathology of vascular dementia Elisabet Englund	77

10 Clinical pathological correlates 85
Lars Gustafson and Ulla Passant

11 Classification and criteria 99
Timo Erkinjuntti

Clinical Features

12 Behavioural neurology of vascular dementia 115
Kjell Martin Moksnes and Anders Wallin

13 Cognition and neuropsychology 131
Tammy M Scott and Marshal F Folstein

Investigations

14 Neuroimaging in vascular dementia 145
John T O'Brien

15 qEEG and dementia with special reference to vascular dementia 165
Ingmar Rosén

Management

16 Medical management 181
Leon Flicker

17 Management of psychiatric disorders 191
David Ames

18 Vascular dementia: consequences for family carers and implications for management 199
Henry Brodaty and Alisa Green

19 The provision of long-term care and the management of behavioural disorders in cerebrovascular disease and dementia 211
Edmond Chiu

20 Prevention 221
Stephen M Davis

Index 235

Contributors

Olafur Aevarsson MD PhD
Landspitalinn-University Hospital
Department of Psychiatry
PO Box 10
IS 121 Reykjavik
ICELAND

David Ames BA MD FRCPsych FRANZCP
Associate Professor of Psychiatry of
Old Age and Consultant Psychiatrist
University of Melbourne Department of
Psychiatry
NorthWestern Health Care Network
Aged Persons Psychiatry Programme
NorthWest Hospital
Parkville, Vic 3052
AUSTRALIA

Henry Brodaty MB BS MD FRACP FRANZCP
Professor of Psychogeriatrics
University of New South Wales and
Director, Academic Department for
Psychogeriatrics
Prince of Wales Hospital
Sydney, NSW 2031
AUSTRALIA

Arne Brun MD PhD
Department of Pathology
University Hospital Lund
SE–221 85 Lund
SWEDEN

Edmond Chiu MBBS DPM FRANZCP AM
Associate Professor in Psychiatry of Old
Age, University of Melbourne and
Director, Aged Psychiatry, Education
and Research
St George's Health Services
Melbourne, Vic 3101
AUSTRALIA

Stephen Davis MD FRACP
Professor and Director of Neurology
Department of Neurology
Royal Melbourne Hospital and
University of Melbourne
Melbourne, Vic 3050
AUSTRALIA

Robin Eastwood MD FRCPC FRCPsych
Professor, Department of Psychiatry
and Public Health
Vice-chair Research, Health Sciences
Center School of Medicine
St Louis University
St Louis, MO 63104
USA

Elisabet Englund MD PhD
Department of Pathology
Division of Neuropathology
University Hospital Lund
SE–221 85 Lund
SWEDEN

Timo Erkinjuntti MD PhD
Chief, Memory Research Unit
Department of Clinical
Neurosciences
Helsinki University Central Hospital
Helsinki
FINLAND

Leon Flicker MB BS PhD FRACP
Professor of Geriatric Medicine
University of Western Australia
Royal Perth Hospital
Perth, WA 6847
AUSTRALIA

Marshal F Folstein MD
Department of Psychiatry
Tufts University School of Medicine
New England Medical Centre
750 Washington Street
Boston, MA 02111
USA

Alisa Green BSc (Psych)
Academic Department for
Psychogeriatrics
Prince of Wales Hospital
Randwick
NSW 2031
AUSTRALIA

Lars Gustafson MD PhD
Department of Psychogeriatrics
University Hospital Lund
SE–221 85 Lund
SWEDEN

Kazuo Hasegawa MD PhD
Vice Executive Director
St Marianna University School of
Medicine
Miyamae-ku
Kawasaki-shi
Kanagawa, 216-8511
JAPAN

Akira Homma MD
Head, Department of Psychiatry
Tokyo Metropolitan Institute of
Gerontology
35-2 Sakaecho
Itabashi-ku
Tokyo 173-0015
JAPAN

Anthony F Jorm PhD DSc
Professor and Deputy Director
National Health and Medical Research
Council
Psychiatric Epidemiology Research
Centre
Australian National University
Canberra, ACT 0200
AUSTRALIA

Kjell Martin Moksnes MD
Head, Department of
Gerontopsychiatry
Clinic of Psychiatry
Ullevaal Hospital
Oslo
NORWAY

John T O'Brien MRCPsych DM
Senior Lecturer in Old Age Psychiatry
Wolfson Research Centre
Institute for the Health of the Elderly
Newcastle General Hospital
Newcastle-upon-Tyne
UK

Ulla Passant MD PhD
Department of Psychogeriatrics
University Hospital Lund
PO Box 638
SE–221 85 Lund
SWEDEN

Ingmar Rosén MD PhD
Division of Clinical Neurophysiology
Department of Clinical Neuroscience
University Hospital Lund
SE–221 85 Lund
SWEDEN

Tammy M Scott PhD
Department of Psychiatry
New England Medical Centre
750 Washington Street
Boston, MA 02111
USA

Yucun Shen MD
Professor of Psychiatry
Institute of Mental Health
Beijing Medical University
51 Hua Yuan Bei Lu
100083 Beijing
People's Republic of China

Ingmar Skoog MD
Department of Psychiatry
Sahlgrenska Hospital
SE–413 45 Göteborg
SWEDEN

Anders Wallin MD PhD
Institute of Clinical Neuroscience
Sahlgrenska University Hospital
SE–431 80 Moelndal
SWEDEN

Xin Yu MD
Consultant Psychiatrist
Institute of Mental Health
Beijing Medical University
51 Hua Yuan Bei Lu
100083 Beijing
People's Republic of China

Introduction

Edmond Chiu

Dementia research has been strongly influenced by the historical distinction between the vascular and degenerative diseases, probably with limiting effects on subclassification in both groups. Alzheimer and Binswanger described the clinical and pathological heterogeneity of dementia caused by vascular disorder. Binswanger was the first to point out the relationship between a slowly progressive, subcortical vascular encephalopathy with local neurological deficits and vascular white matter lesions. In the past 50 years, however, Alzheimer's disease research has dominated the field, pushing dementias with other aetiologies into the background and comparative obscurity. As increasing funds became available for Alzheimer's disease research it increasingly took on a life of its own, to the disadvantage of other dementias.

However, some committed researchers in the area of dementia continued, without the kind of fanfare and media hype which accompanied every small and large 'discovery' in the study of Alzheimer's disease, to labour away in studying clinical, biological, nosological and psychosocial domains.

Epidemiological studies continued to be performed and revealed conflicting patterns of prevalence, with Asian countries like China and Japan showing a larger proportion of dementia of vascular origin than Alzheimer's disease. The attempt to standardize classification brought forward sets of criteria with some international consensus.

Clinicians and pathologists, especially from Lund led by Gustafson and Brun, revealed white matter lesions as important in the pathological process. At the same time they identified the role of hypoperfusion and episodic postural hypotension as significant risk factors. The concept of incomplete white matter infarction was clarified with important clinical and pathological correlations.

Cognitive neuropsychology has made some headway in beginning to clarify the neuropsychological expressions of a heterogeneous subgroup of dementias with vascular aetiology. Such understanding contributes to more rational interpretation of neuropsychiatric expressions, while neuropathology and neuropsychology combine to provide a more focused exploration of disabilities and advance strategies for the management of the ravages of cerebrovascular disease and dementia.

The advances in neuroimaging techniques and quantitative EEG in recent years have provided new tools in the clarification of, by indirect non-invasive methodologies, in vivo abnormalities linked with clinical correlates, thus avoiding problems inherent in post-mortem methods of clinical pathological examination.

Prevention of mortality and the reduction of damaging effects of cerebrovascular disease are becoming increasingly possible and are well supported by quality evidence. Whether such preventions will in future reduce or increase consequent dementia awaits further longitudinal research.

Medical treatment, psychiatric disorders, family care burden and the provision of long-term care are matters which daily confront the clinician and society. Consideration of these aspects is frequently avoided in texts. This volume has deliberately addressed these questions to provide a more holistic view of people who have dementia with a cerebrovascular aetiology.

The chapters in this book provide up-to-date discussions of all these very relevant aspects of cerebrovascular disease and dementia. While the term 'VAD' is used in this text, the editors are conscious that nomenclature may change in the future as vascular factors are now also being increasingly identified with Alzheimer's disease pathology. The use of the title 'Cerebrovascular Disease and Dementia' is an attempt to move the concept away from the restrictive view that currently exists in the dominant categorical nosological system to broader-based aetiological considerations that link cerebrovascular diseases to the resultant morbidity of dementia as a general syndrome.

The editors offer this text with the hope that it encourages each reader to explore further the biopsychosocial domains of patients whose dementia has a background of cerebrovascular disease.

1
Historical overview

Lars Gustafson

Cerebral vascular disease holds a position as a major cause of neurological disability and mental disorder, especially in old age with a wide spectrum of psychiatric manifestations such as delirium, dementia, personality change, affective disorder, hallucinations, paranoia, and other psychotic reactions as well as circumscribed cognitive deficits such as dysphasia, dysmnesia and dyspraxia. This chapter focuses upon the historical background of the distinction and classification of dementia syndromes, caused by vascular lesions of the brain, here called vascular dementia (VAD). Dementia, derived from the Latin '*de mens*', 'without mind' is an acquired clinical syndrome, by definition of long duration and usually progressive. The word dementia has, however, been given different meanings in different contexts. It may denote a clinical syndrome, irrespective of aetiology, but also imply that the aetiology of this syndrome is organic brain disease. Moreover, dementia may be used in a wider sense, describing the underlying brain disease from its early, subtle manifestations to the advanced stage of severe deterioration. Dementia was long considered to be irreversible, although this nihilistic view was open to criticism.[1] Terms such as treatable and reversible dementia and dysmentia[2] have been suggested to emphasize the aetiological and clinical heterogeneity and the possibility of treatment and prevention.

The classification of dementia has developed, based on accumulating evidence of clinicopathological entities, and presumed aetiological factors. Apoplexy, with acute effects on consciousness and motor function, was a well-known clinical phenomenon from antiquity, and so were its sequels, such as paresis and changes of mentation and behaviour. Haemorrhage long remained the dominant pathophysiological explanation of stroke until, in the eighteenth century, a pathological subdivision corresponding to haemorrhage and infarction was offered. The early nineteenth century saw the introduction of the concept of 'softening' and its association to arterial occlusion and infarction in stroke.[3] Attention was also drawn to a prodromal phase of apoplexy with symptoms such as headache and dizziness. The association between apoplexy and cardiac disease was analysed, as was also the relationship between cerebral lesions and cognitive impairment and various emotional and cognitive disturbances. In 1854, in a classification of mental diseases,[4] Baillager separated *paralysie générale* from *démence incoherente* and *démence simple*, the latter two labelled 'incurable diseases'. Kahlbaum, in his influential clinical textbook of 1863,[5] described *vesania progressiva apoplectica,* as well as *dementia paralytica, dementia aquisita,* and *presbyophrenia.* The importance of vascular occlusions in apoplectic dementia (démence apoplectique), was emphasized by Ball and Chambard in 1881,[6] in an encyclopaedia on medical science. Kraepelin,[7] in the 1896 edition of his psychiatric textbook, separated the organic brain syndromes into diffuse and localized brain diseases and dementia was considered to be mainly associated with ageing. This perspective was modified by the work of Alzheimer and others, and in the 1910 edition of his textbook, Kraepelin[8] introduced Alzheimer's disease (AD) as a presenile dementia. Cerebral arteriosclerosis, was, however, considered the major cause of organic dementia, and post-apoplectic and arteriosclerotic dementia were used as synonyms.

Dementia research has been strongly influenced by the historical distinction between vascular and degenerative diseases, probably with limiting effects on the subclassification in both groups. The unitary view of apoplectic and arteriosclerotic dementia was challenged in the late nineteenth century, when new histopathological techniques made it possible to speculate on independent circulatory and degenerative changes behind the development of organic dementia. The contributions of Alzheimer and Binswanger revealed the clinical and pathological heterogeneity of dementia caused by vascular disorder. Binswanger,[9] was the first to point out the relationship between a slowly progressive, subcortical vascular encephalopathy (PSVE), with focal neurological deficits and vascular white matter lesions. The neuropathological account, given by Alzheimer,[10] generally substantiated Binswanger's observations. Alzheimer further developed the subclassification of VAD cerebral disorders into arteriosclerotic brain atrophy, PSVE, dementia apoplectica and perivascular gliosis. Binswanger's disease (BD) and subcortical arteriosclerotic encephalopathy became alternative designations of PSVE. Olzewski,[11] Jellinger and Neumayer[12] and others have reviewed the clinical materials, and further contributed to the clinical and pathological description of BD.[13–18] The term 'Binswanger's disease' has been criticized and a change to a more descriptive term, such as 'leukoaraiosis', has been suggested.[19] The previous opinion that BD is a rare form of dementia has however changed, due to improved radiological diagnosis based on computed tomography (CT) and magnetic resonance imaging (MRI) and post-mortem studies in different countries.[20–23]

The view of dementia as due as to 'chronic, global ischaemia' caused by gradual strangulation of blood supply to the brain was favoured by many, although not without questioning. There is, however, little evidence that hypertension or arteriosclerosis per se lead to cognitive decline, although the probability of reduced reserve capacity due to subclinical brain lesions has been suggested.[24] In 1974, Hachinski et al[25] introduced the term 'multi-infarct dementia' (MID) to stress the relationship between this type of progressive dementia and multiple cerebral infarcts. The clinical picture in MID was similar to the early description of arteriosclerotic brain atrophy and PSVE, by Alzheimer,[10] and in many textbooks thereafter. The ischaemic score (IS) that was originally developed as a clinical tool to aid in the differentiation between MID and AD[26] and to study cerebral blood flow in dementia is based on the classical description of arteriosclerotic psychosis in the textbook *Clinical Psychiatry* by Mayer-Gross et al.[27] The IS has been analysed and modified in a large number of studies,[28] but the original version is still the most widely used diagnostic tool in research and clinical practice.[29,30]

The understanding of cerebrovascular factors in dementia has been influenced by the evolving knowledge of the complex metabolic, chemical and neurogenic control of the cerebral blood flow (CBF) and metabolism.[31,32] Normally, the autoregulation achieves constant blood flow, in spite of marked blood pressure variations, but above and below certain limits the autoregulation breaks down and the CBF follows the systemic blood pressure passively. Hypertension predisposes to different types of arterial lesions and epidemiological studies have found hypertension a risk factor, in both VAD and AD.[33,34] The relationship between hypertension, changes of baroreceptor pharmacological blood pressure reduction and cognitive decline in ageing and dementia is currently under debate.[35,36] Reduction of systolic blood pressure below the autoregulatory range may cause hypoperfusion and ischaemia, especially in border zones and vulnerable areas.[37-39] The importance of changes in the regulation of blood pressure is supported by the increasing prevalence of low and labile blood pressure at a late stage of VAD and AD[40] and a positive association between cognitive performance and blood pressure after the age of 75 has been reported.[41]

Dementia, however, is not a compulsory consequence of stroke.[42,43] It is related to the localization and severity of the ischaemic lesions,[44] and also to the patient's age and the possibility of multiple aetiologies with contributions from trauma, degeneration and nutritional deficiency.[23,43] Tomlinson et al[45] considered a total infarction volume of about 100 ml as the limit beyond which dementia is a regular sequel. However, much smaller volumes of infarction have been reported in VAD, especially when the lesions were bilateral or predominant in the speech dominant hemisphere.[46,47] Dementia is sometimes caused by small and few, even single, infarcts due to the strategic position of the lesion. This type of strategic infarct dementia (SID), an eponym suggested by Brun and Gustafson,[48] may follow from, for example, bilateral thalamic infarction and lesion in the angular gyrus, hippocampus, the cingulate gyrus and basal forebrain.

The interest in the role of white matter lesions in VAD increased greatly during the 1980s because of a series of clinicopathological diagnostic imaging studies of this white matter disease (WMD).[37,49-53] Descriptive terms such as leukoaraiosis (LA) from the Greek *leukos* (white) and *araios* (rarefied), white matter low attenuation (WMLA) leukoencephalopathy and 'periventricular white matter lesions' were introduced for these pathologies detectable with CT and MRI. The histopathological account of these changes, also called 'selective incomplete white matter infarction' (SIWI), showed demyelinization and rarefaction in deep hemispheric regions.[37,51,54] WMD is common in vascular and degenerative dementia, and with increasing prevalence in normal ageing. Two-thirds of all AD cases[37] and almost all MID cases show white matter ischaemic lesions. They also appear in a pure form, often with frontal predominance and clinical similarity to frontotemporal dementia (FTD).[55] The current opinion is that WMD is due to stenosing small vessel disease confined to the white matter in combination with systemic hypotension and heart disease,[56,57] although other vascular and biochemical factors have also been emphasized.[58,59] Against this background it has been suggested that VAD should be redefined, with more emphasis on identification of the vascular mechanisms that contribute to cognitive impairment in dementia.

Previously no simple genetic pattern of inheritance was discerned for cerebrovascular disease and dementia, although close relatives to patients with stroke-associated dementia showed a somewhat higher risk for this disease.[60,61] Familial causes of stroke such as homocysteinuria and Icelandic and Dutch types of amyloidosis of brain vessels have however been identified,[62,63] and linked to specific mutations in chromosome 20 and 21.[64,65] Several families have been described where consecutive generations have had a particular syndrome which is characterized by subcortical ischaemic strokes and identified by MRI, dementia with frontal-type features, recurrent attacks of migraine and mood disturbances. This 'cerebral autosomal dominant arteriopathy with subcortical infarcts and leukoencephalopathy' (CADASIL) has recently been mapped to chromosome 19.[66] It was probably first described as 'Binswanger's disease with a rapid course in two sisters' in 1955,[67] and known by other eponyms, such as hereditary multi-infarct dementia[68] and chronic, familial, vascular encephalopathy. These genetic findings clearly indicate a future approach to classification of VAD and treatment.

The introduction of new techniques for measuring cerebral metabolism and blood flow in the 1960s, and of cranial CT scanning in the late 1970s, made it possible to visualize focal and diffuse brain pathology in dementia. With the 133-xenon clearance technique developed by Lassen and Ingvar[69] it became possible to show the significant correlations between the regional cerebral blood flow (rCBF) and the clinical picture and cognitive impairment, and between ante-mortem rCBF diagnoses and post-mortem neuropathological findings in dementia.[70] More recently, positron emission tomography (PET), single photon emission computerized tomography (SPECT) and MRI have offered three-dimensional functional imaging of organic and non-organic mental diseases. Numerous studies have been performed in patients with stroke and ischaemic brain lesions, for differential diagnosis between VAD and other organic dementias and dementia-like syndromes caused by non-organic mental disease.[71] Most studies have shown a decreased CBF level in organic dementia, but inconsistent results have been reported regarding differences between VAD and degenerative dementia and sometimes striking discrepancies between brain imaging pathology and its clinical consequences. Common findings in VAD are spotty and asymmetrical focal flow pathology and more diffuse white matter flow and metabolic changes. Repeated measurements often reveal variations in the extent and localization of pathology including periods of improvement, indicating the dynamics of infarct development and the functional association between cortical and subcortical structures.[72] Structural and functional abnormalities may or may not be co-localized and the distribution of functional abnormality may exceed that of brain damage shown with neuropathological and morphological brain imaging techniques.[73]

The advances in knowledge of the aetiology, pathogenesis and haemodynamic factors in cerebrovascular disease have gradually led to a more positive attitude to the prevention, treatment and rehabilitation of the various types of VAD, considering the broad spectrum of primary deficits, secondary emotional reactions and various complications to the underlying cerebrovascular disease. Larger longitudinal treatment studies of anticoagulants, antiplatelet agents, neuroprotectives, blood pressure regulating drugs and vascular surgery have been performed. A major problem in these treatment studies, as also in epidemiological studies of VAD, is the difficulty in description and classification of the patient sample. In spite of improved clinical diagnosis with brain imaging, there is an urgent need for pathological evaluation of the ante-mortem clinical diagnosis in these studies. The reduced number of post-mortem examinations reported in most countries has become a serious threat to the evaluation of well-grounded therapeutic trials.

Cardiac disease and arrythmias are powerful risk factors for stroke.[39,74-76] The co-existence of multiple aetiologies, especially the interaction between cerebrovascular and cardiac diseases, in the evolution of VAD was recognized early. The incidence of both types of diseases increases with age, and hypertension and diabetes predispose to both. The reciprocal influence between brain and heart is further indicated by the fact that cardiac arrythmia may result from paroxysmal brain activity.[77] The clinical importance of cardiogenic dementia has been strongly indicated by the establishment of work groups and international trials with a focus on thrombo-embolism in atrial fibrillation.[78,79]

The association between cerebrovascular disease and affective disorder was pointed out early on, and a direct aetiological link was

8 Cerebrovascular Disease and Dementia

suggested by Post,[80] who found a close time relation between the first cerebrovascular incident and the onset of affective symptoms. Folstein et al[81] reported an increased prevalence of depression in stroke patients compared to other patient groups with significant physical disabilities. During the 1980s several studies found evidence that the severity of depression, following stroke, was directly correlated to the closeness of the lesion to the frontal pole.[82] Moreover, a predominance of vascular lesions in the left frontal lobe, the anterior thalamus and hemispheric functional asymmetry in organic affective states was pointed out,[83-85] although mood disorder is also found in patients with other localization of vascular damage. The 'vascular depression' concept has been introduced,[86] emphasizing the clinical importance and the need for further research in this area.

Of clinical and principal interest is a group of unusual dementias, caused by infections and inflammatory vascular disease, some of them treatable and reversible. This group contains such diseases as systemic lupus erythematosus (SLE), giant cell arteritis, polymyalgia rheumatica, polyarteritis nodosa and Bürgers disease. There is clinical evidence of CNS involvement, primarily vascular with degeneration of collagen and inflammatory changes in small arteries and arterioles in 50–70% of all SLE cases, and responsible for the so-called steroid-sensitive dementias.[87,88]

In spite of the early achievements in the subclassification of VAD, most textbooks have favoured a mainly homogeneous concept lately called VAD. In 1988 a classification on clinical and patho-anatomical basis was suggested, adding SID, SIWI and small vessel infarct disease to the repertoire.[48] The responsibility for the principles of diagnostic classifications has been mainly taken over by international and national organizations and work groups. DSM-III-R,[89] published in 1987, recognized the clinical picture and risk factors in MID. The DSM-IV of 1994[90] has kept this unitarian view of MID, now called VAD, with a subclassification based on 'predominant clinical features', such as delirium, delusion or depression. The ICD-10,[91] published in 1993, offers 'vascular (former arteriosclerotic) dementia', which in addition to MID includes such entities as 'VAD of acute onset', 'subcortical VAD', 'mixed cortical and subcortical VAD', 'other VAD' and 'VAD unspecified'. Subcortical VAD with diffuse demyelination may also be called Binswanger's disease. Moreover, the common co-existence with AD is pointed out.

In 1990 (published in English in 1994), a Swedish consensus group developed principles for ante-mortem diagnosis of dementia diseases, according to the predominant clinical features and type and localization of the brain disease.[92]

The first set of criteria for the diagnosis of ischaemic VAD (IVD) was proposed by the state of California's Alzheimer's Disease Diagnostic and Treatment Centers (ADDTC), which in 1992 described probable, possible and definite IVD and mixed dementia.[93] VAD was also defined, in terms of brain imaging, thereby widening the concept to include MID, 'single stroke dementia' and BD. The NINDS-AIREN criteria, developed in 1991 and published 2 years later,[94] elaborated on the causality between cerebrovascular disease and symptoms of dementia. It emphasizes the need for clinical and neuroimaging criteria for early and specific diagnosis of probable, possible and definite VAD with the ambition to facilitate treatment, prevention and epidemiological research.

The number of attempts to provide a lasting classification of mental deterioration, dementia, associated with cerebrovascular disease illustrates the inconsistency and limitations of the present terminology. The validity of the diagnosis VAD is often challenged, and alternatives such as 'vascular cognitive impairment' have been suggested.[95] The different views of the concept of VAD and the presence of vascular factors in almost all types of organic dementia show the need for a flexible multi-dimensional classification system, keeping apart predominant clinical syndromes and predominant aetiology, thereby strongly encouraging aetiology- and treatment-oriented attitudes.[96]

References

1. Critchley M, *The Parietal Lobes* (Edward Arnold: London, 1953).

2. Chiu E, What's in a name—dementia or dysmentia? *Int J Ger Psych* (1994) **9**:1–4.

3. Abercrombie J, *Pathological and Practical Researches on Diseases of the Brain and the Spinal Cord* (Waugh & Innes: Edinburgh, 1828).

4. Baillager M, *Maladies Mentales. Essai de Classification* (Librairie de Victor Masson: Paris, 1854).

5. Kahlbaum K, *Die Gruppirung der Psychischen Krankheiten und die Einteilung der Seelenstörungen* (AW Kafemann: Danzig, 1863).

6. Ball B, Chambard E, Déménce apoplectique. In: Dechambre A, Lereboullet L, eds, *Dictionnaire Encyclopédique des Sciences Médicales* (Masson: Paris, 1881) 581–5.

7. Kraepelin E, *Psychiatrie: Ein Lehrbuch für Studirende und Aerzte*, 5th edn (Verlag von Johann Ambrosius Barth: Leipzig, 1896).

8. Kraepelin E, *Klinische Psychiatri* (Barth: Leipzig, 1910).

9. Binswanger O, Die Abgrenzung der allgemeinen progressiven Paralyse, *Berl Klin Wochenschr* (1894) **31**:1103–5, 1137–9, 1180–6.

10. Alzheimer A, Neuere Arbeiten über die Dementia senilis und die auf atheromatöser Gefässerkrankung basierenden Gehirnkrankheiten, *Monatschr Psychiatrie Neurol* (1898) **3**:101–15.

11. Olzewski J, Subcortical arteriosclerotic encephalopathy; review of the literature on the so-called Binswanger's disease and presentation of two cases, *World Neurol* (1962) **3**:359–75.

12. Jellinger K, Neumayer E, Progressive subcorticale vasculäre Encephalopathie Binswanger, *Arch Psychiatr Nervenkr* (1964) **205**:523–54.

13. Delay J, Brion S, *Les Démences Tardives* (Masson: Paris, 1962).

14. Janota I, Dementia, deep white

matter damage and hypertension: Binswanger's disease, *Psychol Med* (1981) **11**:39–48.

15. Tomonaga M, Yamanouchi H, Tohgi H, Kameyama M, Clinicopathologic study of progressive subcortical vascular encephalopathy (Binswanger type) in the elderly, *J Am Geriatr Soc* (1982) **30**:524–9.

16. Dubas F, Gray F, Roullet E, Escourelle R, Leucoencéphalopathies artériopathiques, *Rev Neurol (Paris)* (1985) **141**:93–108.

17. Ishii N, Nishihara Y, Imamura T, Why do frontal lobe symptoms predominate in vascular dementia with lacunes? *Neurology* (1986) **36**:340–5.

18. Fredriksson K, Brun A, Gustafson L, Pure subcortical arteriosclerotic encephalopathy (Binswanger's disease): a clinicopathologic study. Part 1: Clinical features, *Cerebrovasc Disord* (1992) **2**:87–92.

19. Pantoni L, Garcia JH, The significance of cerebral white matter abnormalities 100 years after Binswanger's report, *Stroke* (1995) **26**:1293–301.

20. Roman GC, The identity of lacunar dementia and Binswanger's disease, *Med Hypotheses* (1985) **16**:389–91.

21. Roman GC, Why not Binswanger's disease? *Ann Neurol* (1988) **45**: 141–2.

22. Bennett DA, Wilson RS, Gilley DW, Fox JH, Clinical diagnosis of Binswanger's disease, *J Neurol, Neurosurg Psychiatry* (1990) **53**:961–5.

23. Brun A, Vascular dementia: pathological findings. In: Burns A, Levy R, eds, *Dementia* (Chapman & Hall: London,1994) 653–63.

24. Salerno J, Grady C, Mentis M et al, Brain metabolic function in older men with chronic essential hypertension, *J Gerontol* (1995) **3**:M147–M154.

25. Hachinski VC, Lassen NA, Marshall J, Multi-infarct dementia. A cause of mental deterioration in the elderly, *Lancet* (1974) **ii**:207–10.

26. Hachinski V C, Iliff L D, Zilkha E et al, Cerebral blood flow in dementia, *Arch Neurol* (1975) **32**:632–7.

27. Mayer-Gross W, Slater E, Roth N, *Clinical Psychiatry*, 2nd edn (Bailliere, Tindall & Carsell: London, 1969).

28. Gustafsson L, Nilsson L, Differential diagnosis of presenile dementia on clinical grounds, *Acta Psychiatr Scand* (1982) **65**:194–209.

29. Dening TR, Berrios GE, The Hachinski Ischemic Score: a reevaluation, *Int J Geriatr Psych* (1992) **7**:585–9.

30. Maroney JT, Bagiella E, Desmond VC, Meta-analysis of the Hachinski Ischemic Score in pathologically verified dementias, *Neurology* (1997) **49**:1096–105.

31. Paulsson O B, Strandgaard S, Edvinsson L, Cerebral autoregulation, *Cerebrovasc Brain Metab Rev* (1990) **2**:161–92.

32. Edvinsson L, McKenzie ET, McCulloch J, *Cerebral Blood Flow and Metabolism* (Raven Press: New York, 1993) 437–45.

33. Skoog I, Andreasson L-A, Landahl S et al, A population-based study on blood pressure and brain atrophy in 85-year-olds, *Hypertension* (1998) **32**:404–9.

34. Skoog I, The relationship between blood pressure and dementia: a review, *Biomed Pharmacother* (1997) **51**:367–75.

35. Bots M L, Grobbee DE, Hofman A, High blood pressure in the elderly, *Epidemiol Rev* (1991) **13**:294–314.

36. Nilsson P, Gullberg G, Ekesbo R et al, No impaired cognitive function in treated patients with mild–moderate hypertension compared to normotensive controls, *Blood Pressure* (1998) **7**:209–13.

37. Brun A, Englund E, A white matter disorder in dementia of the Alzheimer type. A patho-anatomical study, *Ann Neurol* (1986) **19**:253–62.

38. Mentis JM, Salerno J, Horwitz B et al, Reduction of functional neuronal connectivity in long-term treated hypertension, *Stroke* (1994) **25**:601–7.

39. Yamamoto H, Bogousslavsky J, Mechanisms of second and further strokes, *J Neurol Neurosurg Psychiatry* (1998) **64**:771–6.

40. Passant U, Warkentin S, Gustafson L, Orthostatic hypotension and low blood pressure in organic dementia: a study of prevalence and related clinical characteristics, *Int J Geriatr Psychiatry* (1997) **12**:395–403.

41. Breteler MMB, Groebee DE, Hofman A, Blood pressure, hypertension, orthostatic hypotension, and cognitive function in the elderly: the Rotterdam study. In Breteler MMB, ed, *Cognitive Decline in the Elderly. Epidemiologic Studies on Cognitive Function and Dementia*, thesis (Erasmus University, Rotterdam, 1993).

42. Kotila M, Waltimo O, Niemi M-L, Laaksonen R, Dementia after stroke, *Eur Neurol* (1986) **25**:134–40.

43. Nolan KA, Lino MM, Seligmann AW, Blass JP, Absence of vascular dementia in an autopsy series from a dementia clinic, *J Am Geriatr Soc* (1998) **46**:597–604.

44. O'Brien MD, How does cerebrovascular disease cause dementia? *Dementia* (1994) **5**:133–6.

45. Tomlinson BE, Blessed G, Roth M, Observations on the brains of demented old people, *J Neurol Sci* (1970) **11**:205–42.

46. Erkinjuntti T, Haltia M, Palo J, Sulkava R, Accuracy of the clinical diagnosis of vascular dementia: a prospective clinical and postmortem neuropathological study, *J Neurol, Neurosurg Psychiatry* (1988) **51**:1037–44.

47. Ladurner G, Iliff LD, Sager WD, Lechner H, A clinical approach to vascular multiinfarct dementia, *Exp Brain Res* (1982) **5**(Suppl):243–50.

48. Brun A, Gustafson L. Zerebrovaskuläre Erkrankungen. In: Kisker KP, Lander A, Meyer J-E, Muller C, Strömgren E, eds, *Psychiatrie der Gegenwart 6; Organische Psychosen* (Springer: Berlin, Heidelberg, 1988) 253–94.

49. DeReuck J, van der Eecken H, Periventricular leukomalacia in adults: clinicopathological study of four cases *Arch Neurol* (1978) **35**:531 (abstract).

50. Erkinjuntti T, Sipponen JT, Iivanainen M et al, Cerebral NMR and CT imaging in dementia, *J Comput Assist Tomogr* (1984) **8**:614–18.

51. Englund E, Brun A, A white matter disorder: common in dementia of the Alzheimer's type, *J Clin Exp Neuropsychol* (1985) **7**:168–9.

52. Bogousslavsky J, Regli F, Uske A, Leukoencephalopathy in patients with ischemic stroke, *Stroke* (1987) **20**:222–7.

53. Lindgren A, Roijer A, Rudling O et al, Cerebral lesions on magnetic resonance imaging, heart disease, and vascular risk factors in subjects without stroke. A population-based study, *Stroke* (1994) **5**:929–34.

54. Janota I, Mirsen TR, Hachinski VC, Lee DH, Neuropathologic correlates of leuko-araiosis, *Arch Neurol* (1989) **46**:1124–8.

55. Brun A, Gustafson L, Psychopathology and frontal lobe involvement in organic dementia. In: Iqbal K, McLachlan DRC, Winblad B, Wisnewski HM, eds, *Alzheimer's Disease: Basic Mechanisms, Diagnosis and Therapeutic Strategies* (John Wiley & Sons: London, 1991) 27–33.

56. Englund E, Brun A, Gustafson L, A

white matter disease-dementia of Alzheimer's type. Clinical and morphological correlates, *Int J Geriatr Psychiatry* (1989) **4**:87–102.

57. Kawamura J, Meyer JS, Ichijo M et al, Correlations of leuko-araiosis with cerebral atrophy and perfusion in elderly normal subjects and demented patients, *J Neurol Neurosurg Psychiatry* (1993) **56**:182–7.

58. Gottfries CG, Karlson I, Soennerholm L, Senile dementia—a white matter disease? In: Gottfries CG, ed, *Normal Aging, Alzheimer's Disease and Senile Dementia. Aspects of Etiology, Pathogenesis, Diagnosis and Treatment* (Ed de l'Université de Bruxelles: Bruxelles, 1985) 111–18.

59. Wallin A, Gottfries CG, Karlsson I, Svennerholm L, Decreased myelin lipids in Alzheimer's disease and vascular dementia, *Acta Neurol Scand* (1989) **80**:319–23.

60. Åkesson HO. A population study of senile and arteriosclerotic psychoses, *Hum Hered* (1969) **19**:546–66.

61. Jarvik LF, Matsuyama SS, Parental stroke: risk factor for multi-infarct dementia? *Lancet* (1983) **ii**:1025.

62. Gudmundsson G, Hallgrimsson J, Jonasson TA, Bjarason O, Hereditary cerebral hemorrhage with amyloidosis, *Brain* (1972) **95**:387–404.

63. Wattendorff AR, Bots GTAM, Went LN, Endtz LJ, Familial cerebral amyloid angiopathy presenting as recurrent cerebral haemorrhage, *J Neurol Sci* (1982) **55**:121–35.

64. Palsdottir A, Abrahamson M, Thorsteinsson L et al, Mutation in cystatin C amyloid angiopathy: identification of disease causing mutation and specific diagnosis by polymerase chain reaction based analysis, *Hum Genet* (1992) **89**:377–80.

65. Van Broeckhoven C, Haan J, Bakker E et al, The genetic defect in hereditary cerebral hemorrhage with amyloidosis of Dutch type is tightly linked to the B-amyloid gene on chromosome 21, *Science* (1990) **248**:1120–2.

66. Tournier-Lasserve E, Joutel A, Melki J et al, Cerebral autosomal dominant arteriopathy with subcortical infarcts and leukoencephalopathy maps on chromosome 19q12, *Nature Genetics* (1993) **3**:256–9.

67. Van Bogart L, Encéphalopathie sous-corticale progressive (Binswanger) à évolution rapide chez deux soeurs, *Med Hellen* (1955) **24**:961–72.

68. Sourander P, Wålinder J, Hereditary multi-infarct dementia. Morphological and clinical studies of a new disease, *Acta Neuropathol (Berl)* (1977) **39**:247–54.

69. Lassen NA, Ingvar DH, Radioisotopic assessment of regional cerebral blood flow. In: *Progress in Nuclear Medicine* 1 (Karger: Basel) 376–409.

70. Ingvar DH, History of brain imaging in psychiatry, *Dement Geriatr Cogn Disord* (1997) **8**:66–72.

71. Rapaport S, Positron emission tomography in Alzheimer's disease in relation to disease pathogenesis: a critical review, *Cerebrovasc Brain Metab Rev* (1991) **3**:297–335.

72. Risberg J, Gustafson L, Regional cerebral blood flow measurements in the clinical evaluation of demented patients, *Dement Geriatr Cogn Disord* (1997) **8**:92–7.

73. Scheltens P, Barkhof, F, Leys D et al, Histopathologic correlates of white matter changes on MRI in Alzheimer's disease and normal aging, *Neurology* (1995) **45**:883–8.

74. Wolf PA, Dawber TR, Thomas HE, Kannel WB, Epidemiological assessment of chronic atrial fibrillation and risk of stroke: the Framingham study, *Neurology* (1978) **28**:973.

75. Abdon N-J, The sick sinus syndrome: a common diagnostic and therapeutic challenge in the elderly. In: Harris R, ed, *Geriatric Medicine, Lesson 12* (Physicians Programs: New York, 1979).

76. Meyer JS, Mac Clintic K, Rogers RL et al, Aetiological considerations and risk factors for multi-infarct dementia, *J Neurol Neurosurg Psychiatry* (1988) **51**:1489–97.

77. Blumhardt LD, Smith PEM, Owen L, Electrocardiographic accompaniments of temporal lobe epileptic seizures, *Lancet* (1986) **i**:1051–6.

78. Cerebral Embolism Task Force, Cardiogenic brain embolism, *Arch neurol* (1989) **46**:727–43.

79. International Stroke Trial Collaborative Group, The International Stroke Trial (IST): a randomised trial of aspirin, subcutaneous heparin, both, or neither among 19 435 patients with acute ischaemic stroke, *Lancet* (1997) **349**:1569–81.

80. Post F, *The Significance of Affective Symptoms in Old Age. A Follow-up Study of One Hundred Patients* (Oxford University Press: London, 1962).

81. Folstein MF, Maiberger R, McHugh P, Mood disorder as a specific complication of stroke, *J Neurol Neurosurg Psychiatr* (1977) **40**:1018–20.

82. Robinson RG, Szetela B, Mood change following left hemisphere brain injury, *Ann Neurol* (1981) **9**:447–53.

83. Lipsey JR, Robinson RG, Pearlson GD et al, Dexamethasone suppression test and mood following stroke, *Am J Psychiatry* (1985) **142**:318–23.

84. Robinson RG, Kubos KL, Starr LB et al, Mood changes in stroke patients: relationship to lesion location, *Compr Psychiatry* (1983) **24**:555–66.

85. Flor-Henry P, On certain aspects of the localization of the cerebral systems regulating and determining emotion, *Biol Psychiatry* (1979) **14**:677–98.

86. Alexopoulos GS, Meyers BS, Young RC et al, The clinical presentation of 'vascular depression'. *Am J Psychiatry* (1997) **154**:562–5.

87. Chynoweth R, Foley J, Pre-senile dementia responding to steroid therapy, *Br J Psychiatry* (1969) **115**:703–8.

88. Paulsson GW, Steroid-sensitive dementia, *Am J Psychiatry* (1983) **140**:1031–3.

89. DSM-III-R, *Diagnostic and Statistical Manual of Mental Disorders* (American Psychiatric Association: Washington DC, 1987).

90. DSM-IV, *Diagnostic and Statistical Manual of Mental Disorders*. (American Psychiatric Association: Washington DC, 1994).

91. ICD-10, *World Health Organization Tenth Revision of the International Classification of Diseases* (WHO: Geneva, 1992).

92. Wallin A, Brun A, Gustafson L, eds, Swedish consensus on dementia diseases, *Acta Neurol Scand* (1994) **90** (suppl) 1–31.

93. Chiu HC, Victoroff JI, Margolin D, Jagust W, Criteria for the diagnosis of ischemic vascular dementia proposed by the State of California Alzheimer's Disease Diagnostic and Treatment Centers, *Neurology* (1992) **42**:473–80.

94. Roman GC, Tatemichi TK, Erkinjuntti T, Cummingst JL, Vascular dementia: diagnostic criteria for research studies. Report of the NINDS-AIREN International Workshop, *Neurology* (1993) **43**:250–60.

95. Hachinski V, Vascular dementia: a radical redefinition. In: Carlson LA,

Gottfries CG, Winblad B, eds, *Vascular Dementia. Etiological, Pathogenic, Clinical and Treatment Aspects* (Karger: Basel, 1994) 130–132.

96. Essen-Möller E, Suggestions for further improvement of the international classification of mental disorders, *Psychol Med* (1971) **1**:308–11.

2
Epidemiology of vascular dementia in Europe

Ingmar Skoog and Olafur Aevarsson

Dementia may be caused by several different cerebrovascular disorders subsumed under the term vascular dementia (VAD). Although this term is now used in most epidemiological studies, no serious efforts have been made to distinguish between the different types of VAD in these types of studies. Instead, almost all population-based studies on the prevalence and incidence of VAD use the term to describe the special form of VAD related to small and large strokes, often labelled multi-infarct dementia. The only population study that examined VAD related to ischaemic white matter lesions suggested that this may be the most common cause of all dementias.[1] Seventy per cent of demented 85-year-olds in that study had ischaemic white matter lesions compared to 35% in the non-demented group.

Prevalence

VAD related to stroke is generally believed to be the second most common cause of dementia after Alzheimer's disease (AD). As may be seen in Table 2.1, the proportion of demented individuals diagnosed with VAD varies, while there is no substantial difference in the age-stratified prevalence of dementia. The proportion diagnosed with VAD is believed to be lower in Western Europe and among North Americans of European ancestry than in Asia and Eastern Europe.[12,13] One Swedish study[7] reported that a very high proportion of demented 85-year-olds were classified as VADs. The proportion of VAD was higher than previously reported in western countries, and higher than reported in another Swedish study from Stockholm published at about the same time.[2] However, the crude prevalence of AD in the same age group was similar in these two studies (13.0% in Gothenburg vs 11.8% in Stockholm), while the prevalence of VAD differed considerably (14.0% in Gothenburg vs 4.9% in Stockholm). It is not clear whether the difference corresponds to differences in risk factors for VAD between these two Swedish cities, to

Table 2.1 Prevalence of dementia and VAD in Europe.

			All dementias					Proportion (%) with VAD among the demented
	Country	Sex	70–74 years (%)	75–79 years (%)	80–84 years (%)	85–89 years (%)	90+ years (%)	
Fratiglioni et al[2]	Sweden	Men		5	10	14	22	26
		Women		6	10	22	34	24
Ott et al[3]	Holland	Men	2	6	14	28	41	18
		Women	2	6	19	33	41	15
Rocca et al[4]	Italy	Men	4	9	26	43		40
		Women	3	8	11	33		35
O'Connor et al[5]	Britain	All		4	11	19	33	21
Aevarsson et al[6]	Sweden	Men				27[d]/25[e]		44[d]/44[e]
Skoog et al[7]		Women				31[d]/46[e]		44[d]/45[e]
Livingston et al[8]	Britain	Men	2[b]		9[f]			13 (both sexes)
		Women	4[b]		18[f]			
Sulkava et al[9]	Finland	Men	5[a]	8[c]		12[f]		42
		Women	3[a]	12[c]		20[f]		37
Manubens et al[10]	Spain	Men		9	14	24		16
		Women		14	19	26		11
Brayne and Calloway[11]	Britain	Women	0	3				31

a = 65–74, b = 65–80, c = 75–84, d = age 85, e = age 88, f = this age group and above

differences in assigning a diagnosis of VAD in cases of stroke, or to any other methodological factor described below.

The prevalence of dementia increases with age. Most studies find, however, that the prevalence of VAD rises less sharply with age than that of AD,[5,11,13,14] and at very high ages the prevalence of VAD may even level off. Therefore, most studies report that the relative proportion of VAD among the dementias decreases with increasing age, while that of AD increases.[5,9,11,13,15]

The prevalence of AD is generally reported to be higher in women than in men,[4,5,9,12,15–17] especially after age 80. VAD, on the other hand, is reported to be more common in men,[4,5,9,12,13,15,16] especially before the age of 75 years.

There are no indications that the prevalence of VAD decreases, despite the steady decline in stroke incidence and better treatment of hypertension. One reason may be that more patients survive after severe stroke. The paradox may therefore be that better treatment of stroke may lead to a higher prevalence of VAD.

Incidence

Prevalence rates are influenced by disease incidence but also by the duration of the disease. Incidence rates therefore provide a better measure of disease risk. However, very few studies have calculated incidence rates for VAD. The incidence of dementia and VAD is shown in Table 2.2. A meta-analysis regarding age-specific incidence of all dementias including VAD was recently published by Jorm and Jolley.[18] They used a Loess-curve fitting to analyse data from 23 published studies reporting age-specific incidence data. The incidence of dementia increased exponentially with age. However, most of the increase seems to be accounted for by an increase in the incidence of AD. Few incidence studies have analysed VAD separately. The incidence of VAD varies widely between studies, but it seems clear that the incidence of VAD increases less rapidly with age compared to AD. Men tend to have a higher incidence of VAD at younger ages and women tend to have a higher incidence of AD in very old age.

Two large European incidence studies confirm these findings. The Rotterdam study[19] examined 7046 subjects aged 55 years and older with a mean follow-up time of 2.1 years. The incidence of AD increased steeply

Table 2.2 Incidence of dementia.

	Country	Sex	70–74 years	75–79 years	80–84 years	85–89 years	90+ years	Proportion (%) with VAD among the demented
			Rate per 1000 years					
Jorm and Jolley[18]	Europe mild +	All	18	33	60	104	180	
	East Asia mild	All	7	15	33	72		
	Europe moderate	All	6	12	22	38	66	
	USA moderate	All	5	11	18	28		
Ott et al[19]	Holland	Men	5	15	25	29	26	23
		Women	4	18	25	50	77	11
Fratiglioni et al[20]	Sweden	Men		12	33	25	15	38
		Women		20	43	72	87	12
Aevarsson et al[21]	Sweden	Men				90		46
		Women				103		46
Paykel et al[22]	Britain	Men		15	71	29	0	25
Brayne et al[23]		Women		27	36	112	89	(both sexes)
Boothby et al[24]	Britain	All	6	37	39e			24
Copeland et al[25]	Britain	All	4a	12b		29e		21

a = 65–74, b = 75–84, c = age 85, d = age 88, e = this age group and above with age, while that of VAD increased somewhat up to the oldest age categories, where it levelled off. Men had a tendency to develop VAD more often than did women. The Kungsholmen Project[20] examined 1473 individuals aged 75 and above. The incidence of VAD was 2.3 per 1000 person-years for women and 3.1 for men in the age group 75–79, 7.5 for women and 13.7 for men in the age group 80–84, 6.8 for women and 12.3 for men in the age group 85–89, whereas in those above age 90 the figures were 3.9 for women and 0 for men. These figures were much lower than those obtained for AD and the incidence rate increased much more steeply with age in AD than in VAD. As in the other studies, women had a higher incidence of AD in all age groups, while men tended to have a higher incidence of VAD.

Methodological factors affecting the proportion diagnosed with VAD

As described in Table 2.3, several methodological factors may influence the proportion diagnosed with VAD.

(a) Auxiliary examinations

Most epidemiological studies have relied mainly on history to obtain information regarding symptoms of cerebrovascular disease. Three recent European studies[4,7,8] used detailed clinical diagnostic procedures, including CT scanning in some cases, on subjects diagnosed as demented in population surveys. The relative proportion of VAD was higher than previously reported in two of these studies.[4,7] In a 3-year follow-up of the 85-year-olds examined by Skoog et al,[7] the proportion of VAD increased from 47% at age 85 to 54% at age 88, despite a higher mortality rate in VAD than in other dementias.[6] One reason for the increased proportion of VAD was that new episodes of focal neurological symptoms and signs and new infarcts on CT scans were detected during the follow-up in demented individuals with a cause of dementia other than vascular at the age of 85. Diagnosis changed to VAD in nine out of 31 cases with a diagnosis of AD at age 85. Thus, the more information that is gathered (for example, from close informants, medical records or brain imaging) and the longer the subjects are followed, the more cerebrovascular factors are likely to be found. It could be argued whether the classification in these cases should be mixed dementia or AD. However, the new episodes could be an expression of previously silent cerebrovascular disease, which might have already contributed to the dementia at baseline. Cerebrovascular diseases may also increase the possibility that individuals with Alzheimer lesions in their brains will express a dementia syndrome.[26] Because of the difficulties in distinguish-

Table 2.3 Causes for differences between studies in the proportion diagnosed with VAD.

The amount of information collected
Differential mortality
  Screening
  Prevalence day
Inclusion of institutionalized individuals
Diagnostic criteria and their application
Clinical similarities between AD and VAD
Cognitive decline after severe stroke
  Dementia or not?
  AD, VAD or mixed?

ing between VAD and AD, it has been suggested that the term AD with cerebrovascular disease should be used to describe this category.[27,28]

(b) Differential mortality

The mortality rate is higher in VAD than in AD,[29] which may influence the relative proportion diagnosed with VAD in population studies. Many population studies use a screening procedure to identify individuals with dementia. In those screened positive a more comprehensive examination is performed to diagnose the type of dementia. The time between screening and actual examination may strongly affect the proportions of different types of dementia due to the higher mortality rate in VAD. Even in studies not using a screening procedure, the relative proportion of VAD will be affected by differential mortality. Most studies select a certain prevalence day and include all people that are alive at that date. The actual examinations are, however, generally performed some time after that date. During this time, those with high mortality (for example, VAD) may be disproportionately more often lost due to death.[7] This may be especially important in the very old where the mortality rate is high, and may be one explanation for the findings that the frequency of VAD rises less sharply with age than that of AD.

(c) Inclusion of institutionalized individuals

Many population studies do not examine individuals in institutions. This may be especially important at high ages where the institutionalization rate is high. Individuals with VAD are reported to have a higher institutionalization rate than those with AD.[7,30] It may be that individuals with VAD suffer more often from other handicaps, such as paresis or aphasia. Studies not including institutionalized individuals may thus yield lower relative proportions of VAD.

20   Cerebrovascular Disease and Dementia

The importance of these factors is shown in Table 2.4, where a comparison between the Gothenburg study[7] and the East Boston study[31] is performed. The Gothenburg study had a comparably high proportion with VAD, while the East Boston one had the opposite. In contrast to the Gothenburg study, the East Boston study used a screening procedure, did not include brain imaging in the diagnoses and did not include institutionalized individuals. To compensate for the 16 months' interval between screening and examination in the East Boston study, all individuals who died during the 16 months after examination were excluded from the Gothenburg study in Table 2.3. Second, diagnoses in Gothenburg were recalculated without using information from CT scans and, finally, all individuals in institutions were excluded. By this approach the proportion of VAD in Gothenburg decreased from 47 to 25%.

(d) Diagnostic criteria

In epidemiological studies the criteria for VAD are mainly based on the presence of significant stroke or cerebrovascular disease. The National Institute of Neurological Disorders and Stroke and the Association Internationale pour la Recherche et l'Enseignement en Neurosciences (NINDS-AIREN criteria)[32] suggest that a diagnosis of 'possible' VAD may be made in the presence of dementia with focal neurological signs if brain imaging studies are missing or in the absence of a clear temporal relationship between dementia and stroke. Thus, by using these criteria, the dementias will often be divided into one group with and one without stroke. The temporal relationship between stroke and onset of dementia is often used to strengthen the possibility that the two disorders are aetiologically related. The NINDS-AIREN criteria[32] suggest a limit of 3 months for the onset of dementia after stroke. This is difficult to apply in population studies, in which dementia has often had its onset many years before

Table 2.4   A comparison between the East Boston study and the Gothenburg study regarding the proportion diagnosed with vascular dementia.

	East Boston[31]	Gothenburg[7]
Alzheimer's disease	84	43
Vascular dementia	4	48
Including institutions	No	Yes
Screening	Yes	No
Interval from screening to examination	16 months	0
CT scan	No	Yes
After modifications		
Alzheimer's disease	84	61
Vascular dementia	4	25

examination and where exact onset of dementia and stroke may be difficult to determine. Most criteria leave much room for the researcher to decide when a stroke is related to the dementia. In studies using brain imaging the NINDS-AIREN criteria suggest that a diagnosis of probable VAD requires that focal signs consistent with stroke *and* relevant cerebrovascular disease by brain imaging should be present. In the study by Skoog et al,[7] the use of the NINDS-AIREN criteria for probable VAD, requiring a history of stroke *and* brain imaging findings of infarcts, yielded a proportion of 13% for VAD, while the use of the possible VAD criteria gave a proportion of 47%.

Wetterling et al[33] applied different criteria to 167 elderly patients admitted with probable dementia. Forty-five were classified as VAD according to DSM-IV, 21 according to ICD-10, 12 according to NINDS-AIREN criteria and 23 according to the criteria of the State of California Alzheimer's Disease Diagnostic and Treatment Centers (ADDTC). Only five cases met criteria for VAD in all diagnostic guidelines. This study illustrates that the proportion of different forms of dementia reported in the literature relies heavily on the criteria used.

(e) Similarities in the clinical expression of AD and VAD

It is possible that VAD may be underdiagnosed and AD may be overdiagnosed in population studies because of the similarities in the clinical expression of these disorders. First, VAD may have an insidious onset and gradual course[34-36] and may be mistaken for AD. Second, many infarctions are clinically silent, without evidence of stroke or focal neurological symptoms and signs.[36,37] Third, even if CT has been used many infarcts are not detectable by CT,[34,38-41] and cerebral areas can be damaged and non-functional although CT scan imaging remains normal.[42]

(f) Stroke

It is not always clear whether individuals with dementia symptoms after one or two major strokes are included in the demented group. It is possible that some population studies have not diagnosed individuals with severe cognitive impairment after a major stroke as having dementia. Furthermore, a diagnosis of dementia may be especially difficult to perform in stroke patients suffering from severe aphasia. Thus, if individuals with severe stroke are excluded already at the stage of classification as dementia or not, this may explain why the proportion of VAD is often far lower than would be expected considering the frequency of stroke in the population.

In cases who are already classified as demented and have a history of cerebrovascular disease, it is often difficult to determine whether the dementia was caused by the cerebrovascular disease. Often it is up to the investigator's judgment to decide whether a stroke has caused the dementia, contributed to it or is just there by coincidence. This distinction is often difficult to make at autopsy. Depending on the investigator's beliefs, these cases will be classified as VAD, mixed dementia or AD.

Vascular factors in AD

Several population studies from Europe have recently reported that vascular risk factors may also be important in AD.[42-47] Indeed, the recent finding from the Syst-Eur trial[48] that treatment of isolated systolic hypertension reduces the incidence of dementia by 50% emphasized vascular risk factors as possible targets for prevention. Finally, as already mentioned, other types of VAD than the form associated with stroke, such as white matter dementia, have generally not been examined in population studies. All this indicates that not only the frequency of VAD (that is cerebrovascular disease causing dementia) but also the frequency of vascular risk factors for dementia have been underestimated during the last decades.

References

1. Skoog I, Palmertz B, Andreasson L-A, The prevalence of white matter lesions on computed tomography of the brain in demented and non-demented 85-year-olds, *J Geriatr Psychiatry Neurol* (1994) **7**:169–75.
2. Fratiglioni L, Grut M, Forsell Y et al, Prevalence of Alzheimer's disease and other dementias in an elderly urban population: relationship with age, sex and education, *Neurology* (1991) **41**:1886–92.
3. Ott A, Breteler MMB, van Harskamp F et al, Prevalence of Alzheimer's disease and vascular dementia: association with education. The Rotterdam Study, *Br Med J* (1995) **310**:970–3.
4. Rocca WA, Bonaiuto S, Lippi A et al, Prevalence of clinically diagnosed Alzheimer's disease and other dementing disorders: a door-to-door survey in Appignano, Macerata Province, Italy, *Neurology* (1990) **40**:626–31.
5. O'Connor DW, Pollitt PA, Hyde JB et al, The prevalence of dementia as measured by the Cambridge Mental Disorders of the Elderly Examination, *Acta Psychiatr Scand* (1989) **79**:190–8.
6. Aevarsson O, Skoog I, Dementia disorders in a birth cohort followed from age 85 to 88. The influence of mortality, non-response and diagnostic change on prevalence, *Int Psychogeriatr* (1997) **9**:11–23.
7. Skoog I, Nilsson L, Palmertz B et al, Svanborg A, A population-based study of dementia in 85-year-olds, *New Engl J Med* (1993) **328**:153–8.
8. Livingston G, Sax K, Willison J, Blizard B, Mann A, The Gospel Oak study stage II: the diagnosis of dementia in the community, *Psychol Med* (1990) **20**:881–91.

9. Sulkava R, Wikström J, Aromaa A et al, Prevalence of severe dementia in Finland, *Neurology* (1985) **35**:1025–9.

10. Manubens JM, Martinez-Lage JM, Lacruz F et al, Prevalence of Alzheimer's disease and other dementing disorders in Pamplona, Spain, *Neuroepidemiology* (1995) **14**:155–64.

11. Brayne C, Calloway P, An epidemiological study of dementia in a rural population of elderly women, *Br J Psychiatry* (1989) **155**:214–19.

12. Jorm AF, Korten AE, Henderson AS, The prevalence of dementia: a quantitative integration of the literature, *Acta Psychiatr Scand* (1987) **76**:465–79.

13. Rocca WA, Hofman A, Brayne C et al, The prevalence of vascular dementia in Europe: facts and fragments from 1980–1990 studies, *Ann Neurol* (1991) **30**:817–24.

14. Åkesson HO, A population study of senile and arteriosclerotic psychoses, *Hum Hered* (1969) **19**:546–66.

15. Magnússon H, Mental health of octogenarians in Iceland. An epidemiological study, *Acta Psychiatr Scand (Suppl)* (1989) **79**:1–112.

16. Kay DWK, Beamish P, Roth M, Old age mental disorders in Newcastle upon Tyne. Part I: A study of prevalence, *Br J Psychiatry* (1964) **110**:146–58.

17. Mölsä PK, Marttila R, Rinne UK, Epidemiology of dementia in a Finnish population, *Acta Neurol Scand* (1982) **65**:541–52.

18. Jorm AF, Jolley D, The incidence of dementia: a meta-analysis, *Neurology* (1998) **51**:728–33.

19. Ott A, Breteler MMB, van Harskamp F et al, Incidence and risk of dementia. The Rotterdam Study, *Am J Epidemiol* (1998) **147**:574–80.

20. Fratiglioni L, Viitanen M, von Strauss E et al, Very old women at highest risk of dementia and Alzheimer's disease: incidence data from the Kungsholmen Project, Stockholm, *Neurology* (1997) **48**:132–8.

21. Aevarsson O, Skoog I, A population-based study on the incidence of dementia disorders between 85 and 88 years of age, *J Am Geriatr Soc* (1996) **44**:1455–60.

22. Paykel ES, Brayne C, Huppert FA et al, Incidence of dementia in a population older than 75 years in the United Kingdom, *Arch Gen Psychiatry* (1994) **51**:325–32.

23. Brayne C, Gill C, Huppert FA et al, Incidence of clinically diagnosed subtypes of dementia in an elderly population. Cambridge Project of Later Life, *Br J Psychiatry* (1995) **167**:255–62.

24. Boothby H, Blizard R, Livingston G, Mann AH, The Gospel Oak Study stage III: the incidence of dementia, *Psychol Med* (1994) **24**:89–95.

25. Copeland JRM, Davidson IA, Dewey ME et al, Alzheimer's disease, other dementias, depression and pseudodementia: prevalence, incidence and three-year outcome in Liverpool, *Br J Psychiatr* (1992) **161**:230–9.

26. Snowdon DA, Greiner LH, Mortimer JA et al, Brain infarction and the clinical expression of Alzheimer disease. The Nun Study, *JAMA* (1997) **277**:813–17.

27. Slooter AJ, Tang MX, van Duijn CM et al, Apolipoprotein E epsilon4 and the risk of dementia with stroke. A population-based investigation, *JAMA* (1997) **277**:818–21.

28. Skoog I, Risk factors for vascular dementia. A review, *Dementia* (1994) **5**:137–44.

29. Aevarsson O, Svanborg A, Skoog I, Seven-year survival after age 85

years. Relation to Alzheimer disease and vascular dementia, *Arch Neurol* (1998) **55**:1226–32.

30. Fratiglioni L, Forsell Y, Torres HA, Winblad B, Severity of dementia and institutionalization in the elderly: prevalence data from an urban area in Sweden, *Neuroepidemiology* (1994) **13**:79–88.

31. Evans DK, Funkenstein H, Albert MS et al, Prevalence of Alzheimer's disease in a community population of older persons. Higher than previously reported, *JAMA* (1989) **262**:2551–6.

32. Román GC, Tatemichi TK, Erkinjuntti T et al, Vascular dementia: diagnostic criteria for research studies. Report of the NINDS-AIREN international workshop, *Neurology* (1993) **43**:250–60.

33. Wetterling T, Kanitz R-D, Borgis K-J, Comparison of different diagnostic criteria for vascular dementia (ADDTC, DSM-IV, ICD-10, NINDS-AIREN), *Stroke* (1996) **27**:30–6.

34. Erkinjuntti T, Sulkava R, Diagnosis of multi-infarct dementia, *Alzheimer Dis Assoc Disord* (1991) **5**:112–21.

35. Fischer P, Gatterer G, Marterer A et al, Course characteristics in the differentiation of dementia of the Alzheimer type and multi-infarct dementia, *Acta Psychiatr Scand* (1990) **81**:551–3.

36. O'Brien M, Vascular dementia is underdiagnosed, *Arch Neurol* (1988) **45**:797–8.

37. Del Ser T, Bermejo F, Portera A et al, Vascular dementia. A clinicopathological study, *J Neurol Sci* (1990) **96**:1–17.

38. Forette F, Boller F, Hypertension and the risk of dementia in the elderly, *Am J Med* (1991) **90**(Suppl 3A):14–19.

39. Mohr JP, Caplan LR, Melski JW et al, The Harvard cooperative stroke registry: a prospective registry, *Neurology* (1978) **28**:754–62.

40. Radue E-W, Du Boulay GH, Harrison MJ, Thomas DJ, Comparison of angiographic and CT findings between patients with multi-infarct dementia and those with dementia due to primary neuronal degeneration, *Neuroradiology* (1978) **16**:113–15.

41. Werdelin L, Juhler M, The course of transient ischemic attacks, *Neurology* (1988) **38**:677–80.

42. Harsch HH, Tikofsky RS, Collier BD, Single photon emission computed tomography imaging in vascular stroke, *Arch Neurol* (1988) **45**:375–6.

43. Ott A, Slooter AJ, Hofman A et al, Smoking and risk of dementia and Alzheimer's disease in a population-based cohort study: the Rotterdam Study, *Lancet* (1998) **351**:1840–3.

44. Ott A, Breteler MMB, de Bruyne MC et al, Atrial fibrillation and dementia in a population-based study. The Rotterdam Study, *Stroke* (1997) **28**:316–21.

45. Ott A, Stolk RP, Hofman A et al, Association of diabetes mellitus and dementia: the Rotterdam Study, *Diabetologia* (1996) **39**:1392–7.

46. Hofman A, Ott A, Breteler MMB et al, Atherosclerosis, apolipoprotein E, and the prevalence of dementia and Alzheimer's disease in the Rotterdam Study, *Lancet* (1997) **349**:151–4.

47. Skoog I, Lernfelt B, Landahl S et al, A 15-year longitudinal study on blood pressure and dementia, *Lancet* (1996) **347**:1141–5.

48. Forette F, Seux M-L, Staessen JA et al, Prevention of dementia in randomised double-blind placebo-controlled Systolic Hypertension in Europe (syst-Eur) trial, *Lancet* (1998) **352**:1347–51.

3
Epidemiology of vascular dementia in North America

Robin Eastwood

History

Earlier,[1] we noted studies of historical interest in reviewing the epidemiology of dementia in North America. The early mental hospital studies dealt mainly with such diagnostic categories as senile psychoses and cerebral arteriosclerosis. Studies in Massachusetts and New York state early this century suggested that cerebral arteriosclerosis was increasing.[2-4] These authors recognized that there were nosocomial effects and that the differential diagnosis of these disorders is often difficult and that the conditions may frequently coexist.

More recently, community cross-sectional studies[5,6] showed that Alzheimer's disease (AD) and cognitive impairment were more prevalent than previously reported. Longitudinal studies obviously give more interesting information than cross-sectional studies, like incidence and risk factor data. One example was a New York study of volunteers,[7] which looked at the incidence of dementia over a 5-year period. Fifty-six cases out of 434 subjects, all 75–85 years on entry, developed dementia with 32 (57%) meeting diagnostic criteria for AD and 15 (27%) for multi-infarct dementia (MID) or mixed dementia; 8 (14%) had other disorders or were undiagnosed. The observed incidence of dementia was 3.53 per 100 person years at risk and for AD alone was about 2 per 100 person-years at risk. Risk factors for MID and mixed dementia were diabetes, left ventricular hypertrophy and a history of stroke. So recent community studies say that AD and MID are the most common dementias, with AD the most prevalent in North America. However, as noted by Landis and Page[4] and Katzman et al,[7] AD and MID may be coincident. This complicates the calculation of estimated rates and investigation of risk factors. Lately, Rockwood[8] pointed out that mixed dementia occurs more commonly than expected by chance alone. There may be a spectrum of disease from pure AD to pure vascular dementia (VAD) (see Classification).

Classification

Before leaving past and recent history, there is a need for an historical perspective on diagnosis. A Canadian conference[9] on Diagnosis of Vascular Dementia: Consortium of Canadian Centers for Clinical Cognitive Research Consensus Statement is as good a place to start as any. First it was thought that there was more interest in VAD today. During the twentieth century there had been an initial interest in 'hardening of the arteries' producing chronic hypoperfusion, but interest waned when AD became au courant in the mid and late century. What was left was a belief in North America that VAD was the second most common dementia, at around 10–20% of all dementias. Hachinski, who has had such a significant role in this field, developed the terms multi-infarct dementia (MID) and leukoariosis, and the Hachinski scale, to separate AD and MID. In 1992 moreover, he made a 'call for action against the vascular dementias'.[10] It was realized that the term 'multi-infarct dementia' was too limited and that conceptually the term 'vascular dementia' or VAD was an improvement. This allowed for such mechanisms as single, strategic strokes, small vessel disease and white matter changes, hypoperfusion and other non-stroke cardiovascular causes. Nevertheless, the tussle between the cerebral infarct argument and the hypoperfusion viewpoint has so far not been settled.

Since several sets of criteria for VAD existed before and after the conference, they had to be examined first prior to going on. These were:

- The Hachinski ischaemic score[11]
- The ICD-9 definition of arteriosclerotic dementia[12]
- The ICD-10 definition of VAD[13]
- The DSM-III and DSM-III-R definition of multi-infarct dementia[14]
- The CAMDEX definition of multi-infarct/VAD[15]
- The VAD criteria of Erkinjuntti[16]
- The California Alzheimer Treatment Centers definition[17]
- American/European Consensus Group (NINDS)/AIREN definition[18]

The conference decided to concentrate on the last two.

These sets of criteria are 'conceptually similar but differ in detail' and are each rooted in the multiple infarct model for VAD and the AD model for cognitive impairment. In consequence, they require dementia to be present, vascular brain lesions to be present and a temporal link between the two. Brain imaging is a requirement, although this can be relaxed if only CT is available and if multiple cortical lesions are evident clinically. White matter changes are supportive but not diagnostic. While each set has definite, probable and possible categories, critics have suggested that improvements would be primary (without stroke) and secondary (stroke with secondary dementia). Neuropsychology is desirable but of limited use, particularly with small subcortical infarcts, silent infarcts and white matter changes. Of brain imaging types, MRI is preferable to CT brain scan in terms of sensitivity, but discovering an infarct accidentally may be complicated since the lesion may be silent or comorbidity to another dementia diagnosis. Specificity is notably worse with MRI and perivascular rarefaction and other non-ischaemic causes of hypodense lesions appear to be indistinguishable from ischaemic ones. Neuropathology is normally a 'gold standard' but since VAD is a syndrome rather than a disease, correlating vascular changes and cognitive changes may not be easy.

Vascular cognitive impairment

Subsequently, the term 'vascular cognitive impairment' has been suggested. Bowler et al[19] examined 96 patients who had had only a TIA or minor stroke and there was no clinical evidence of AD, depression or other causes of cognitive disorder. All were examined, given an MRI and neuropsychological testing. Only 53 had cognitive decline (44 memory, 18 language, seven praxis, seven orientation, five arithmetic, four executive function, 12 reasoning and two visuospatial function), these being mostly subcortical and executive. Atrophy proved to be the best correlate of cognitive loss on imaging; neuropsychological testing separated VAD from AD; gradual onset was more likely than sudden onset; improvement was seen in less than half of the patients.

In an earlier article, Bowler and Hachinski[20] made the following important point:

> 'the concept of vascular dementia continues to be confused. Unfortunately it has acquired diagnostic criteria that liken it to Alzheimer's Disease ... These criteria have several flaws. Most importantly they do not permit the diagnosis until sufficient cognitive impairment has occurred to impair daily activities.'

Furthermore, cerebrovascular disease can be treated and should be treated as early as possible. But unfortunately hitherto all of the diagnostic criteria see VAD as a single entity. This makes it hard to designate aetiologies.

With this in mind, Bowler and Hachinski recommended the term 'vascular cognitive impairment' or VCI. This includes all cases of VAD except those caused by large artery stroke. VCI, therefore, is to be limited to 'cases where there is little physical disability and impaired cognition is the predominant clinical problem'. The authors pointed out that while 8% of those over 65 have dementia, some 9–38% of these dementias, depending on the study, are vascular in origin. Males generally predominate. (Conversely, 56% of dementias are vascular in Japan.)

Longitudinal studies

This then takes us to several longitudinal studies carried out in the USA on VAD. Clearly VCI is a recent concept and it behoves us to look at prior data from longitudinal studies of the so-called 'vascular dementia'.

Tatemichi et al,[21] from Columbia, New York, determined the prevalence of dementia in patients over 60 with acute ischaemic stroke. They did this because, while cerebrovascular disease in pure or mixed form is thought to cause 30–40% of all dementias, nosocomial problems meant that the true risk was not known. So 927 patients with acute ischaemic stroke from the stroke databank cohort were measured. Of 726 testable patients, 116 or 16% were demented as ascertained by a neurologist. No neuropsychological tests were given and the study was recognized as being an exploratory effort. All the diagnoses were clinical judgments. Coming to risk factors, the prevalence of dementia was related to age, reduced alertness, aphasia and hemi-neglect but not to gender, race, handedness, education level or employment status prior to the stroke. Previous stroke and previous myocardial infarction were also related to stroke but not hypertension, diabetes mellitus, atrial fibrillation and previous use of antithrombotic drugs. Prevalence was most linked to infarcts following large vessel disease. The authors use the generic term 'dementia' and, in actuality, over a third of their cases were vascular, over one-third were AD and a quarter were mixed. From CT findings, it was shown that the number of old and new lesions, cortical atrophy and hydrocephalus were significantly associated with prevalence but not infarct volume. Regarding site, dementia was more frequent when the lesion was in the occipital, tempero-occipital and tempero-parietal areas. Incidence was determined on 610 patients not demented at stroke onset and was found to be 5.4% for a 60-year-old and 10.4% for a 90-year-old. Age, but not gender, previous stroke and cortical atrophy were risk factors at stroke onset.

Two years later, the same group[22] asked the following research question: Does cerebrovascular disease increase the risk of dementia and, if so, to what extent? They repeated their previous study but added refinements. The subjects were examined in much more detail and were rated on the clinical dementia rating (CDR) scale. There had to be a temporal link between the dementia syndrome and stroke. Of the 297 subjects enrolled, 251 (84.5%) were testable and examined at 3 months. Using DSM-III-R criteria, 66 patients (26.3%) proved to be demented. Stroke caused about half and, as a complication of AD, about another third. Compared to stroke-free controls the risk of dementia in the stroke group was nine times greater. Risk factors were age, less education and to some extent being non-white. The rate means that in 1988 there were almost half a million Americans with stroke and dementia.

Two years later, in 1994, the same group[23] then asked the question: Is there a delayed dementia following well-defined stroke, the incidence of which is greater than in a control group? The patients were from the previous study with a longer follow-up. Those without dementia in the 1992 paper were followed up for 4 years or until death if earlier (18.4%). Over 4 years, 36 went on to develop dementia (incidence rate of 8.4 cases per 100 person-years) compared to eight or an incidence of 1.3 in the controls (all AD). The authors noted that, even after adjusting for key variables and allowing for potential biases, the incidence of dementia in the stroke group was exceptionally high. Most were mild with a CDR of 1. Eight had new strokes. Eight had significant medical comorbidity. A few had smooth deteriorations as found in AD. Expressed differently, about one-third became demented following stroke, giving a relative risk of 5.5. Older age at stroke, fewer years of education and a low score on the MMSE were significantly related. So the authors said:

'We conclude that ischemic stroke in elderly persons increases the long-term risk of developing dementia by approximately five fold compared to those without stroke. Age, education, and baseline intellectual function contribute independently to that risk' *and* 'our results are at least consistent with the thesis that a stroke may accelerate the cognitive consequences of aging, including the effects of Alzheimer's Disease.'

Slooter et al[24] examined the role of apolipoprotein E genotypes in dementia and stroke and found that APOE ϵ4 was more common than in normal controls. The attributable risk of APOE ϵ4 among dementia patients with stroke was 41% overall, 33% among those with VAD and 44% among those with AD and cerebrovascular disease. This may imply a common genetic susceptibility. In the well-known Nun study (Snowden et al[25]) post-mortem data showed that those who met the neuropathological criteria for AD *and* had brain infarcts had poorer cognition and higher prevalence of dementia in life, particularly if the infarcts were in the basal ganglia, thalamus or deep white matter. Conversely, in those not meeting the criteria for AD, the presence of lacunar infarcts was not particularly relevant.

It has to be remembered that North America, like Gaul, has three parts: the USA, Canada and Mexico, which are all different. Similarly the main ethnic groups in the USA—Caucasian, African-American, Hispanic-American and Asian-American—are also different.

First, comparison of stroke incidence worldwide shows modest variation.[26] Second, cerebrovascular disease in the USA started to increase in the 1980s, especially in older people, men and African-Americans.[27] The increase may have been due to better detection by neuro-imaging. In earlier decades, the stroke incidence had decreased, thought to be due to better treatment of hypertension.[28] There are ethnic difference:[29]

African-, Japanese- and Chinese-Americans have more intra-cranial and Caucasians more extra-cranial cerebrovascular disease. There also appears to be a persistent 'stroke belt' in the southern USA. Risk factors are older age, male sex, black race, lower socioeconomic status, heart disease, hypertension, diabetes, smoking, alcohol and diet.[29] Better living standards, reduced smoking and drinking and better diet have helped lower rates, but have been offset by better detection, increase in longevity and better survival from coronary heart disease. In contrast,[30] older Hispanics have lower rates thought to be due to lower blood pressure, and this is true also of Native Americans.[31] By comparison,[32] Canada has one of the lowest death rates from cerebrovascular disease. However, in both the USA and Canada the rates are comparable for cerebrovascular disease, which in each country is the third leading cause of death.[33] Finally, a recent survey showed that the overall incidence rate for first ever and recurrent stroke (excluding TIAs) was 411 per 100 000 among blacks and 179 per 100 000 among whites for all age groups except for those over 75 years.[34] This gave 731 100 first ever or recurrent strokes in the USA in 1996.

In conclusion, more attention has been paid recently to the condition we call 'vascular dementia' in North America. This mirrors the consideration that was given to this type of disorder at the beginning of the twentieth century. Considerable, even excessive, attention has been given to nomenclature. The most recent term 'vascular cognitive impairment' is currently being aired.

Vital longitudinal studies tell us that cerebrovascular disease has identified risk factors. There is no doubt that stroke causes dementia greatly in excess of normal expectation, both in the short term and the long term on follow-up. Similarly, we know that there are gender and racial differences in the incidence of stroke in the USA, with African-Americans having the highest rates.

References

1. Eastwood MR, Rifat SL, Roberts D, The epidemiology of dementia in North America, *Eur Arch Psychiatry Clin Neurosci* (1991) **240**: 207–11.

2. Elkind H, Taylor M, The alleged increase in the incidence of the major psychoses, *Am J Psychiatry* (1936) **92**:817–25.

3. Malzberg B, Prevalence of mental diseases among urban and rural population of New York State, *Psychiatr Q* (1935) **9**:55–87.

4. Landis C, Page PD, *Modern Society and Mental Disorder* (Farrar & Rhinehart: New York, 1938).

5. Pfeffer RI, Afifi AA, Chance JM, Prevalence of Alzheimer's disease in a retirement community, *Am J Epidemiol* (1987) **125**:420–35.

6. Evans DA, Funkenstein HH, Albert MS et al, Prevalence of Alzheimer's disease in a community population of older persons, *JAMA* (1989) **262**:2551–6.

7. Katzman R, Aronson M, Fuld P et al,

Development of dementing illnesses in an 8-year-old volunteer cohort, *Ann Neurol* (1989) **25**:317–24.

8. Rockwood K, Editorial, Lessons from mixed dementia, *Int Psychogeriatrics* (1997) **9**:245–9.

9. Rockwood K, Parhad I, Hachinski V et al, Diagnosis of vascular dementia: Consortium of Canadian Centres for Clinical Cognitive Research concensus statement, *Can J Neurol Sci* (1994) **21**: 358–64.

10. Hachinski V, Preventable senility: a call for action against the vascular dementias, *Lancet* (1992) **340**:645–8.

11. Hachinski VC, Iliff LD, Zilhka E et al, Cerebral blood flow in dementia, *Arch Neurol* (1975) **32**:632–7.

12. World Health Organization, *Manual of the International Statistical Classification of Diseases, Injuries and Causes of Death*, 9th rev (World Health Organization: Geneva, 1989).

13. World Health Organization, *Manual of the International Statistical Classification of Diseases, Injuries and Causes of Death*, 10th rev (World Health Organization: Geneva, 1989). (Typescript document MNH/MEP/87.1, 25–31.)

14. American Psychiatric Association, *Diagnostic and Statistical Manual*, 3rd edn (American Psychiatric Association: Washington, 1987).

15. Roth M, Huppert FA, Tym E, Mountjoy CW (eds), *CAMDEX: The Cambridge Examination for Mental Disorders of the Elderly* (Cambridge University Press: Cambridge, 1988).

16. Erkinjuntti T, Sulkava R, Diagnosis of multi-infarct dementia, *Alzheimer Dis Assoc Dis* (1991) **5**:112–21.

17. Chui HC, Victoroff JI, Margolin D et al, Criteria for the diagnosis of ischemic vascular dementia proposed by the State of California Alzheimer's Disease Diagnostic and Treatment Centers, *Neurology* (1990) **42**:473–80.

18. Roman GC, Tatemichi TK, Erkinjuntti T et al, Vascular dementia: diagnostic criteria for research studies. Report of the NINDS-AIREN International Workshop, *Neurology* (1993) **43**:250–60.

19. Bowler JV, Hachinski V, Steenhuis R, Lee D, Vascular cognitive impairment: clinical, neuropsychological, and imaging findings in early vascular dementia, Poster presented at The Challenge of Stroke, *Lancet* conference, Montreal, Canada, 1998.

20. Bowler JV, Hachinski V, Vascular cognitive impairment: a new approach to vascular dementia, *Bailliére's Clin Neurol* (1995) **4**: 357–76.

21. Tatemichi TK, Foulkes MA, Mohr JP et al, Dementia in stroke survivors in the Stroke Data Bank cohort. Prevalence, incidence, risk factors, and computed tomographic findings, *Stroke* (1990) **21**:858–66.

22. Tatemichi TK, Desmond DW, Mayeux R et al, Dementia after stroke: baseline frequency, risks, and clinical features in a hospitalized cohort, *Neurology* (1992) **42**:1185–93.

23. Tatemichi TK, Paik M, Bagiella E et al, Risk of dementia after stroke in a hospitalized cohort: results of a longitudinal study, *Neurology* (1994) **44**:1885–91.

24. Slooter AJC, Tang M, van Dujin CM et al, Apolipoprotein E ϵ4 and the risk of dementia with stroke. A population-based investigation, *JAMA* (1997) **277**:818–21.

25. Snowdon DA, Greiner LH, Mortimer JA et al, Brain infarction and the clinical expression of Alzheimer disease: the Nun study. *JAMA* (1997) **277**:813–17.

26. Alter M, Zhang ZX, Sobel E et al, Standardized incidence ratios of stroke: a worldwide review, *Neuroepidemiology* (1986) **5**:148–58.
27. Gillum RF, Cerebrovascular disease morbidity in the United States, 1970–1983. Age, sex, region, and vascular surgery, *Stroke* (1986) **17**:656–61.
28. Higgins M, Thom T, Trends in stroke risk factors in the United States, *Ann Epidemiol* (1993) **3**: 550–4.
29. Feldmann E, Daneault N, Kwan E et al, Chinese-white differences in the distribution of occlusive cerebrovascular disease, *Neurology* (1990) **40**:1541–5.
30. Gillum RF, Epidemiology of stroke in Hispanic Americans, *Stroke* (1995) **26**:1707–12.
31. Gillum RF, The epidemiology of stroke in native Americans, *Stroke* (1995) **26**:514–21.
32. Petrasovits A, Nair C, Epidemiology of stroke in Canada, *Health Rep* (1994) **6**:39–44.
33. Feinleib M, Ingstar L, Rosenberg H et al, Time trends, cohort effects, and geographic patterns in stroke mortality, *Ann Epidemiol* (1993) **3**:458–65.
34. Broderick J, Brott T, Kothari R et al, The Greater Cincinnati/Northern Kentucky Stroke Study: preliminary first-ever and total incidence rates of stroke among blacks, *Stroke* (1998) **29**:415–21.

4
Epidemiology of vascular dementia in Japan

Akira Homma and Kazuo Hasegawa

Introduction

According to a recent report from the Statistics Bureau, the Prime Minister's Office, Japan,[1] the proportion of the aged over 65 years was 16.2% of the total population in 1998. The National Institute of Population and Social Security Research[2] has estimated that the proportion of the aged population will be 22% in 2010, and 28% in 2030. It is predicted that the percentage of the 'old–old' population (over 75 years) will continue to increase rapidly until the year 2020. The number of the aged with dementia will increase concomitantly. It has been reported that approximately 70–80% of the aged with dementia are living in the community.[3]

Local governments in Japan have been greatly concerned with the various problems of the aged because of the rapid increase in their number and they have conducted investigations of living conditions and the need for welfare services, especially for disabled elderly persons with dementia. It is probable that the backgrounds for these surveys differed considerably from those in other countries. In the last two decades, 37 surveys on dementia in the community have been conducted in Japan. Methodological features of epidemiological surveys on dementia and some recent results on the change of prevalence rates of vascular dementia (VAD) will be described here.

Methodological features of surveys in Japan

Investigations have been undertaken nationwide. In some areas surveys have been repeated. In all surveys, clinical diagnoses were made through interviews by psychiatrists on door-to-door visits. Japan offers special advantages for epidemiological studies. All residents eligible for the surveys are registered in the office of the local government. This system makes it easy to select subjects by random sampling with government approval. However, the system has the drawback that financial sponsorship from local governments conducting surveys is limited by the stipulation that surveys must be completed within 1 fiscal year. For this reason, a large, population-based incidence study is difficult to conduct in Japan.

A decrease in the response rate of the surveys has been noted. In 1980 the response rate to a secondary door-to-door survey by psychiatrists in the Tokyo metropolis was as high as 96.8%, while in 1988 it was 91.6%[4] In 1995 it was 69.6%,[5] indicating a decrease of 27.2 points. The response rates in the screening surveys were 90.0% in 1980, 90.9% in 1988 and 86.7% in 1995. In the Kanagawa prefecture, adjacent to the Tokyo metropolis, epidemiological surveys have been conducted three times. The response rates of the secondary surveys were 83.7% in 1982, 74.0% in 1985 and 78.0% in 1993.[4,6] Those of the screening surveys were 96.1, 76.1 and 85.2%, respectively.[4,6]

There is, no doubt, great concern about the problems of the aged. However, it seems that the concern is not always accompanied by an increased understanding of elderly people for epidemiological surveys, even by their care-givers. As will be mentioned later, the above tendency to decrease the response rate to surveys may be reflected in the low frequency in use of welfare services for the aged. This may mean a change is required in the attitude of the public, including elderly people, to personal information. Increasing the awareness of the elderly and care-givers about mental illness in later life is essential for epidemiological surveys, especially when a psychometric test is employed as a screening instrument.

Another characteristic of Japanese surveys is that two-step procedures have been used in all surveys except for the two surveys conducted in the Tochigi prefecture and in the Fukui prefecture (Katsuyama City). Elderly Japanese people are not accustomed to being recruited or asked to be volunteers for research purposes. It has been considered difficult to administer even a simple psychometric test to the elderly in a screening survey. Consequently, the subjects with suspected dementia have been screened mainly on the basis of information concerning activities of daily living (ADLs), and behavioural symptoms of dementia obtained from their relatives. Although such a screening procedure is not efficient, it seems unlikely to overlook cases with suspected dementia.

In 1992, an epidemiological survey was conducted into dementia among the elderly living in the community.[6] Criteria included ADL, past medical histories, present physical status, degree of care required, mental and physical decline as judged by the relatives, and behavioral symptoms (Table 4.1). No psychometric examinations were included as a screening instrument. Five thousand randomly selected subjects from approximately 350 000 elderly persons in the Kanagawa prefecture were subjected to the screening survey with these criteria. From this population 408 elderly people with suspected dementia were identified, and out of these, 116 were diagnosed as demented in the secondary survey by psychiatrists using a semi-structured interview form. The form included demographic variables, a conventional ADL scale, previous histories for physical and mental illnesses, present physical status and findings by physical examinations, check list of personality change, Global Deterioration scale, NM scale (a behaviour rating scale to assess severity of dementia), N-ADL scale, frequency and severity of current psychiatric symptoms and behavioural disorders (46 items), onset of dementia, initial symptoms of dementia, Hasegawa dementia scale—revised which is a simple psychometric scale similar to Mini-Mental State, AD and VAD check list for DSM-III-R and AD for NINCDS-ADRDA criteria, psychiatric diagnosis, and several items about the care, including physical and psychological stress of primary care-givers. This interview form is 28 pages long and takes approximately 1 hour to complete. No cases with suspected dementia were found in 102 randomly selected subjects in the rest of the total sample, thus there were approximately 4600 subjects without suspected dementia. The results confirmed that the screening criteria were likely to be valid and practical, taking into account the reluctant attitude of the Japanese elderly in such surveys.

From 1993 to 1995, the feasibility of a psychometric test called CASI, the Cognitive Abilities Screening Instrument,[7] was examined in a

Table 4.1 Screening criteria for the elderly with suspected dementia in the Kanagawa survey – 1992.

I. Both A and B
    A. General activity or mobility less than getting out independently
    B One of the following:
        1. Marked physical decline
        2. Marked mental decline
        3. Concomitant cerebral vascular disorders
        4. Previous episode of cerebral vascular disorders
        5. Care required: Always or occasionally
        6. Assistance required in eating
        7. Assistance required in dressing
        8. Assistance required in bathing
        9. Assistance required in urinating
        10. Assistance required in excreting
II. In cases with neither A nor B, one of the following:
    1. Getting lost
    2. Delusions
    3. Rejecting bathing or dressing with no reason
    4. Marked forgetfulness (meals, etc.)
    5. Doing/saying that where he/she lives is not really his/her home
    6. Misidentification of his/her spouse or children
    7. Nocturnal confusion
    8. Confusing night time with daytime
    9. Hallucinations

community sample. CASI has been developed for use as a screening instrument for the demented elderly in multi-national epidemiological surveys. CASI has nine subscales:

- long-term memory
- short-term memory
- attention
- concentration/mental manipulation
- orientation
- visual construction
- abstraction and judgment
- list-generating fluency
- language.

The total score has a range from 0, representing maximal impairment, to 100, corresponding to no impairment. If such a psychometric test as a screening instrument of dementia was acceptable and feasible in a community population, it might be desirable to use such an instrument in a multi-national epidemiological study. This was an aim of the study.

CASI was administered to 1800 people randomly selected from approximately 33 000 aged more than 65 years in Machida City, which is located in the west suburbs of the Tokyo metropolis. The total population of the city was approximately 330 000. The response rates in the screening survey decreased with age from 85.2% in the 65–74 years age group to 73.7% in the 75–84 years age group and 69.2% in the 85 years and over range. There were no remarkable differences in the number of the subjects who refused to participate among the three age groups of the study. However, the number of the subjects who were admitted or institutionalized increased with age. This finding might be the reason for the decreasing response rate with increasing age in the screening survey.

The rates of valid response to CASI administration also decreased with age, probably for similar reasons: 95.1% in the 65–74 years age group, 89.6% in the 75–84 years age group, and 80.0% in those aged 85 years or more. These findings suggest that the use of CASI is less feasible in the very old population living in the community of Japan. Three criteria were used to screen the subjects with dementia. The first criterion was that the subjects had CASI scores of less than 77. The second was that their CASI scores were either invalid or could not be rated due to marked visual or auditory impairment or other reasons. The third criterion was that the subjects required care from their family members. A number of the screened subjects who were found to have suspected dementia were included in the secondary survey to confirm the validity of the screening criteria. Most of the elderly subjected to the secondary survey were the individuals whose CASI scores were less than 77. A psychiatrist visited them individually on a door-to-door basis to make psychiatric diagnoses. The psychiatric interview questionnaire consisted mostly of the Consortium to Establish a Registry of Alzheimer's Disease (CERAD) assessment packets. The response rate of the secondary survey was the lowest, 70%, in the youngest age group, and the rate increased with age. The reason might be that ADL in the oldest age group was the most impaired, so that many of them stayed at home.

On the basis of the results of the psychiatric interviews, calculations were made of the sensitivity and specificity of CASI in distinguishing between those with and without dementia. Using the cut-off scores of 77 and 78, sensitivity and specificity in the three age groups were as follows: 1.0 and 0.7 in the 65–74 years age group, 1.0 and 0.49 in the 75–84 years age group, and 0.94 and 0.34 in those aged 85 years and over. The sensitivity and specificity were quite satisfactory in the 65–74 years age group. However, the specificity, in particular, in the other two age groups was not satisfactory. In the 65–74 and the 75–84 years age groups, the highest score of the subject with dementia was 73. Using the cut-off scores of 73 and 74, the sensitivity and specificity were 1.0 and 0.86 in the 65–74 years age group, 1.0 and 0.67 in the 75–84 years age group, and 0.89 and 0.50 in the 85 years and over age group. The specificity in the 85 years and over age group was still unsatisfactory.

In the distribution of the CASI score in the 65–84 years age group, the score in the demented group ranged from 19 to 73 and that in the elderly without dementia from 43 to 99. However, the distribution of the score in the 85 years and over age group was somewhat different from that in the 65–84 years age group: the score ranged from 0 to 83 in the dementia group and from 0 to 95 in the group without dementia. This difference seems to explain the low specificity in the 85 years and over age group.

Table 4.2 shows the mean scores of CASI subscales in the three age

Table 4.2 Mean scores ± SD in subscales of CASI for the elderly without dementia according to the three age groups.

Subscales	65–74 (N = 71)	75–84 (N = 110)	More than 85 (N = 137)
Long-term memory	9.8 ± 0.7	9.7 ± 0.7	9.6 ± 1.6
Short-term memory	7.7 ± 2.7	6.4 ± 3.5	5.5 ± 3.2
Attention	6.8 ± 1.6	6.3 ± 1.7	5.6 ± 2.1
Concentration/mental manipulation	7.8 ± 2.4	7.2 ± 2.5	6.2 ± 2.8
Orientation	17.2 ± 1.6	16.5 ± 2.6	15.0 ± 4.0
Visual construction	9.4 ± 1.9	9.2 ± 2.0	8.6 ± 3.2
Abstraction and judgement	7.8 ± 2.7	7.8 ± 3.0	7.1 ± 3.1
List-generating fluency	6.8 ± 2.4	6.3 ± 2.0	5.8 ± 2.4
Language	9.5 ± 1.1	9.4 ± 1.1	9.2 ± 1.8
Total score	82.3 ± 10.2	78.8 ± 12.2	72.6 ± 14.9

groups without dementia. There were significant differences between the 75–84 years and the 85 years and over age groups with respect to the subscales of recent memory, attention, concentration, and orientation. Thus it is possible that impairment of attention and/or concentration in the very old age group could have influenced the performance in CASI. In addition, there were no significant differences between the three groups in educational years and in the proportion of the elderly with clinical dementia rating (CDR) of 0.5.[8] However, the ADL score in the 85 years and over age group was significantly lower than that in the 65–84 years age group. The decreased ADL in the very old age group seems to be a major factor in decreased concentration and attention. These findings are another indication that CASI may not be feasible in the very elderly, at least in the community of Japan.

These findings indicate that a screening procedure using behavioural symptoms may be useful, at least in a Japanese community sample. However, we have little experience in using a brief psychometric test such as the Mini-Mental State,[9] which requires a much shorter administration time than CASI in a community sample. Further studies are needed to confirm what kind of screening criteria will be the best in a Japanese community sample.

Prevalence rate of VAD in Japan

As shown in Table 4.3, 37 epidemiological surveys on age-associated dementia have been conducted in the community. In all surveys, the subjects were the elderly aged over 65 years. The overall prevalence rates of dementia ranged from 3.1 to 7.3%, with marked variation. The institutionalized and the admitted elderly were included in the survey in the Tochigi and Toyama prefectures, and in Fukuoka City. The prevalence rates were 5.5, 5.7, and 4.7%, respectively, among the subjects. The prevalence rates were not always correlated with the locations where the elderly lived. The prevalence rates of VAD varied from 1.1% in the Yamanashi prefecture to 3.0% in the Tochigi prefecture. The higher prevalence rates were not found in the surveys which included the institutionalized and the admitted elderly. This observed variation is due in part to the differences in study design, inclusion criteria, sample characteristics, and the definition and diagnostic criteria used, although no one factor can account for all of the variance.[10]

However, a trend is seen when the 37 surveys are divided into two groups: 26 surveys conducted before 1989 and 11 conducted after 1990. In the surveys conducted before 1989, the relative predominance of Alzheimer-type dementia (AD) was reported in four surveys (15.4%), while in the latter group the results of the seven surveys (72.7%) showed

Table 4.3   Prevalence rates of age-associated dementia in the community in Japan.

Area investigated	Year	Number of subjects	Prevalence rate (%)	Aetiological diagnosis AD	Aetiological diagnosis VAD	VAD/AD
Hokkaido	1986	9274	3.4	1.2	1.5	1.3
Akita Yuwa Town	1984	1144	7.3	1.2	2.5	2.1
Gumma pref.	1992	2242	3.0	1.4	1.2	0.8
Chiba pref.	1987	5000	3.2	1.8	1.2	0.7
Tochigi pref.	1990	2016*	5.5*	0.9*	3.0*	3.2*
Tokyo metropolis	1973	4716	4.5	1.2	2.7	2.3
Tokyo metropolis	1980	4502	4.6	0.6	1.7	2.9
Tokyo metropolis	1988	4586	4.0	0.9	1.3	1.3
Tokyo metropolis	1995	4343	4.1	1.8	1.2	0.7
Yokohama City	1982	2287	4.8	1.0	1.7	1.6
Yokohama City	1990	4550	3.7	1.7	1.5	0.9
Kanagawa pref.	1982	1507	4.8	1.2	2.0	1.7
Kanagawa pref.	1987	2232	4.9	2.0	2.0	1.0
Kanagawa pref.	1992	4259	3.8	1.8	1.5	0.8
Kawasaki City+	1985	1607	4.7	1.5	2.2	1.5
Yamanashi pref.	1985	2509	3.1	1.4	1.1	0.8
Nagano pref.	1987	1923	5.7	1.9	2.7	1.4
Niigata pref. (3 areas)	1983	2511	3.5	1.1	1.9	1.8
Niigata Yamato Town	1989	2446	7.9	1.2	5.0	4.3
Toyama pref.	1982	913	5.6	2.7	1.6	0.6
Toyama pref.	1985	1327	4.5	2.6	1.7	0.8
Fukui Katsuyama City	1990	5160	5.0	2.0	1.8	0.9
Toyama pref.	1990	1550*	5.7*	2.5*	2.2*	0.9*
Aichi pref.	1983	3106	5.8	2.4	2.8	1.1
Aichi pref.	1990	2992	4.7	2.0	2.4	1.2
Aichi pref.	1996	3302	4.8	2.8	1.8	0.6
Gifu pref. (3 areas)	1983	1649	3.5	0.9	1.6	1.7
Osaka-fu	1983	1844	4.3	1.6	2.3	1.4
Nara Yagi Town	1956	696	4.5	2.2	2.3	1.1
Hiroshima pref.	1991	5000	4.5	2.1	1.4	0.7
Tottori Ooyama Town	1982	1236	4.4	1.8	2.2	1.2
Fukuoka City	1984	3883	3.4	1.3	1.5	1.2
Fukuoka City	1991	5269*	4.7*	1.4*	2.3*	1.6*
Fukuoka Hoshino Village	1983	782	3.5	1.0	1.7	1.7
Fukuoka Hisayama Town	1985	887	6.7	1.4	2.4	1.8
Okinawa Sashiki Village	1975	708	3.8	1.0	2.5	2.4
Okinawa pref.	1991	3524	7.0	3.3	2.2	0.7

* institutionalized & admitted subjects included, AD: Alzheimer-type dementia, VAD: vascular dementia

that AD was more predominant than VAD. In these surveys, the prevalence rates of VAD ranged from 1.2% in the Tokyo metropolis to 2.2% in the Okinawa prefecture (1.7% on average). In contrast, those of AD varied from 1.7% in Yokohama City to 3.3% in the Okinawa prefecture (2.3% on average). As pointed out by Homma,[11] and Graves et al,[12] VAD has been a major cause of dementing illnesses in the elderly in Japan, while the composition of dementia subtypes seems to have changed recently.

In contrast to AD, it is quite difficult to compare the epidemiological results on VAD cross-nationally because of the lack of a common diagnostic criterion. Recently Graves and associates[13] conducted an epidemiological survey for the Japanese-American population in Washington State. The prevalence rates of VAD and AD were reported to be 1.4% and 3.5%, respectively. In comparison with the averaged prevalence rates in Japan, the predominant prevalence of VAD was revealed and the difference in the prevalence rate for VAD between Japan and the USA was smaller than that for AD. It is possible that the prevalence rate of VAD is less susceptible to environmental factors than that of AD. Figure 4.1 shows age-specific prevalence rates of VAD and AD in Tokyo metropolis and King County. A survey in Tokyo metropolis in 1996 used diagnostic criteria identical to those of the survey in King County.[14] It is shown that although age-specific prevalence rates of VAD and AD in Japan are slightly lower than those in the USA, the overall tendency seems quite similar.

Change of prevalence rates in Tokyo metropolis

Since 1974, four large-scale epidemiological surveys have been conducted in the Tokyo metropolis to investigate the prevalence rate of age-associated dementia. The initial survey was done in 1974. At that time, the overall prevalence rate of age-associated dementia was 4.5% among approximately 650 000 elderly residents aged over 65. The second sur-

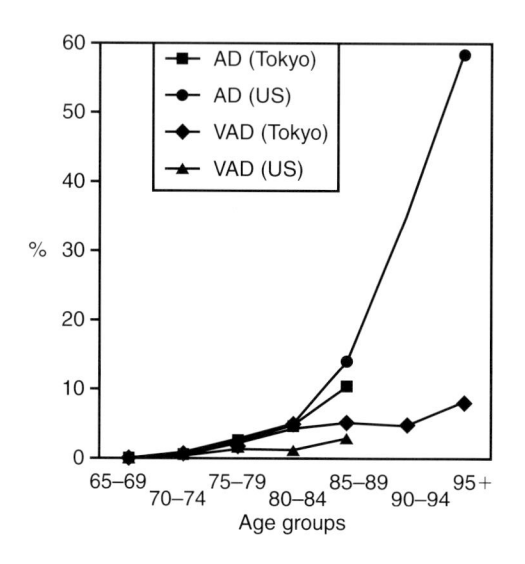

Figure 4.1

Age-specific prevalence rates of VAD and AD in the Tokyo metropolis, Japan and King County, Washington State, USA.

vey was conducted in 1980 and the prevalence rate was 4.6% among 870 000 elderly people. The third survey carried out in 1988 disclosed that the overall prevalence rate was 4.0% among 1 110 000 old people. The prevalence rate in the fourth survey conducted in 1995 was 4.1% out of approximately 1 490 000 aged people. As expected, the prevalence rate of dementia increased with age in the four surveys. Age-specific prevalence rates in the recent three surveys are indicated in Figure 4.2. There appears to be little difference in the age-specific prevalence rates of dementia in the Tokyo metropolis.

However, when the results of these three surveys are compared, a few points should be noted. The proportion of mild dementia among the elderly with dementia was 41.9, 48.1, and 30.9%, respectively, in the three surveys. That of moderate dementia was 24.7, 24.4, and 32.5%, respectively. That of severe or very severe dementia was 33.4, 27.6, and 36.8%, respectively. Although the tendency is not pronounced, it seems that the proportion of severe or very severe dementia is slightly increased and that of mild dementia decreased. As to the subtypes of dementia, the proportion with a mild degree of AD was 4, 10.8, and 20.8%, respectively in the three surveys. That of moderate AD was 8.0, 32.4, and 35.8%, respectively. That of severe or very severe AD was 88.0, 56.7, and 43.2%, respectively. It seems that the severity of AD in the community is becoming mild to some extent. In contrast, the proportion of those with a mild degree of VAD was 41.7, 53.1, and 27.0%, respectively. That of moderate dementia was 27.8, 28.6, and 27.0%, respectively. That of severe or very severe dementia was 31.5, 28.3, and 45.9%, respectively. Apparently the proportion with severe or very severe dementia has increased. This finding may be a recent characteristic of the elderly with dementia in Japan.

A more remarkable finding occurred in the change of disease-specific prevalence rates. Previously it had been well known that patients with

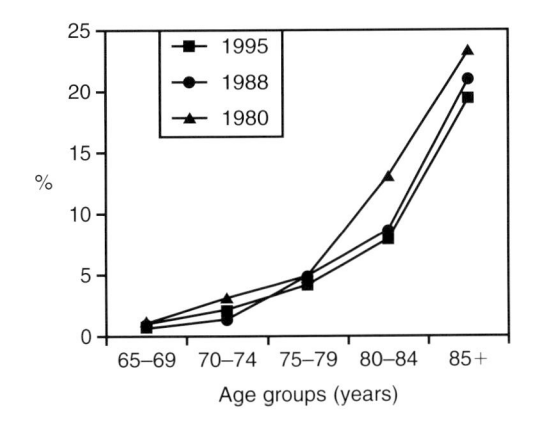

Figure 4.2

Comparison of age-specific prevalence rates in the Tokyo metropolis, 1980–1995.

VAD were more common than those with AD in Japan. For instance, the prevalence rates of AD and VAD were 0.6% and 1.7% in 1980, and 0.9% and 1.3% in 1988. However, in the 1995 survey, the prevalence of AD was 1.8% and that of VAD was 1.2%. It seems that the prevalence rate of AD increased and that of VAD decreased. In the 1995 survey, the ratios of AD and VAD seem almost the same as those found in western countries. However, it should be noted that the prevalence rate of other and unspecified dementia decreased with the change of the prevalence rates of AD and VAD in the surveys of 1980, 1988, and 1995 (Figure 4.3). In particular, when it is considered that there was no actual difference in the age-specific prevalence rates of dementia in 1980, 1988, and 1995 (Figure 4.2), and also that there was no marked difference in the prevalence rates of VAD, it seems most likely that the increase in the prevalence rate of AD represents an actual increase. This is the second characteristic finding in the recent surveys in the Tokyo metropolis. However, very similar tendencies were found in the other surveys, as mentioned earlier.

Procedural and associated socio-medical demographic factors in the surveys in the Tokyo metropolis

First, the decreased prevalence rate of unspecified dementia in 1995 might have been the result of the diagnostic procedure in that survey. In the previous surveys in the Tokyo metropolis, four or five highly experi-

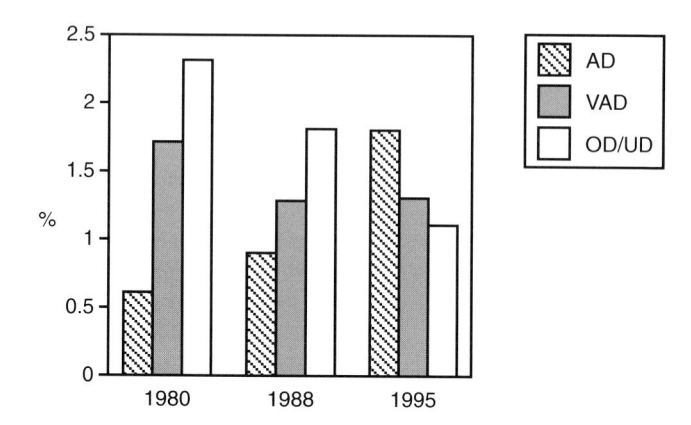

Figure 4.3
Comparison of disease-specific prevalence rates in the Tokyo metropolis, 1980–1995.
AD; Alzheimer's dementia: VAD; vascular dementia: OD; other dementia: UD; unclassified dementia

Table 4.4 Changes of socio-medical demographic factors in the Tokyo metropolis: 1980–1995.

Socio-medical demographic factors	1980	1988	1995
Elderly population with more than 65 years old	871 000	1 101 000	1 486 560
Old–old population with more than 75 years old	286 000	419 000	574 111
Old–old population/elderly population (%)	32.8	38.1	38.6
Proportion (%) of the elderly with			
Good ADL	79.6	82.7	82.3
Bedridden	3.5	2.9	1.7
Proportion (%) of the elderly with stroke history	7.2	6.4	3.2
Mortality from cerebrovascular disorders per 100 000	109.0	86.4	70.8*
Nursing home beds per elderly population (%)	0.62	0.88	1.3
Prevalence rate (%) of the elderly with dementia in nursing homes	—	56.9	54.3
Prevalence rate (%) of AD in nursing homes	—	23.7	19.8
Prevalence rate (%) of VAD in nursing homes	—	19.2	28.9

ADL: activities of daily living, AD: Alzheimer-type dementia, VAD: vascular dementia
* 1993

enced psychiatrists visited the elderly individually on a door-to-door basis. Psychiatric diagnoses were made on the basis of their clinical impressions. However, in the 1995 survey, as many as 19 psychiatrists visited the elderly. Thus in the secondary survey, a semi-structured interview form including diagnostic criteria based on DSM-III-R[15] and the CERAD assessment packet[16] was employed to increase agreement in the diagnosis among the psychiatrists. This was the most important procedural change in the 1995 survey, compared with the previous surveys in the Tokyo metropolis. As a result, it seems that the proportion of unspecified dementia was decreased.

In addition to the procedure of the survey, socio-medical background factors should be considered. Although the prevalence rate of dementia did not increase in 1988 and 1995 in the Tokyo metropolis, the increased size of the aged population caused the increase in the elderly with dementia. At the same time, the number of beds in nursing homes increased from 10 800 to 19 900 in 8 years. Thus it seems likely that more of the elderly with dementia might have been institutionalized.

The third issue that should be considered is that the elderly admitted to medical facilities were not included in the study, although the institutionalized elderly were also investigated to examine the prevalence rates of dementia at the same time. Taking into account that the elderly admitted to the medical facilities represent quite a high risk of dementia, a complete survey including medical facilities is needed in the future.

Incidence studies of age-associated dementia in Japan

There are few reported studies in Japan on the incidence rates of age-associated dementia, especially disease-specific incidence rates. Miyanaga et al[17] reported an overall incidence rate of 1.8%, that of AD 0.5%, and that of VAD 1.0% in 2255 elderly people aged 65 years and over in Yamato town, Niigata prefecture. In this report, the incidence rate of VAD was still higher than that of AD. In the USA, incidence rates of VAD and AD were 0.9 and 2.0%, respectively,[18] and in France they were 0.7 and 1.6%, respectively.[19] It seems interesting that differences between incidence rates of VAD are smaller than for AD, although it is difficult to compare the results due to the difference in age distribution of the subjects. It is not possible to examine a change of incidence rates in Japan because of the lack of published information. A multi-national survey in genetically identical populations is required to confirm the role of environmental factors in the change of incidence rates, as reported in the KAME project on the prevalence rates of dementia in King County, Washington State.[13]

Summary

In this chapter, the prevalence rates of age-associated dementia and some methodological features of the surveys in Japan have been described. A recent possible increase in the prevalence rate of AD and a relative decrease in that of VAD was also indicated in three recent surveys in the Tokyo metropolis. In addition, it is possible that the trend of an increased prevalence rate of AD in Japan is attributable to a change in environmental factors, taking into account the results of multi-site epidemiological surveys on dementia for genetically identical populations. An incidence survey with a similar methodology to such a prevalence study is required to confirm a trend of changing incidence rates for dementia.

References

1. Statistical Bureau, Prime Minister's Office, *Monthly Report of the Estimate of the Population* (Statistical Bureau, Prime Minister's Office: Tokyo, 1998) (in Japanese).
2. National Institute of Population and Social Security Research, *Projection of the Population in Japan* (National Institute of Population and Social Security Research: Tokyo, 1998) (in Japanese).
3. Karasawa A, Prevalence of dementia among the elderly in Japan, *Biomed Therap* (1988) **13**:598–601 (in Japanese).
4. Homma A, Epidemiology and risk factors of age-associated dementia, *Clin Psychiatry* (1992) **21**: 1877–87 (in Japanese).
5. Department of Welfare, Tokyo metropolis, *A Report on Health and Living Condition of the Elderly in Tokyo Metropolis* (Department of Welfare, Tokyo metropolis: Tokyo, 1992) (in Japanese).
6. Imai Y, Homma A, Hasegawa K et al, An epidemiological study on dementia in Kanagawa prefecture, *Jpn J Geriatr Psychiatry* (1994) **5**:855–62 (in Japanese).
7. Teng EL, Hasegawa K, Homma A et al, The Cognitive Abilities Screening Instrument (CASI): a practical test for cross-cultural epidemiological studies of dementia, *Int Psychogeriatr* (1994) **6**: 45–58.
8. Hughes CP, Berg L, Danziger WL et al, A new clinical scale for the staging of dementia, *Br J Psychiatry* (1982) **140**:566–72.
9. Folstein MF, Folstein SE, McHugh PR, 'Mini-Mental State'; a practical method for grading the cognitive state for the clinician, *J Psychiatr Res* (1975) **12**:189–98.
10. Jorm AF, Korten AE, Henderson AS, The prevalence of dementia: a quantitative integration of the literature, *Acta Psychiatr Scand* (1987) **76**:465–79.
11. Homma A, Mental illness in elderly persons in Japan. In: Copeland JRM, Abou-Saleh MT, Blazer DG, eds, *Principles and Practice of Geriatric Psychiatry* (Wiley & Sons: Chichester, 1994) pp. 859–63.
12. Graves AB, Larson EB, White LR et al, Opportunities and challenges in international collaborative epidemiologic research fo dementia and its subtypes: studies between Japan and the US, *Int Psychogeriatr* (1994) **6**:209–23.
13. Graves AB, Larson EB, Edland SD et al, Prevalence of dementia and its subtypes in the Japanese American population of King County, Washington State: the Kame Project, *Am J Epidemiology* (1996) **144**:760–71.
14. Larson EB, McCurry SM, Graves AB et al, Standardization of the clinical diagnosis of the dementia syndrome and its subtypes in a cross-national study: the Ni-Hon-Sea Experience, *J Gerontol* (1998) **53A**:M313–M319.
15. American Psychiatric Association, *Diagnostic and Statistical Manual of Mental Disorders*, 3rd edn (American Psychiatric Association: Washington, DC, 1987).
16. Morris C, Heyman A, Mohs RC et al, The Consortium to Establish a Registry for Alzheimer's Disease (CERAD). Part I: clinical and neuropsychological assessment of Alzheimer's disease, *Neurology* (1989) **39**:1159–65.
17. Miyanaga K, Yonemura K, Kuroiwa T et al, An epidemiological study on dementia in Yamato town, *Jpn J Geriatr Psychiatr* (1994) **5**:323–32 (in Japanese).

18. Katzman R, Aronson M, Fuld P et al, Development of dementing illnesses in an 80-year-old volunteer cohort, *Ann Neurol* (1989) **25**: 317–24.

19. Forette F, Amery A, Staessen J et al, Is prevention of vascular dementia possible? The Syst-Eur Vascular Dementia Project, *Ag Milano* (1991) **3**:373–82.

5
Epidemiology of vascular dementia in China

Yucun Shen and Xin Yu

The problems of ageing in China

The rate of ageing is accelerating in recent years while the proportion and absolute number of elderly people in the total population is increasing (Table 5.1). The life expectancy of Chinese people reached 70 years by 1993. Now there are more than 100 million people aged over 60 in China. It is predicted that the elderly will comprise 10.81% of the population in the year 2000 (Table 5.2), this means there will be 129 million elderly.[1] In Beijing and Shanghai, one in five residents will be elderly.

Due to the implementation of the one child per family policy, the rate of the ageing process in China is accelerating faster and faster. China will become an elderly nation by the end of this century, but professional and social infrastructures have not been organized to meet the challenge of the aging problem.

The 1% sampling survey showed that the average family size in 1995 was 3.7, a 0.3 reduction compared to the 1990 national population survey.[2] Thus, in China, the traditionally valued extended family in which three or even four generations live together is weakened. There are many attributions for this change. First, with the fast growth of the population density, living conditions are deteriorating, especially in urban areas. The

Table 5.1 Data from four population surveys in China.

Population survey	Aged population (million)	Total population (million)	Aged/total population (%)
1953	41.54	567.44	7.32
1964	42.20	694.58	6.08
1982	76.65	1003.79	7.64
1990	98.21	1143.33	8.59

Table 5.2 Prediction of the ageing population in China.

	1985	1990	1995	2000	2025	2050
Total population in China (million)	1049.00	1143.33	1197.00	1270.00	1498.00	1547.00
Aged population (million)	86.00	98.21	116.0	129.00	264.00	331.00
Aged/total population (%)	8.20	8.59	9.69	10.18	17.63	21.40

standard apartments, which were built by the government, obviously cannot accommodate a large family. (These types of apartments are virtually the same all over China.) Second, the accelerating industrialization process and relatively loose political control in the last 20 years made mobility both necessary and easy. Young people, especially from rural areas, tend to move away from their parents' home town, to try to find jobs in cities. Third, the family planning policy inevitably influences family size. Furthermore, in the final quarter of this century, many unpredicted changes occurred in China. For the first time in thousands of years the authority of the elderly is being questioned. Traditional values are being challenged. The elderly are most vulnerable to these changes, especially when they are living on limited pensions while their children enjoy the fruits of the market economy. 'Reverence to the elderly' is repeatedly emphasized in the media, not because the Chinese are still proud of it but because it is felt that this virtue is threatened by social reform. However, Chinese traditional values are struggling to survive in these tremendous social reforms. Numerous elderly people are still playing important roles in family life. They are the main force binding the whole family closely together and contribute a lot to both society and their family by looking after their grandchildren. Furthermore, some senior citizens (most of them well educated) are still very active in social and political life, even in the academic world. Thus they raise an important issue: what can Chinese society do for the welfare of the elderly, and what can the elderly continue to contribute to Chinese society?

With the astonishing change in society and public health, Chinese psychiatrists also face a great challenge never before met. In 1997, at the time of writing, there are 485 psychiatric hospitals all over China, which can offer 107 362 beds; 13 912 doctors are working in psychiatric hospitals. Unfortunately, facilities for elderly patients are very limited. Accurate statistical figures are not available, but it is estimated that fewer than 10% of beds in each psychiatric hospital serve the elderly. Qualified geriatric psychiatrists are even fewer, proportionally.

In view of the urgency of health service facilities for the elderly, nursing homes and hospices for the elderly have been established in both rural and urban areas in the last 5 years. Some of them are funded by local government, some of them are run privately for profit. Most of them mainly admit the elderly without care-givers or elderly patients with terminal illnesses. They all face similar problems: shortage of expertise and of policy guidance. Sometimes they even face a shortage of patients as, under the influence of the old Chinese tradition, the elderly are not willing to go into nursing homes because they believe it is for the childless, and their children are not willing to send their parents to nursing homes because they are afraid of 'losing face'.

Epidemiological studies of vascular dementia (VAD) in China—review

Useful information about the epidemiology of VAD was not available until the last 20 years. The first Chinese psychiatric diagnostic criteria were published in 1957, and did not include 'vascular dementia'. In 1980, the first version of a psychiatric textbook edited by Beijing Medical College mentioned Alzheimer's disease (AD) under 'senile dementia', and VAD under mental disorder due to cerebral VAD.

A search of the literature published before 1980 for epidemiological studies on VAD did not generate any valuable data, with only a few case reports related to 'dementia symptoms after severe strokes'.

The first study which met with all requirements of epidemiological research was conducted in 1982, led by the Institute of Mental Health, Beijing Medical University. This study adopted a standard sampling method, a survey instrument whose validity and reliability were tested, and ICD-9 used as diagnostic criteria. Twelve areas with 51 982 people were involved in this study. The survey found that the lifetime prevalence rate of 'senile dementia' was 0.29% (in 38 136 people aged 15 and over) and that of 'mental disorders induced by cerebral vascular disease' was 0.50%. However, no data on VAD are available since cases were included in the category of 'mental disorders induced by cerebral vascular disease'.[3]

Incidence rate of VAD

In epidemiological research, an incidence study often offers useful information about the disease, especially the risk factors. However, incidence research needs not only more funding but also a high standard of expertise. For these reasons, incidence research on VAD is relatively rare in China. So far, only two incidence studies on VAD have been conducted here.

In 1989, Shen et al completed a 3-year follow-up study on dementia in an urban community of Beijing,[4] in which 812 people aged over 60 who did not have dementia by Mini Mental State Examination (MMSE) evaluation were followed up for 3 years. MMSE was used to detect possible cases. DSM-III was adopted for diagnostic criteria and DDDS (Dementia Differential Diagnostic Schedule) for differential diagnosis. During the 3-year period, seven elderly people developed moderate to severe dementia, and six were diagnosed as having mild dementia. The average annual incidence rate of total dementia was 5.6‰. In the seven moderate to severe dementia patients, three were classified as having VAD. It was estimated that the VAD incidence rate was 1.23‰. The classification in six mild dementia patients was not available. Further analysis demonstrated that low education level, previous unemployment and reduced physical mobility were possible risk factors for the development of dementia. However, the relatively small sample made this analysis less useful.

The Mental Health Center of Shanghai and the University of California, San Diego, collaborated on a study of dementia in an urban community of Shanghai, where 1970 elderly people aged 65 and over who did not have dementia at the baseline were followed up for 5 years. The incidence rate of dementia was 1.15%. In new dementia cases, there were more patients with AD than with VAD (one-quarter of total dementia patients). The incidence rate in females was slightly higher than that in males (1.27% vs 0.98%). It was also higher in the older age group (65–69 years old: 0.68%; 80–84: 3.37%) and in illiterate elderly when compared to educated subjects. This survey was conducted by the application of ADRC laboratory tests and CT examination to differentiate VAD and AD, so the results were relatively reliable.

Prevalence rate of VAD in China

In 1986 the first epidemiological study of age-related dementia on a population aged 60 and over was conducted in China in an urban area of Beijing.[5] In this study, 1090 elderly people were screened by MMSE, the suspected cases were interviewed by psychiatrists, DSM-III was adopted for diagnostic criteria, and DDDS for differential diagnosis. Fourteen cases of dementia of moderate and severe degree were identified, with prevalence rates of 1.28% (≥60) and 1.82% (≥65), respectively. Among these 14 cases of dementia, eight were VAD, three were PDD, and one was due to carbon monoxide intoxication.

Table 5.3 lists results of other studies on the prevalence rate of VAD. Gao et al[9] reported that the incidence rate of VAD in the same area was 0.17%. However, the author did not provide any information about how this figure was arrived at. This study also suggested that the VAD was more prevalent in urban areas than that in rural areas.

All the studies listed in Table 5.3 demonstrated that dementia was more prevalent in older age and in illiterate groups. All studies except that of Zhang et al[10] showed that the prevalence rate of VAD in women was higher than that in men. Zhang et al[6] also indicated that loss of spouse and lower economical status were more common in dementia patients.

It is very interesting to point out that the two studies conducted in Shanghai showed a difference in the ratio of prevalence rates between VAD and AD compared to studies carried out in Beijing (with the exception of the study of Zhang et al[10]): the prevalence rate of VAD was lower than that of AD in Shanghai, and higher than that of AD in Beijing.

Other relevant factors and problems in epidemiological studies on VAD in China

As the majority of the demented elderly are currently taken care of by their families in China, some researchers conducted studies which focused on the burden and health/psychological status of care-givers. A pilot study conducted in 1990 by Li et al[11] showed that 50% of care-givers were spouses of demented patients. Relative's stress scale and SCL-90 assessments indicated that care-givers reported higher stress levels and more negative feelings such as depression, anxiety, hostility, and paranoia compared to a control group. Although female care-givers reported more stress in caring for demented patients, they reported fewer negative symptoms than male care-givers. The author proposed that females in China were expected to undertake more household work and were more liable to accept the role of care-giver.

Another study completed more recently in Shanghai[12] reported that 56% of care-givers were children of demented patients and 30% were spouses. The severity of dementia, impairment of ability of daily life and gender were correlated to the psychological status of the care-givers. Care-givers reported more negative responses when they looked after male, severely demented and more disabled elderly people.

Table 5.3 Prevalence rates of VAD in China.

Author	Year	Location	Population	Diagnostic criteria	Differential diagnostic instruments	Results: VDA (Alzheimer's disease)
Li et al[5]	1989	Beijing, urban area	1090 (>60)	DSM-III	DDDS	0.83% (0.37%)
Zhang et al[6]	1990	Shanghai, urban area	5055 (>55)	DSM-III-R	NINCDS-ADRDA Hachinski ischaemic scale	>55:0.74% (1.50%) >65:1.26% (2.90)
Wu et al[7]	1992	Beijing, urban community	966 (average age 67.8)	Hesegawa dementia scale	No	0.93% (0%)
Chen et al[8]	1992	Beijing, urban community	5172 (average age 68.9 ± 6.6)	DSM-III	DDDS	0.50% (0.2%)
Gao et al[9]	1993	Shanghai, both rural and urban areas	3779 (rural/urban: 2560/1219)	DSM-III-R	Hachinski ischaemic scale	0.85% (3.15%)
Zhang et al[10]	1998	Beijing, urban area	1243	DSM-III-R	Hachinski ischaemic scale	0.96% (1.37%)

One study analysed the mortality rate of VAD in follow-up.[13] The annual mortality rate of VAD was 25.7% and in the group over 75 years old the estimated relative risk contributing to all kinds of dementia was the highest one in all causes of death.

The epidemiological studies on VAD conducted in China so far have several problems:

- Comparisons are difficult because of the use of different diagnostic criteria and screening instruments.
- The sample size was often too small.
- Most of the studies were conducted in urban areas and limited to Beijing or Shanghai.

One very important issue to consider in the evaluation of epidemiological data on VAD is the homogeneity of subjects. Since China is a huge country, it encompasses a diverse range of geographical characteristics. The demographic features of the Chinese people, including physical complexions, dialects, customs, and diets, vary considerably according to geographical area. The Chinese are more heterogeneous than was previously supposed. This difference is reflected in the epidemiology of environment-related diseases. For example, hypertension is generally considered a risk factor for VAD. An investigation on the prevalence rate of hypertension in the elderly in different places in China indicated that the incidence rate of hypertension in Beijing was much higher than that in Shanghai.[14] Another study indicated that the incidence rate of hypertension was higher in northern China.[15] (Beijing is located in northern China and Shanghai in the south.) A possible explanation for these differences is that the salt intake is different between north and south: people in the northern part of China usually take more salt in their diet than their southern counterparts. However, many other factors still need to be investigated. It is too difficult to answer all questions before a nationwide epidemiological investigation is conducted.

References

1. Lu Z, Current status of elderly and its development tendency in China, *Chin J Geriatr* (1994) **14**:194–8.
2. Chinese National Statistical Bureau, *Statistical Report on 1995 1% Sampling Survey of China* (Chinese National Statistical Bureau, 1996).
3. Twelve Areas Epidemiological Investigation on Mental Disorders Coordinating Group, The summary of prevalence rates of various mental disorders from 12 areas' epidemiological investigation, *Chin J Neurol Psychiatry* (1986) **19**:80–2.
4. Shen Y, Li G, Li SR et al, The

3 years follow-up study on elderly dementia in urban area of Beijing, *Chin Mental Health J* (1994) **8**: 165–6.
5. Li G, Shen YC, Chen C et al, An epidemiological survey of age-related dementia in an urban area of Beijing, *Acta Psychiatr Scand* (1989) **79**:557–63.
6. Zhang M, Katzman R, Liu W et al, Prevalence study on dementia and Alzheimer's disease, *Chin J Med* (1990) **70**:424–8.
7. Wu Z, Meng JM, Wang ML, An epidemiological survey of dementia in the elderly in Changchun Street Areas of Beijing, *J Chin Geriatr Med* (1992) **22**:131–3.
8. Chen CK, Shen YC, Li SR et al, The investigation on prevalence rate of elderly dementia in urban area of Beijing, *Chin Mental Health J* (1992) **6**:49–52.
9. Gao ZX, Liu FG, Fang YS et al, A study of morbidity rate of senile dementia among aged in urban and rural areas, *J Neurol Psychiatry China* (1993) **26**:209–11.
10. Zhang JL, Zhang HH, Tao GS et al, An epidemiological study on senile dementia among 1390 elderly people in Haidian district, Beijing, *Chin J Epidemiol* (1998) **19**:18–20.
11. Li YT, Chen CH, Luo HC et al, The psychological well-being of caregivers of elderly dementia, *Chin Mental Health J* (1990) **4**:1–5.
12. Wu WY, Zhong MY, He YL et al, A study on well-being and related factors of caregivers of dementia patients, *Chin Mental Health J* (1995) **9**:49–52.
13. Zhu ZQ, Zhang MY, Katzman R et al, Mortality of dementia and other medical conditions in five-year follow-up survey in community, *Chin J Psych* (1997) **30**:231–4.
14. Wang WZ, Fang XH, Wu SP et al, A community-based survey on hypertension in the elderly in seven cities of China, *Chin J Geriatr* (1996) **15**:332–5.
15. Wu XG, Wu YF, Zhou BF et al, The incidence of hypertension and associated factors in 10 population groups of China, *Natl Med J China* (1996) **76**:24–9.

6
Epidemiology: meta-analysis

Anthony F Jorm

Meta-analysis is simply the use of statistical methods to aid a review of the literature. Meta-analysis has been applied in a number of reviews of the epidemiology of dementia to estimate prevalence rates, incidence rates and the strength of risk factors. Most of this work has been focused on the dementia syndrome or on Alzheimer's disease (AD), with much less done on vascular dementia (VAD). The reasons for the dearth of work on VAD relate primarily to inadequacies in the data available. The results of a meta-analysis are only as good as the data it is based on. In considering the results of meta-analyses on VAD, there are important limitations on the available data which must be borne in mind:

1. The diagnosis of VAD has changed considerably over time. Earlier studies used the term 'arterioscerotic dementia', which was eventually replaced by 'multi-infarct dementia' and then 'vascular dementia'. Diagnostic criteria were not available for the early studies and have gradually evolved over time. For this reason, earlier studies are difficult to compare with more recent ones.
2. The diagnosis of VAD was originally based on clinical examination, but more recently brain imaging techniques have played an important role. Such techniques are often not feasible in field surveys, so that the diagnosis of VAD in epidemiological studies is generally more basic than in clinical studies. The development of new technology has led to VAD being split into various subtypes, but these are seldom distinguised in epidemiological studies.
3. Because both cerebrovascular disease and AD become more common with age, they are frequently found to co-occur, particularly in the very elderly. Whereas clinical studies can select out relatively pure types by excluding these mixed dementias, epidemiological studies of representative samples must include them. Most epidemiological studies attempt to force all subjects into a pure category, but some allow a residual mixed category. If there is a mixed category, it is not clear whether they should be grouped with VAD for the purposes of a meta-analysis or kept separate. Pooling them has the disadvantage that any associations found may really be attributable to co-morbid

AD, whereas excluding them may lead to an underestimation of the occurrence of VAD.

When considering the results of the meta-analyses described below, these important limitations of the data must be kept in mind.

Prevalence of VAD

The first meta-analysis of dementia prevalence was reported by Jorm et al in 1987.[1] They analysed 47 prevalence studies, including 22 which gave age-specific rates. They found that while the prevalence rates differed significantly from study to study, they varied with age in a surprisingly consistent manner. Specifically, the prevalence of dementia was found to increase exponentially up to age 95, with a doubling in prevalence for every 5.1 years of age [95% confidence interval (CI): 4.8–5.4 years]. There were too few data after age 95 for any conclusions to be drawn. However, it is not possible for prevalence to continue rising exponentially to extreme ages because rates would soon exceed the possible maximum of 100%. At higher ages, a logistic model may be more appropriate than an exponential one because it has a theoretical upper limit of 100%.[2]

Of the 22 studies which were used to fit the exponential model for dementia prevalence, only seven provided data on AD and VADs. When an attempt was made to fit an exponential model to data from these seven studies, the VAD data from one study did not fit. However, when this study was excluded, the model gave a satisfactory fit. Prevalence rates for VAD were found to double every 5.3 years of age (95% CI: 4.6–6.3), while those of AD doubled every 4.5 years (95% CI: 4.0–5.0). In other words, the exponential rise with age was steeper for AD than for VAD.

In the meta-analysis by Jorm et al,[1] the relative importance of AD and VAD was found to differ by sex and by country. When sex differences were examined, prevalence rates for AD showed a significantly higher female rate, while for VAD there was no significant sex difference. When national differences were examined, VAD was found to be more prevalent than AD in Japanese and Russian studies, there was no difference in Finnish and North American studies, while British and Scandinavian studies found AD to be more prevalent.

The national differences found in the meta-analysis could have been due to differences in diagnostic practice across countries, particularly in view of the rudimentary diagnostic procedures that are often used in field surveys. However, the case for cross-national differences can be strengthened by examining data from other sorts of studies. Clinical studies provide a more rigorous diagnosis, but at the expense of representativeness.

Neuropathological studies provide the 'gold standard' diagnosis, but the cases coming to autopsy are even less representative. Nevertheless, if clinical and neuropathological studies from various sources provide similar findings to prevalence surveys, we can have more confidence in the results. To check for such consistency, Jorm later carried out a semi-quantitative analysis of the relative occurrence of AD and VAD in various regions of the world.[3] There was consistent evidence that AD is more common than VAD in Britain and North America and, to a lesser extent, in Scandinavia. In the rest of Europe and in Australia, the evidence also favoured a higher occurrence of AD, with the exception of Russian prevalence studies which reported more VAD. However, Russian neuropathological studies have found that VAD is considerably overdiagnosed there at the expense of AD. Consequently, it was concluded that AD predominates in countries with largely Caucasian populations. In East Asia the picture was quite different, with both prevalence and neuropathological studies fairly consistently reporting a higher prevalence of vascular than AD.

Although a number of other meta-analyses have been carried out on dementia prevalence, these have either dealt with dementia as a syndrome[4-6] or with AD.[7-9] The only attempt to cover VAD was the EURODEM project which pooled prevalence data from western European studies published between 1980 and 1990.[10] However, this attempt was hampered by the limited amount of data available and the lack of common diagnostic criteria. The only conclusions that could be drawn were that prevalence rises steeply with age, it is generally higher in men, and AD is generally more common than VAD.

Incidence of VAD

While prevalence rates are useful for planning services, incidence rates are better for studying risk factors. This is because differences between groups in prevalence may be due to differences in either the duration of the disease or in incidence. Because they require longitudinal data, incidence studies are much less frequently carried out than prevalence studies. Only very recently have enough incidence studies become available to permit a meta-analysis. Two meta-analyses of dementia incidence have recently been published,[11,12] but only one of these specifically examined VAD.[11]

Jorm and Jolley analysed the data from 23 studies which reported age-specific incidence data. Eleven of these studies gave data on VAD and 14 on AD. The data were analysed using Loess curve fitting. This method uses local neighbourhoods to find curves that best fit the data. Loess curves make no assumptions about the form of the incidence curve, unlike parametric methods that assume either an exponential or logistic curve. However, if log incidence is plotted against age, and the Loess curve forms a straight line, this implies that the rise in incidence with age is exponential.

When the data on all dementias were analysed, the Loess curve relating log incidence to age was found to be linear, implying an exponential rise. However, there were few data on persons over the age of 90, so what happens in extreme old age remains an open question. Figure 6.1 shows the data on VAD. Although the Loess curves are basically straight lines, the data points show considerable variability, reflecting the problems of assessing VAD in field surveys. As would be expected, studies assessing mild+ VAD tend to show higher incidence rates than those assessing moderate+ VAD. Figure 6.1 also shows an interesting sex

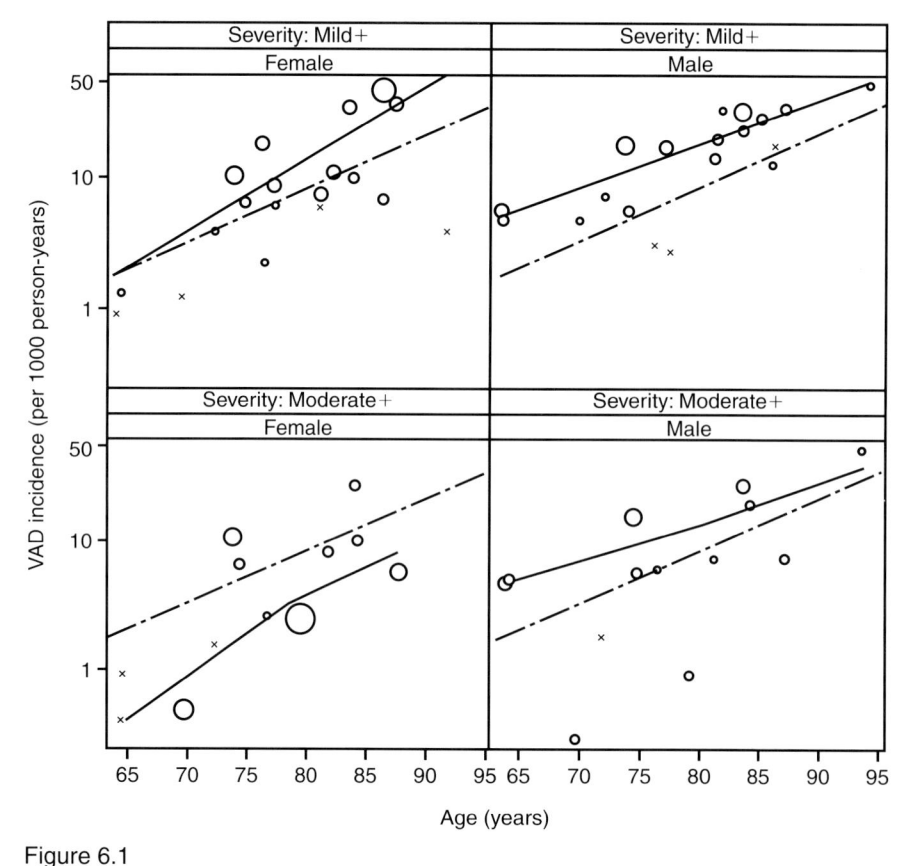

Figure 6.1

Loess curves of log incidence by sex. The solid line is the Loess curve. The dashed line is for visual reference in making comparison across panels. The circles are data points from the various studies, with the area of the circle proportional to the weight of the point. Very small circles are shown by an X to make them more visible.

difference, with steeper incidence curves for females. Males have a higher incidence at younger ages, but females tend to catch up at older ages. The higher incidence in males at younger ages may reflect the effects of smoking, with only non-smokers surviving to very old age.

Figure 6.2 shows the findings for Europe compared to East Asia (no data were available for other regions). The European studies are divided according to whether they assessed mild+ or moderate+ VAD. By contrast, the East Asia studies only assessed mild+ dementia. The incidence of mild+ VAD did not differ significantly between Europe and East Asia.

Similar analyses were carried out for AD. Again, the rise with age appeared to be exponential up to age 90, although it tended to be

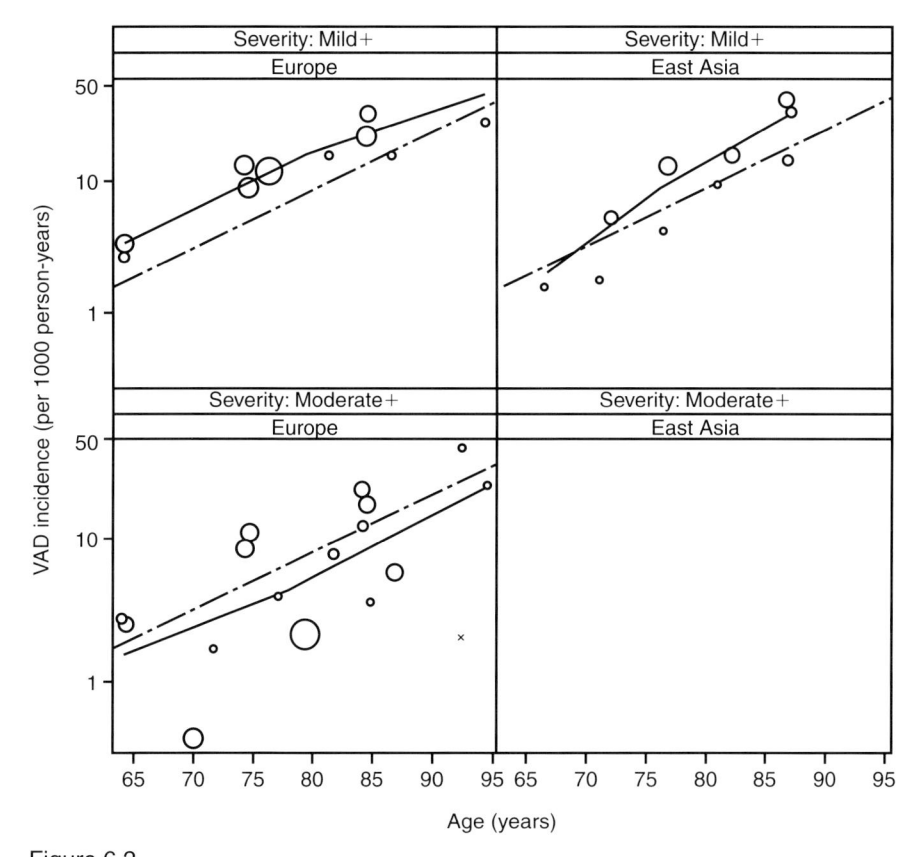

Figure 6.2

Loess curves of log incidence by region. The solid line is the Loess curve. The dashed line is for visual reference in making comparison across panels. The circles are data points from the various studies, with the area of the circle proportional to the weight of the point. Very small circles are shown by an X to make them more visible.

steeper for AD than for VAD. There was no sex difference at younger ages, but females tended to have a higher incidence at the older ages. The incidence of AD tended to be lower in East Asian countries at younger ages, but this regional difference disappeared at the older ages.

Conclusions

Although meta-analysis has provided some useful summaries of epidemiological findings on global dementia and AD, limitations of the available data make it difficult to draw firm conclusions about VAD. However, the following tentative conclusions can be offered:

1. The prevalence and incidence of VAD rise approximately exponentially with age, at least until age 90.
2. The occurrence of VAD rises less steeply with age than for AD.
3. Cerebrovascular disease is a relatively more important cause of dementia for males than for females.
4. Cerebrovascular disease is a relatively more important cause of dementia in East Asian than in Western countries.

Any advance in the epidemiology of VAD beyond these basic conclusions will rest on the development of valid diagnostic methods which are feasible in field surveys and which can be applied consistently in different studies.

References

1. Jorm AF, Korten AE, Henderson AS, The prevalence of dementia: a quantitative integration of the literature, *Acta Psychiatr Scand* (1987) **76**:465–79.
2. Dewey M, How should prevalence be modelled? *Acta Psychiatr Scand* (1991) **84**:246–9.
3. Jorm AF, Cross-national comparisons of the occurrence of Alzheimer's and vascular dementias, *Eur Arch Psychiatr Clin Neurosci* (1991) **240**:218–22.
4. Hofman A, Rocca WA, Brayne C et al, The prevalence of dementia in Europe: a collaborative study of 1980–1990 findings, *Int J Epidemiol* (1991) **20**:736–48.
5. Ritchie K, Kildea D, Robine J-M, The relationship between age and the prevalence of senile dementia: a meta-analysis of recent data, *Int J Epidemiol* (1992) **21**:763–9.
6. Ritchie K, Kildea D, Is senile dementia 'age-related' or 'ageing-related'?—evidence from meta-analysis of dementia prevalence in the oldest old, *Lancet* (1995) **346**:931–4.
7. Rocca WA, Hofman A, Brayne C et al, Frequency and distribution of Alzheimer's disease in Europe: a collaborative study of 1980–1990 findings, *Ann Neurol* 1991; **30**:381–90.
8. Corrada M, Brookmeyer R, Kawas C, Sources of variability in prevalence rates of Alzheimer's dis-

ease, *Int J Epidemiol* (1995) **24**:1000-1005.

9. United States General Accounting Office, *Alzheimer's Disease: Estimates of Prevalence in the United States* (United States General Accounting Office: Washington DC, 1998).

10. Rocca WA, Hofman A, Brayne C et al, The prevalence of vascular dementia in Europe: facts and fragments from 1980–1990 studies, *Ann Neurol* (1991) **30**:817–24.

11. Jorm AF, Jolley D, The incidence of dementia: a meta-analysis. *Neurology* (1998) **51**:728–33.

12. Gao S, Hendrie HC, Hall KS, Hui S, The relationship between age, sex, and the incidence of dementia and Alzheimer disease, *Arch Gen Psychiatry* (1998) **55**:809–15.

7
The epidemiology of vascular dementia: an overview and commentary

Anthony F Jorm

The first four chapters in this section have summarized the evidence on the epidemiology of vascular dementia (VAD) in different regions of the world, while the last chapter in the section summarizes the results of meta-analyses involving all countries from which data are available. The purpose of the present chapter is to provide an integration and commentary on these varied contributions. The chapter identifies common themes raised in the previous chapters as well as areas of difference.

Diagnostic criteria and methods

At the present time, epidemiologists are unable to give anything like definitive prevalence and incidence rates for VAD by age, sex and region. There are many reasons for this, but probably the most important is that there is no consensus on what diagnostic criteria should be used and how they should be implemented in field surveys. As pointed out by Eastwood, the classification and terminology have changed from chronic hypoperfusion, to multi-infarct dementia (due to large and small strokes), to the broader concept of VAD (which incorporates other types of cerebrovascular disease associated with dementia) to vascular cognitive impairment (which incorporates milder states of impairment). As well as this change in terminology over time, there are quite varied diagnostic criteria competing at each point in time. As Skoog and Aevarsson have discussed, even in clinical samples the rates can vary considerably depending on the criteria.

There are other sources of methodological variation which are particularly important in epidemiological field studies. The existing criteria are designed primarily for use in clinical research where a wide range of investigations is possible. However, some types of investigation (for example brain imaging) are difficult to implement within the constraints of field studies. This has meant that most studies of VAD have in fact focused on multi-infarct dementia and ignored ischaemic white matter lesions (Skoog and Aevarsson). The more clinical investigations carried out when making a diagnosis, the higher the relative prevalence of VAD (Skoog and Aevarsson). There are also problems in making judgments about the aetiological significance of cerebrovascular lesions: the historical information available about onset may be limited, VAD may have an insidious onset in some cases, mimicking Alzheimer's disease (AD), and infarctions may be clinically silent (Skoog and Aevarsson).

There are also regional differences in diagnostic approach, which may be seen even where the same diagnostic criteria are being used. Homma and Hasegawa point out that elderly Japanese do not like psychometric screening tests, so researchers must rely on relatives' reports of activities of daily living and behavioural changes. On the other hand, in other countries there may be difficulty in finding a suitable informant because of a weaker cultural commitment to caring for elderly relatives.

Cultural differences in patterns of aged care can have an effect in another way, through national differences in rates of nursing home placement. Nursing home residents are often omitted from epidemiological field studies. Even within a single region, some studies include nursing home residents and others do not (Skoog and Aevarsson; Homma and Hasegawa). The rate of nursing home placement may also vary over time, making historical comparisons difficult (Homma and Hasegawa). However, whether these differences in sampling substantially affect prevalence and incidence rates is difficult to determine because other methodological differences have a masking effect (Homma and Hasegawa).

Prevalence

Despite the noise contributed by all these methodological differences, it is possible to come to some conclusions. Not surprisingly, the prevalence of VAD increases steeply with age, although the increase appears to be less steep for VAD than for AD (Skoog and Aevarsson; Jorm).

There are also likely to be sex differences. Early studies showed a higher crude prevalence of VAD in men than women, and the converse for AD (Jorm). However, recent studies give a more refined picture of sex differences: the prevalence of AD is higher in women, especially after age 80, while VAD is more common in men, especially before 75 (Skoog and Aevarsson).

For epidemiologists, incidence studies are preferable to prevalence studies. The reason is that prevalence may differ between groups because of incidence differences or because of survival differences. The mortality in VAD has been reported as very high in both Europe and China (Skoog and Aevarsson; Shen and Yu), implying that VAD may appear a bigger contributor to dementia incidence than to dementia prevalence.

Incidence

Incidence studies are unfortunately rare. Barriers to doing an incidence study include not only the greater resources required, but the short-term research funding policies in some countries (Homma and Hasegawa; Shen and Yu).

As with prevalence, the rates vary greatly from study to study, undoubtedly due to methodological differences (Jorm). Nevertheless, we can say that incidence rises steeply with age in an exponential fashion, at least up to age 90 (Jorm). Incidence also appears to rise less steeply for VAD than for AD, consistent with the data on prevalence (Aevarsson and Skoog; Jorm), showing that survival differences do not account for this effect. Sex differences are also similar for prevalence and incidence. Men tend to have a higher incidence of VAD at younger ages, and women a higher incidence of AD at higher ages (Aevarsson and Skoog; Jorm).

Are there true regional differences?

There is considerable interest in whether incidence or prevalence rates differ between regions. Such a difference implies a different profile of risk factors between the regions. There may be some risk factors that vary more between regions than within regions and that can only be feasibly identified by cross-regional comparisons.

A meta-analysis of early prevalence studies found that AD was the most common dementing disease in some countries, while in others such as Japan and Russia, VAD was more common (Jorm). Later evidence suggested that the predominance of VAD in Russian studies was due to different diagnostic practices. However, the Japanese pattern of dementia continues to arouse epidemiological interest. As discussed below, this pattern may be changing, with Japan becoming more like Caucasian populations in having a predominance of AD. The data on cross-national differences in incidence are more sparse. A meta-analysis of the available studies found no difference in VAD incidence between Europe and East Asia (Jorm). By contrast, the incidence of AD was lower in East Asia, at least in the young old. The difference disappeared with age as the East Asian countries caught up.

There may also be regional and ethnic differences within countries. In China, for example, the prevalence of VAD may be higher in urban areas and in Beijing compared to Shanghai (Shen and Yu). Consistent with this observation, the prevalence of hypertension is higher in Beijing, perhaps because of the higher salt intake (Shen and Yu). In the USA, there are certain regions with a higher stroke risk, although whether the VAD rates also differ is unknown (Eastwood). Furthermore, there are ethnic differences: African, Japanese and Chinese Americans having more intracranial and Caucasians more extracranial cerebrovascular disease (Eastwood).

The study of regional and ethnic differences is made difficult because of the many methodological differences between studies. There is a clear need for studies which attempt to use identical methodology with different groups (Homma and Hasegawa; Jorm). Homma and Hasegawa point to the KAME Project in Washington state, USA, which examines dementia in Japanese Americans, as the sort of project that needs to be extended across countries.

Are there historical changes?

It is very difficult to judge whether the prevalence or incidence of VAD has changed, for several reasons. Very little information was available 20 years ago (Shen and Yu) and, even where historical data are available, the changes in classification and diagnostic methods make direct comparison difficult. Even societal changes like declining participation rates in epidemiological studies can have an effect (Homma and Hasegawa).

Nevertheless, despite a decline in stroke incidence and better treatment of hypertension, the limited evidence available from Europe does not support any decline in prevalence (Skoog and Aevarsson). There could be other factors at work that offset these gains, such as better treatment of stroke leading to longer survival and better detection (Skoog and Aevarsson; Eastwood). On the other hand, prevalence studies in Japan show an historical trend in the relative prevalence of VAD and AD. In studies carried out before 1989, VAD tended to predominate, whereas in more recent studies, AD has become dominant (Homma and Hasegawa). In a series of prevalence studies carried out in Tokyo, overall rates of dementia did not change, while VAD decreased and AD increased (Homma and Hasegawa). However, there were inevitable changes in assessment methods over time which complicate comparisons, and the number of nursing home beds also increased. Homma and Hasegawa speculate that there has been an historical change in exposure to environmental risk factors for AD. As with the study of regional differences, serial studies using identical methodology are needed before we will know whether dementia prevalence or incidence is changing.

Ageing of the population

One conclusion that probably no one would disagree with is that the ageing of the population will lead to a rapid increase in the number of VAD cases. This rapid increase is already apparent in more developed countries like Japan (Homma and Hasegawa), but will be increasingly apparent in the less developed countries like China in the next century (Shen and Yu).

8
The neuropathology of vascular dementia

Arne Brun

Introduction

Although cerebrovascular lesions often cause dementia in cooperation with other brain changes, they also do so on their own as shown by the pathology of proven cases of pure vascular disease with dementia. The clinical profile of the cases varies: with or without neurological deficits and with or without stepwise progression. Hence it is difficult to justify the use of 'dementia' of the cerebrovascular type, and it also fails to cover cardiac and hypotensive–hypoperfusive forms. Vascular cognitive impairment, as recently suggested by Bowler and Hachinski,[1] does not seem to solve the problem. Stroke dementia and cerebrovascular dementia suffer from the same weaknesses. Other confounding disorders may also blur the picture. To the pathologist none of these difficulties apply, but in mixed cases the weight of each component may, when pronounced, cause evaluation difficulties—something that of course also bothers the clinician. The term 'vascular dementia' (VAD) might better cover the subject since it may be taken to include the cardiac and hypotensive–hypoperfusive forms as well.[2]

Ageing is a confounding factor

One of the most common confounding factors in VAD is the ageing process, which can be described as a combination of degenerative and cerebrovascular changes among which the latter may be difficult to single out from the vascular dementing disease itself. In the literature the dementia under consideration is usually described as VAD or VAD plus other disorders, but VAD plus ageing is rarely considered. The importance of ageing is emphasized by the finding that VAD is the most common form of organic dementia after the age of 85.[3] This may be due to the fact that normal ageing, with its degenerative and small, silent vascular lesions, can be viewed as predisposing to dementia due to a reduction of brain reserve capacity, bringing the individual closer to the level of insufficiency that requires only minor lesions for dementia to result.

Among the degenerative ageing changes, senile plaques and neurofibrillary tangles are the most obvious. The latter are particularly pronounced in the entorhinal area of the hippocampus, an area vital to memory processing. There is also an amyloid angiopathy, sometimes as severe as that seen in Alzheimer's disease (AD), in which it can vary considerably in severity. More important, however, is a progressive loss of synapses in the cortex, often amounting to as much as 40–50% in the oldest cases.[4]

The vascular lesions are mainly expressed as a varying number of minute infarcts in the grey and white matter or large periventricular white matter incomplete infarcts, shown as white matter lucensies on imaging. When sufficiently pronounced, these lesions seem to cooperate to produce a dementia typical for the aged and which may therefore be termed 'dementia of the senium' or 'summational dementia',[5] since none or few of these small lesions are demonstrable and no single lesion can be held responsible and thus no conventional label can be applied. Before this stage is reached, however, the reduced reserve capacity may cooperate with any other kind of lesion or disease to produce dementia, which then appears to progress more quickly in the aged than in the younger patient with greater reserve capacity. Thus the more advanced the age, the less severe the lesion required to cause dementia. This then also means that even a minor stroke may seem to cause dementia, resulting in a clinical mislabelling of the condition since the stroke would not have resulted in dementia in a younger patient with greater reserve capacity. Further neuronal stress, for example in connection with narcosis, or functionally important deficiency states such as for vitamin B_{12}, and failing function of other organs, such as an ageing heart, would tend to produce cognitive impairment, temporarily or definitely.

Patho-anatomical classification of VAD

A simple basis for patho-anatomical classification of VAD is the size of the vessel responsible.[6] This approach is rational since the large vessels comprising the carotid, circle of Willis and its main branches and larger meningeal arteries are afflicted mainly with the consequences of common arteriosclerosis with atheromatous lesions, whereas the small vessels of arteriolar size mainly suffer from hypertensive angiopathy and fibrohyaline arteriolosclerosis. This results in a different lesion pattern that combines with a difference in infarct size. From this it also follows that large and small vessel disease may appear separately, resulting in pure large or small vessel dementia as demonstrated on extensive neuropathological examination. In one study, when all types of VAD were considered, almost half of them were of the pure type.[6]

In addition, reduction in oxygen and/or glucose can produce brain lesions, either global (apallic or semiapallic syndromes) or focal due to special local metabolic demands (regional selective vulnerability) or to regional haemodynamic conditions (border zone infarction and selective incomplete white matter infarcts). Venous occlusions may also cause large infarcts. A last group is formed by meningeal and brain haemorrhages. Against this background a neuropathological classification of VAD, modified from Brun and Gustafson,[7] is proposed (Table 8.1).

Large vessel dementia

Multi-infarct dementia (MID), a term introduced by Hachinski et al,[8] was originally meant to cover the whole field of VAD but is now mostly used to designate dementia due to large infarcts and in the present classification named large vessel dementia, caused mainly by thromboembolism originating from atherosclerotic lesions in the large vessels. However, a cardiac origin is also stressed, for example by the Cerebral Embolism Task Force,[9] giving rise to the term cardiac dementia, also applicable, in

Table 8.1.   Neuropathological classification of VAD.

1   Large vessel dementia
    Multi-infarct dementia (MID): Multiple large infarcts, cortical and subcortical, usually with perifocal incomplete infarcts, especially in white matter
    Strategic infarct dementia (SID): Restricted, few infarcts in functionally important, mostly subcortical brain regions (thalamus, basal ganglia, basal forebrain, ACA and MCA territories, angular gyrus)

2   Small vessel dementia
    Subcortical infarct dementia
        Binswanger's disease
        Lacunar state:
            Multiple small lacunar infarcts with large perifocal incomplete infarcts, especially in white matter
    Cortical and subcortical infarct dementia
        Hypertensive and arteriolosclerotic angiopathy
        Amyloid angiopathy, sometimes with haemorrhages
        Collagen vascular disease
        Hereditary forms
        Venous occlusion (large or small vessels)

3   Hypoxic-ischaemic/hypoperfusive dementia
    Diffuse hypoxic-ischaemic encephalopathy or restricted due to regional selective vulnerability
    Incomplete white matter infarcts
    Border zone infarcts

4   Haemorrhagic dementia
        Subdural haemorrhage
        Subarachnoid haemorrhage
        Cerebral haemorrhage

particular, to hypoperfusive dementia through other mechanisms. The occlusion of the larger vessels results in large infarcts involving cortex and white matter and also central grey and brain stem structures. In an extensive neuropathological study of 175 cases of dementia,[6] this was found to be the smallest group comprising 15% of all the VAD cases. This may explain the finding by Hulette et al,[10] who only investigated MID cases, that 'pure' VAD in general is very uncommon. A significant part of the infarct pathology, especially in the white matter, was the perifocal incomplete infarct, often involving larger areas than the complete infarct. Here the tissue damage decreased in a peripheral direction from the complete infarct centre, in grey matter within a narrow zone but in the white matter in wide areas. This is a penumbra zone,[11] not fully appreciated on brain imaging, particularly CT, and it thus makes up an often undiscovered or poorly identified correlate to the functional brain deficit. This zone deserves attention in view of the possible benefits of treatment supporting flow and metabolism, with the aim to prevent further growth of the penumbra zone together with incorporation of the original penumbra zone in the complete infarct, as discussed by Back et al.[12] In the grey matter such incomplete infarcts are also named selective neuronal loss,[13] and in the experience of the present author often best observed in hippocampal anoxic damage.

Strategic infarct dementia (SID) is a special type of large vessel dementia, due to a few but topographically important infarcts, and in this sense it is the opposite to MID. This concept was introduced in 1988,[7] and has since been increasingly used to denote a dementia caused by few or single, often restricted infarcts but with a strategic location in functionally important regions. One of the best known examples is bilateral anterior thalamic infarcts producing dementia of a frontal type. This places special emphasis on the role of brain imaging in dementia diagnosis as illustrated by a case clinically diagnosed as AD without CT lesions but with a thalamic strategic infarct shown on MR, which prompted a revision of the diagnosis to strategic VAD.[14]

Small vessel dementia

Small vessel dementia is due to obstruction of vessels of arteriolar size, namely mainly intracerebral vessels, sometimes due to microemboli from heart valves or atheromatous large vessel lesions, particularly carotid stenosis, and special vessel diseases such as collagen diseases,[15] amyloid angiopathies, especially the haemorrhagic familial forms, and hereditary angiopathies. The major cause is, however, hypertensive angiopathy which may assume two forms: cortical plus subcortical and purely subcortical referred to as Binswanger's disease (BD) or PSVE. Lacunar state may be regarded as a milder form of the latter. The two varieties are basically similar, showing small infarcts of lacunar size up to 10–15 mm in diameter. Esiri et al[16] referred to small vessel dementia as microvascular disease and found it to be the most common variety in their neuropathological study. Small vessel disease was also reported by Akiguchi et al[17] to be the leading form of VAD in Japan. This is in agreement with our finding that small vessel disease accounts for 33% of cases of pure or mixed VAD. Of these cases, almost half the number were of the pure type, predominately BD, making this disorder an important subgroup of VAD, accounting for a fourth of pure VAD.[6]

Subcortical infarct dementia
Binswanger's disease was initially characterized pathologically by Alzheimer and is marked by lacunar infarcts usually measuring 5–10 mm in diameter and situated in the brain stem and central grey nuclei but above all in the frontal white matter, sparing the cortex. In the white matter the lacunes are surrounded by wide areas of partial loss of myelin and oligodendroglial cells accompanied by a mild astrocytic gliosis causing an extensive cortical undermining. This change impresses as the main structural substrate for the functional deficit explaining frontal symptoms, gait and incontinence problems. The small lacunes are most probably of minor importance. The loss of white matter is reflected in a widening of the frontal ventricular horns. This change has the character of an incomplete white matter infarct which, at least in part, is demonstrable on brain imaging. It can be assumed to evolve due to repeated episodes of ischaemia in a penumbra zone around the lacunes which in combination with the relative discreteness of the damage on each occasion explains the clinical character of a progressive disorder. Many of these cases suffer from hypertension. Absence of hypertension should raise the suspicion of CADASIL (cerebral autosomal dominant arteriopathy with subcortical infarcts and leukoencephalopathy).[1] In CADASIL the angiopathy is less florid than in BD, characterized by fibrohyaline arteriosclerosis. This condition is dominantly hereditary and the gene localized to chromosome 19 though distinct from the ApoE gene.[18] It could be regarded as a disorder in a Binswanger spectrum but without hypertension.[19] In contrast to some authors,[20] others[21,22] consider BD to be a well-defined disorder and an important cause of VAD, particularly in the older age groups. This stresses the necessity of whole brain sections for the full evaluation of the disease pattern. Also, looking at all age groups BD is rather common, comprising the dominant variety of pure small vessel dementia in one study.[6]

Cortical and subcortical infarct dementia
Cortical plus subcortical infarct dementia is regularly associated with hypertension and arteriolosclerosis. The vascular level and size involved

is somewhat more varied than in BD and hence the infarcts show a greater variation in size, although they are largely in the lacunar range. The complications of hypertensive angiopathy are more prominent here, with mural and perivascular haemorrhages and microaneurysms, and the lesions are less frontally accentuated than in BD. Other rarer causes of small vessel dementia are collagen vascular disease, hereditary angiopathies such as familial amyloid angiopathy, CADASIL, hereditary multi-infarct dementia and glycosaminoglycan angiopathy. A combination of large and small vessel disease with large and small infarcts surprisingly accounted for only 22% of VAD in one study.[6]

Venous occlusions
As a cause of VAD, venous occlusions are rare due to the limited survival rate after such incidents, which are rare in themselves.

Hypoxic-ischaemic hypoperfusive dementia

Hypoxic-hypoperfusive dementia is here defined as dementia due not to focal cessation of flow, as in preceding forms of VAD, but to a temporary reduction of flow or substrate supply below the level necessary for neural structural integrity for a period of time long enough to damage brain tissue. A chronic ischaemic state appears unphysiological in itself, in agreement with Bowler et al[1] and as a cause of brain damage, in view of the existence of autoregulatory mechanisms and the possibility of variation in oxygen extraction. These factors, which are general rather than focal, produce global anoxic encephalopathy or focal lesions due to selective vulnerability such as border zone infarcts, both of which are, however, uncommon causes of VAD. The larger group here is one with incomplete infarcts of the white matter in particular. This group is roughly of the same size as small vessel VAD,[6] and is treated in a separate chapter of this volume.

Haemorrhagic dementia

Haemorrhage with dementia is included here since it is clearly related to vascular disease and also causes secondary ischaemic anoxic lesions. It is unusual, however, but may be seen after subdural and subarachnoid as well as intracerebral haemorrhage.

References

1. Bowler J, Hachinski V, Vascular dementia. In: Ginsberg MD, Bogousslavsky J, eds, *Cerebrovascular Disease: Pathophysiology, Diagnosis and Management* (Blackwell Science: Berlin, 1998) 1126–44.
2. O'Brien MD, How does cerebrovascular disease cause dementia? In: Hartmann A, Kuschinsky W, Hoyer S, eds, *Cerebral Ischaemia and Dementia* (Springer Verlag: Berlin).
3. Amar K, Wilcock G, Vascular dementia. Fortnightly review, *BMJ* (1996) **312**:227–31.
4. Liu X, Ericsson C, Brun A, Cortical synaptic changes and gliosis in normal ageing, Alzheimer's disease and frontal lobe degeneration, *Dementia* (1996) **7**:128–34.
5. Brun A, Gustafson L, Mårtensson SM, Ericsson C, Neuropathology of late life, *Dementia* (1992) **3**: 125–30.
6. Brun A, Pathology and pathophysiology of cerebrovascular dementia: pure subgroups of obstructive and hypoperfusive etiology, *Dementia* (1994) **5**:145–7.
7. Brun A, Gustafson L, Zerebrovaskuläre E. In: Kisker KP, Lauter H, Meyer J-E, Muller C, Strömgren E, eds, *Psychiatrie der Gegenwart 6* (Springer: Berlin, 1988) 253–95.
8. Hachinski V, Lassen NA, Marshall J, Multiinfarct dementia: a cause of mental deterioration in the elderly, *Lancet* (1974) **ii**:207–10.
9. Cerebral Embolism Task Force, Cardiogenic brain embolism, *Arch Neurol* (1989) **46**:727–43.
10. Hulette C, Nochlin D, McKeel MD et al, Clinical–neuropathologic findings in multi-infarct dementia: a report of six autopsied cases, *Neurology* (1997) **48**:668–72.
11. Astrup J, Siesjö BK, Symon L, Thresholds in cerebral ischemia—the ischemic penumbra, *Stroke* (1981) **12**:723–5.
12. Back T, Nedergaard M, Ginsberg MD, The ischemic penumbra. Pathophysiology and relevance of spreading depression-like phenomena. In: Ginsberg MD, Bogousslavsky J, eds, *Cerebrovascular Disease: Pathophysiology, Diagnosis and Management* (Blackwell Science: Berlin, 1998) 276–86.
13. Weiller C, Chollet F, Frackowiak RSJ, Physiologic aspects of functional recovery from stroke. In: Ginsberg MD, Bogousslavsky J, eds, *Cerebrovascular Disease: Pathophysiology, Diagnosis and Management* (Blackwell Science: Berlin, 1998) 2057–66.
14. Wolf R, Orszagh M, März W, Case study. Revision of an Alzheimer's diagnosis in a patient with an almost normal CT scan: why strategic vascular lesions may be overlooked, *Alzheimer's Res* (1997) **3**:73–6.
15. Lishman WA, Cerebrovascular disorders. In: Lishman WA, ed, *Organic Psychiatry. The Psychological Consequences of Cerebral Disorder*, 3rd edn (Blackwell Science: Berlin, 1997) 375–430.
16. Esiri MM, Wilcock GK, Morris JH, Neuropathological assessment of the lesions of significance in vascular dementia, *J Neurol Neurosurg Psych* (1997) **63**: 749–53.
17. Akiguchi L, Tomimoto H, Suenaga T et al, Alterations in glia and axons in the brains of Binswanger's disease patients, *Stroke* (1997) **28**:1423–9.
18. Tournier-Lasserve E, Joutel A, Melki J et al, Cerebral autosomal dominant arteriopathy with subcortical infarcts and leukoen-

cephalopathy maps on chromosome 19q12, *Nat Genet* (1993) **3**:256–9.
19. Hedera P, Friedland R, Cerebral autosomal dominant arteriopathy with subcortical, infarcts and leukoencephalopathy: study of two American families with predominant dementia, *J Neurol Sci* (1997) **146**:27–33.
20. Pantoni L, Garcia JH, The significance of cerebral white matter abnormalities 100 years after Binswanger's report. A review, *Stroke* (1995) **26**:1293–301.
21. Roman G, From UBOs to Binswanger's disease. Impact of magnetic resonance imaging on vascular dementia research, *Stroke* (1996) **27**:1269–73.
22. Caplan LR, Binswanger's disease: revisited, *Neurology* (1995) **45**:626–33.

9
White matter pathology of vascular dementia

Elisabet Englund

Introduction

The cerebral white matter is often affected by structural pathological changes in cerebrovascular disease and vascular dementia (VAD). The high prevalence of histopathologically proven white matter involvement in VAD[1–3] indicates that damage to this part of the brain is of major importance in the clinical expression of dementia, an impact that has been underestimated previously.

This chapter describes the presentation of morphological white matter changes in different forms of VAD and compares these changes with the structural white matter appearance in mixed neurodegenerative and vascular dementia as well as with that of normal aging. Secondly, pathogenesis of the white matter pathology in VAD is discussed. The last part draws some diagnostic and differential conclusions on white matter disease from the combination of radiological and pathological findings.

White matter changes found in VAD

On a regional tissue level, the structural changes constituting cerebral white matter disease (WMD) appear in two forms which often occur in combination, although either form may dominate the picture. These are focal and diffuse changes, respectively.[4]

Focal changes

The focal white matter lesions are represented by large cavitating, medium-sized or minor infarcts with cystic or lacunar formation. Whereas the fresh/recent infarct often retains the necrotic material, cyst formation and lacunar infarcts provide the evidence of older damage of at least several weeks, where the tissue has 'settled' after the incident and there has been both passage and clearing of macrophages.

The large cystic infarcts can reach a diameter of over 20 mm and may extend from the central white matter to be combined with infarction in the adjacent cortex, shown as glial scarring and often extensive indentation of the latter towards the underlying cyst. Fibrillary astrocytes and a meshwork of glial fibrillar detritus may build up the lining of the cyst. A few remaining macrophages may contain pigment of haemosiderin as evidence of a previous extravasation of blood. Traces of very mild blood–brain barrier disruption may be detected by immunohistochemical staining for albumin in the perivascular tissue. Localized reactive astrocytosis and microglial activation are also indications of such a process.

The medium-sized and particularly small focal white matter infarcts of a few millimetres in diameter are often accompanied by lacunes in the basal ganglia, particularly in the thalamus and putamen.

Blood vessels of all calibres are pathologically altered by arteriosclerosis and/or hypertension as well as by other possible and varying stressors. The degree of vascular pathology is highly variable and may also be regionally or focally accentuated, with sparing of large domains.

Diffuse changes

Diffuse white matter pathology of cerebrovascular disease and VAD is characterized by an attenuation and reduction of tissue components without complete loss of any of the elements. Hence within a specific region, the number of axons, myelin sheaths and oligodendrocytic nuclei is reduced, but adjoined by the presence of limited reactive glia, mainly fibrillary astrocytes and macrophages. It constitutes the picture of subtotal ischaemic necrosis, or incomplete white matter infarction (IWI).[5]

Diffuse and focal changes

One frequently appearing form of diffuse pathology is represented in the perifocal tissue around the complete white matter infarcts, whether they be cavitating or scarred—thus diffuse and focal changes often occur in combination.

The diffuse pathology exhibits a spectrum of degrees of histopathological severity from the scarred border of the completely devitalized infarct centre to the better preserved periphery at some distance from the infarct midpoint. The periphery merges with the surrounding normal white matter at a distance from the infarct, that is variable due to localization and specific preconditions in each situation.

On cut brain sections, the perifocal diffuse white matter pathology generally covers an area much (10- to 100-fold) larger than that of the complete infarct, hence with a corresponding huge dominance over the latter in terms of volume. The structural changes here are those found in individuals with large-vessel disease and small-vessel disease,[2] respectively and in combination.

Diffuse pathology alone

Another form of diffuse pathology appears as the sole white matter pathology and is not associated with focal lesions/complete infarcts. It is seen in a subgroup of VAD subjects in which there are no other associated pathological tissue changes in either grey or white matter, but a central arteriolopathy.[6] It has the character of a stenosing fibrohyaline sclerosis affecting many of the arterioles, leaving the veins unremarkable. The arterioles show a wall thickened by acellular fibrohyaline material, collagen replacement of the smooth muscle layer and reduction of the luminal width to all but complete occlusion. This arteriolopathy is sometimes, though not unconditionally, accompanied by small-vessel pathology of the hypertensive type, but it is not invariably or particularly prevalent in cases with large-vessel arteriosclerosis. The arterioles engaged are generally seen within the region of attenuated white matter, but are sometimes extended beyond the borders of detectable tissue changes.

In this situation, the entire pathology thus consists of diffuse white matter attenuation with subtotal loss of tissue elements a mild glial reaction and arteriolosclerosis, but no complete infarct. It represents the selective incomplete white matter infarction (SIWI).[7] Macroscopically it is difficult to detect, but may on fresh-cut sections of relatively severe cases reveal a sunken white matter appearance and a slightly greyish discolouring. The pathology here corresponds with non-infarct/hypoperfused disease, most often with a distinct component of small-vessel disease.[6]

White matter changes in forms of mixed dementia

Mixed dementia generally means AD-VAD: a prominent Alzheimer encephalopathy (AE) with the appearance of a considerable amount of focal infarcts. In AD-VAD, the white matter pathology is mainly diffuse *and* focal, as described above. Diagnostic efforts may be complicated in the situation of 'co-operating pathologies', for example in cases where a very mild AE concurs with minor vascular lesions, which alone would not have triggered symptoms and signs of dementia.[6,8]

The following types of dementia are not classically mixed but are often of a 'combined' type.

AD-SIWI

Diffuse white matter pathology or SIWI of the same form as above, at least identical on a light microscopical level, is also found in AD as a disorder that concurs with the grey matter degeneration of this disease.[6, 7] It is seen in over 50% of Alzheimer cases, with a slight increase in prevalence with advanced age. All combinations of severity of the grey and white matter pathology are seen, for example severe cortical AE with mild (or no) WMD as well as prominent WMD in a brain with relatively mild AE—to a level where the mildest component is close to the level judged to be normal for age. SIWI may be found in the frontal as well as all other regions, along with a stenosing arteriolosclerosis accentuated in the deep, central strata, but generally sparing the subcortical u-fibres.[7]

FTD-SIWI

Among the frontotemporal dementias (FTD)—frontal lobe degeneration of non-Alzheimer type and Pick´s disease—diffuse white matter changes (SIWI) also appear, but to a lesser degree and in rather fewer cases. Except for such situations, FTD is not considered to be a mixed form of dementia. A similar, yet different form of diffuse pathology is often more striking in FTD cases: that is a relatively dense astrocytic gliosis along with moderate loss of myelin, paralleling the extent of detectable cortical degeneration. The latter WMD is regionally associated with the cortical degeneration and hence accentuated in the frontal and temporal lobes, where it engages all parts of the white matter including the subcortical u-fibres.[6] It may be difficult to differentiate from a vascular component by imaging methods.[9]

White matter changes in normal ageing

The process of aging causes subtle and minor structural changes in the white matter,[6, 10] with a subsequent enlargement of the ventricular system. A regionally non-specific shrinkage of the brain also includes a mild decrease of myelinated tracts. Radiologically, CT and MRI findings of white matter changes in normal aging are well known,[11, 12] and the morphologic correlates include mild demyelination and gliosis .[13,14] A limited periventricular loss of myelin is found in mentally well-preserved elderly,[6] but also widespread arteriolosclerosis and dilated perivascular spaces.[13] A cribriform state[15] connotes the presence of numerous widened perivascular spaces around slightly sclerotic arterioles, often with mild hypertension in normally aged individuals. Although it is not a recognized pathologic condition corresponding to defined clinical symptoms, it is observed to be prominent in a few individuals who retrospectively appear to have been mildly demented, but who were never diagnostically evaluated.[6]

Wallerian degeneration

In any brain subject to cortical or subcortical grey matter damage, secondary or Wallerian degeneration occurs.[16] It is a slow process of tissue regression emanating from the damaged neuron through anterograde axonal breakdown and subsequent devitalization of myelin. It is most readily discernible in cases with severe neurodegenerative disease, such as advanced AD or FTD, and may be differentiated from the other pathologic processes by its accentuation adjacent to the most pronounced cortical-neuronal damage.[4,9]

Pathogenesis

A complete white matter infarct is the result of a relatively abrupt ischaemia within a defined region. The size of an infarct in part relates to the (central parts of) territorial borders of the supplying artery, which in the white matter is often an end artery. Following *vessel occlusion*, the lacunar form of small infarct develops. In the *non-occlusive* situation, a rapid and profound hypoperfusion, for example of haemodynamic causes, may result in a complete border-zone infarct.

Incomplete white matter infarction evolves over a long time. When prominent enough to be detected microscopically, it is a stabilized condition without trace of the active ischaemic or hypoxic process (oedema, focalized gliosis and myelin breakdown) that may have occurred previously. Albeit only partially, the pathology of incomplete infarction by definition involves all tissue components. Due to the presence of associated vasculopathy associated in many cases with the absence of other brain pathology, these white matter changes are concluded to emanate from hypoxic-ischaemic events in the brain. As support to this conclusion, clinical signs of suboptimal cerebral perfusion, often due to mild cardiac failure and recurrently low/insufficient systemic blood pressure,[17] are frequently present.

Haemodynamic factors are important in the pathogenesis of VAD and as such are probably underestimated.[18] A cerebral vasculature already compromised by arteriosclerosis, hypertensive arteriolopathy, and denervation angiopathy,[6] will not adjust adequately to haemodynamic flow changes, hence possibly opening the gates for recurrent episodes of hypoperfusion. Insufficiently compensated hypoperfusion, either by the effects of previous hypertension or by systemic hypotension or both, will be followed by regional cerebral ischaemia. The cerebral white matter is highly vulnerable to ischaemia, as shown in numerous clinical and clinicopathological correlative studies and in an experimental study on rat brain.[19] A selective, at least accentuated damage in oligodendrocytes was demonstrated after brief experimental rat brain ischaemia,[20] and suggested to be mediated through glutamate and free radical toxicity. In humans, an accumulating amount of evidence on the links between white matter pathology and blood pressure abnormalities in dementia was recently reviewed.[21]

Diagnosis and differentiation

As a central part of the ischaemic white matter pathology with infarcts, the perifocal diffuse white matter pathology is one of the most common types of vascular-ischaemic tissue damage in the brain, especially in those demented in whom the structural changes develop rather progressively and over a long time. Clinically, diffuse WMD gradually undercuts the cortex of the involved area, whether being predominantly frontal, occipital or homogeneous. Due to the organization of white matter with widely spread fibre tracts connecting with large neocortical areas, both anatomical and functional isolation of these may be insidious and very slow. The clinical detection of WMD naturally depends on the affected region per se and the expressiveness of the cortical area being undercut in each situation, as well as on speed of progression. Radiologically, it may pass undetected due to its gradual transition to/merging with the adjacent normal tissue and thereby indistinct borders. Also post mortem, the diffuse changes are histopathologically difficult to detect and to delineate without coronary whole-brain sections, particularly considering the effects of aging and the concurrence with Wallerian degeneration. The neuropathological WMD in VAD is the morphological equivalent to some of all radiologically identified WMD, which in many other conditions such as primary degenerative dementia, post-traumatic encephalopathy, prion disease, metabolic and toxic disorders corresponds to different histopathological entities in spite of an apparent similarity with imaging techniques.

Small but crucial differences may help to differentiate among the conditions considered in the various cases. For example:

- In imaging of widespread WMD, the presence of even very discrete focal white matter lesions speaks in favour of a vascular origin and small-vessel disease, while a completely homogeneous MRI pathology of the white matter may reflect SIWI *or* non-ischaemic WMD.
- Patchy and confluent lesions are not necessarily of different origin, but instead are often closely related, emanating from the same vascular-ischaemic incident.

- A slightly irregular, asymmetric pattern favours VAD.
- Radiologically seen cortical atrophy *and* subjacent WMD indicates neurodegenerative disease with associated white matter change, as in FTD.[9,22]
- Lack of cortical atrophy, sparing of subcortical u-fibres and central/deep, eg frontal homogeneous WMD may reflect pure SIWI, which is not uncommon.[6]

It is an urgent task to standardize the nomenclature among research groups and between different professional disciplines with regard to macroanatomical and microscopical definitions.[9] The terms 'deep' versus 'central' and 'subcortical' white matter may at times have different implications, which has the potential to complicate or confound correlative efforts in the study of white matter pathologies.

References

1. Roman GC, Tatemichi TK, Erkinjuntti T et al, Vascular dementia: diagnostic criteria for research studies. Report of the NINDS-AIREN international workshop. *Neurology* (1993) **43**:250–60.

2. Brun A, Pathology and pathophysiology of cerebrovascular dementia: pure subgroups of obstructive and hypoperfusive etiology. *Dementia* (1994) **5**:145–7.

3. Tomimoto H, Akiguchi I, Wakita H et al, Regressive changes of astroglia in white matter lesions in cerebrovascular disease and Alzheimer´s disease patients. *Acta Neuropathol* (1997) **94**:146–52.

4. Englund E, Neuropathology of white matter changes in Alzheimer´s disease and vascular dementia. *Dement Geriatr Cogn Disord* (1998) **9**(Suppl1):6–12.

5. Englund E, Brun A, Persson B, Correlations between histopathologic white matter changes and proton MR relaxation times in dementia. *Alzheimer Dis Assoc Disord* (1987) **1**:156–70.

6. Englund E, Neuropathology of white matter disease: parenchymal changes. In: Pantoni L, Inzitari D, Wallin A, eds, *The Matter of White Matter. Clinical and Pathophysiological Aspects of White Matter Disease Related to Cognitive Decline and Vascular Dementia* (ICG Publications: Dordrecht, 1999) in press.

7. Brun A, Englund E, A white matter disorder in dementia of Alzheimer type: a pathoanatomical study. *Ann Neurol* (1986) **19**:253–62.

8. Pasquier F, Leys D, Why are stroke patients prone to develop dementia? *J Neurol* (1997) **244**:135–42.

9. Larsson E-M, Passant U, Sundgren P et al, Magnetic resonance imaging and histopathology in frontotemporal dementia. *Dement Geriatr Cogn Disord* (1999) in press.

10. Miller AKH, Alston RL, Corsellis JAN, Variation with age in the volumes of grey and white matter in the cerebral hemispheres of man:

measurements with an image analyser. *Neuropath Appl Neurobiol* (1980) **6**:119–32.

11. Kobari M, Meyer JS, Ichijo M, Oravez WT, Leukoaraiosis: correlation of MR and CT findings with blood flow, atrophy and cognition. *Am J Neuroradiol* (1990) **11**:273–81.

12. Scheltens P, Barkhof F, Leys D et al, Histopathologic correlates of white matter changes on MRI in Alzheimer's disease and normal aging. *Neurology* (1995) **45**:883–8.

13. Van Swieten JC, Van den Hout JHW, Van Ketel BA et al, Periventricular lesions in the white matter on magnetic resonance imaging in the elderly. A morphometric correlation with arteriolosclerosis and dilated perivascular spaces. *Brain* (1991) **114**:761–74.

14. Grafton ST, Sumi SM, Stimac GK et al, Comparison of postmortem magnetic resonance imaging and neuropathological findings in the cerebral white matter. *Arch Neurol* (1991) **48**:293–8.

15. Blackwood W, Vascular disease of the central nervous system. In: Greenfield JC, Blackwood W, McMenemy WH et al, eds, *Neuropathology*, 1st edn (Edward Arnold: London, 1958) 67–131.

16. Kreutzberg GW, Blakemore WF, Graeber MB, Cellular pathology of the central nervous system. In: Graham DI, Lantos PL, eds, *Greenfield's Neuropathology*, 6th edn (Arnold: London, 1997) 85–156.

17. Englund E, Brun A, Gustafson L, A white matter disease in dementia of Alzheimer's type—clinical and neuropathological correlates. *Int J Ger Psychiatry* (1989) **4**:87–102.

18. Moroney JT, Bagiella E, Desmond DW et al, Risk factors for incident dementia after stroke. Role of hypoxic and ischemic disorders. *Stroke* (1996) **27**:1283–9.

19. Pantoni L, Garcia JH, Gutierrez JA, Cerebral white matter is highly vulnerable to ischemia. *Stroke* (1996) **27**:1641–7.

20. Petito CK, Olarte JP, Roberts B et al, Selective glial vulnerability following transient global ischemia in rat brain. *J Neuropathol Exp Neurol* (1998) **57**:231–8.

21. Skoog I, A review on blood pressure and ischaemic white matter lesions. *Dement Geriatr Cogn Disord* (1998) **9**(Suppl 1):13–19.

22. Kitagaki H, Mori E, Hirono N et al, Alteration of white matter MR signal intensity in frontotemporal dementia. *Am J Neuroradiol* (1997) **18**:367–78.

10
Clinical pathological correlates

Lars Gustafson and Ulla Passant

Introduction

The clinical manifestations of cerebrovascular disease are varied and complex as are their relationships to the type and localization of the vascular lesion. Stroke may not only give rise to circumscribed, delineated neurological and psychological impairments but also global changes of mentation and behaviour. The symptoms, however, may not only be the result of the vascular brain lesion but also of concomitant somatic disorders some of which, such as cardiac disease, blood pressure pathology and diabetes, are well-known risk factors for cerebrovascular disease. Previous mental and physical health, medication, alcohol consumption and socio-economic conditions may also play an important role. In the psychiatric field, there is usually a mixture of symptoms, some of which can be interpreted as primary deficits related to the organic damage and dysfunction, while others may be regarded as secondary adaptive (compensatory as well as protective) or insufficiency reactions to the brain damage.[1,2] However, no mental symptoms in and of themselves are pathognomonic of vascular dementia (VAD) or any other type of dementia. It is the symptom constellation, the timing of their appearance and the clinical course that are important. Therefore, a symptom may be interpreted differently in different contexts, and the clinical diagnosis of VAD should rely on a broad assessment of both psychiatric and neurological features. Analyses of the association between the clinical picture and brain pathology often show an inconsistency and a lack of correlations. This has been explained by inconclusive evaluations of the brain damage and the fact that individuals differ in their mental reactions to identical or very similar brain pathology.[3] On this basis it is obvious that the effect of an insult may be difficult to predict, with regard to both resulting tissue injury and its functional consequences. However, the development of brain imaging techniques and a careful correlation of the results to post-mortem findings are gradually offering new insights into this field. This chapter will deal with the pathological correlates to certain clinical features in VAD.

Disease onset and progress

Mental deterioration and neurological deficits may develop rapidly or slowly as a result of single or repeated cerebrovascular lesions. An abrupt onset and episodic worsening, with a clouding of consciousness and disorientation, associated with focal symptoms and signs indicative of cerebrovascular disease, have been noted in fewer than 50% of the cases. The cognitive decline following a single stroke may remain unchanged, but more characteristic is a gradual recovery, which, however, seldom reaches the pre-stroke functional level. Such episodic deterioration following a remittent or markedly fluctuating course may in retrospect be described as a stepwise downhill progression. Recurrent strokes are most often of the same type, aetiology and localization as a first stroke,[4] which almost always indicates the region at risk. However, clinical onset of VAD may be preceded by 'little strokes' in neurologically silent areas of the brain.[5] Recent CT and MRI findings of subclinical ischaemic lesions, most prevalent in the white matter, support this hypothesis. The subclinical, 'silent' stroke may be caused by blood pressure drops, cardiac insufficiency and any critical somatic condition. Such lesions, as well as subclinical Alzheimer's disease (AD) changes, may sometimes explain an unexpected rapid onset of severe dementia following a few small mainly subcortical strategic infarcts.[6,7] The most prevalent types of VAD, however, show a more gradual intellectual decline, sometimes accompanied by an outbreak of depression, paranoia and other mental disturbances.

Our present view of clinico-pathological correlations in VAD is based on studies of individual cases and patient groups, more recently substantiated by structural and functional brain imaging. It is often possible to recognize symptoms and signs which clearly indicate the localization of the vascular damage and the brain vessels involved. The pathological examination should, however, also consider the impact of other non-vascular types of brain disease, and the possibility of dementia as an effect of summation of lesions of different type and localization.[6,7]

Frontal lobe traits

Vascular frontal and frontal-subcortical syndromes which may mimic degenerative frontal or frontotemporal lobar dementia are of special interest.[8] Vascular dementia with frontal features may be caused by frontal cortical infarcts, bilateral thalamic infarcts,[9–12] bilateral caudate infarcts,[13] Binswanger's disease[14–17] and incomplete white matter infarctions found in the frontal lobes only.[18] Thus, the vascular lesions may directly involve a frontal lobe or work by rejection or projection to frontal structures. The clinical picture caused by these lesions is dominated by changes of personality and behaviour with signs of disinhibition, lack of insight, emotional levelling, euphoria, depressed mood and apathy. There is often a mental slowing, impaired attention and impaired executive functions, memory failure, and neurologically, gait problems, primitive reflexes and urinary incontinence. The characteristic shuffling, small-stepped gait is related to interruptions of thalamocortical and corticospinal connections. Urinary incontinence is associated with lesions in the superior frontal gyrus, anterior cingulate gyrus and the white matter in between.[19] The combination of progressive dementia, incontinence, gait disturbance and ventricular dilatation on CT and MRI in Binswanger's disease may sometimes lead to the diagnosis of hydrocephalic dementia.[20] Thalamic strokes and vascular lesions and malformations in the caudate nuclei may sometimes produce choreoatheloic movements, thereby mimicking Huntington's disease.[21]

Parietal lobe lesions

Cognitive impairment and dementia are more likely to develop as a result of strokes within the dominant hemisphere, bilateral vascular lesions and when thalamic structures are involved.[22] The clinical picture caused by infarction in the angular artery territory roughly corresponding to the temporoparietal association cortex is of special interest. The central role of parietal lobe lesions in dementia conditions was pointed out by Critchley.[23] Left-sided lesions in this area are associated with the Gerstmann syndrome, dyscalculia, dysgrafia, right–left disorientation and finger dysgnosia.[24] The consistency of this clustering has been criticized,[25] but an 'enlarged' Gerstmann syndrome, including dyspraxia, sensory aphasia and anomic aphasia, shows a strong similarity to the focal temporoparietal symptom pattern typical of AD. Vascular lesions involving or undercutting the angular gyrus in the speech dominant hemisphere may therefore be misinterpreted as AD when the clinical course is progressive. The Gerstmann syndrome may also be caused by other lesions.[26] The symptom constellation of the enlarged syndrome is strongly related to the severity of the dementia syndrome.[27]

Clinical fluctuations

Certain features such as fluctuating course, stepwise deterioration and confusional episodes with clouding of consciousness are prevalent in cerebrovascular disease and VAD. Stepwise deterioration and fluctuating course were the two items of the Hachinski Ischemic Score[28] which most clearly distinguished mutli-infarct dementia (MID) from AD in a recent study of 312 pathologically verified dementia cases.[29] Variations in the severity of symptoms within a day and between days as well as typical episodic return to a relatively efficient level,[30] as described in VAD, indicate the complexity and variability of cerebral circulatory conditions. The episodic improvement in cerebrovascular disease indicates the potential viability of dysfunctional regions bordering on the complete infarction, the ischaemic penumbra.[31,32] There is possibly an injury gradient between dead central and undamaged peripheral tissues. This type of lesion is also found in degenerative dementia with hypoperfusive periods associated with failing cardiovascular functions. Nocturnal confusion (observed in all types of dementia and delirium), another item in the Ischemic Score, is probably too unspecific to have any stronger discriminative diagnostic value.[33,34] The clinical fluctuations in VAD are to some extent predictable since they appear in association with psychological and somatic strain.

Acute stroke and ischaemic attacks are often accompanied by delirious episodes, and the course of VAD is characterized by confusional episodes. The incidence of these confusional episodes is mainly unknown. Acute confusional states have been reported in 25–48% of stroke patients.[35,36] Precipitating factors such as cognitive decline, medication, infections and other somatic disorders have been identified. The type and localization of the vascular lesions seem to play an important role. Extensive and haemorrhagic lesions, focal lesions, especially in left posterior and right middle cerebral artery territories, and in right hemisphere superficial, hippocampal and thalamic vascular lesions have been associated with confusional states.[35–39] Agitated delirium accompanied by visual hallucinosis has been reported in patients with unilateral and bilateral vascular lesions in the middle temporal gyrus, especially in the right hemisphere,[40] in the mesial temporal, parietal and occipital lobes[41,42] and thalamus.[43] The characteristic fluctuating consciousness in delirium is associated with large and right hemisphere lesions and with vertebro-basilar insufficiency.[44] The aetiology of delirium is usually multifactorial. Vascular lesions decrease the resistance to delirium caused by any type of somatic and psychological stress including sleep and sensory deprivation. Increased vulnerability due to subclinical ischaemic lesions, especially in precentral areas, and an interaction with drugs also contribute to the high risk of confusional episodes in late onset AD and Lewy body dementia.[45,46]

Occlusion and insufficiency of the vertebro-basilar arteries may give a large variety of symptoms which are sometimes difficult to differentiate from other organic and functional mental disorders. The variation of symptoms is explained by the different structures supplied by these arteries. Vertebro-basilar insufficiency is more common in patients who are relatively hypotensive and systemic hypotension might precipitate ischaemia.[47,48] The majority of patients who suffer infarction in the vertebro-basilar territory show symptoms such as drop attacks, episodic vertigo and diplopia accompanied by nystagmus. A clouding of consciousness has been reported in 30% of these patients, possibly due to the involvement of the reticular activating system. This clouding of consciousness may be associated with illusions and hallucinatory experiences, sometimes described as beautiful and dreamlike. Transient or permanent cognitive impairment especially memory failure is prevalent when hippocampus, the mamillary bodies and thalamic structures are involved.[49,50] Infarcts in the area of the posterior cerebral artery have been related to psychomotor slowing, inertia and emotional lability.[51]

Affective symptoms

The association between affective symptoms and cerebrovascular disorders was first pointed out by Kraeppelin in 1904.[52] Post[53] found a close time relation between the first cerebrovascular incidence and the onset of affective symptoms. The likelihood that elderly depressives have an increased risk of developing cerebrovascular disease has been substantiated by MRI, which showed a high prevalence of silent cerebral infarction in patients with presenile and senile major depression.[54] Different types of emotional disturbances such as increased sentimentality and tearfulness and inappropriate uncontrolled laughter have been described. Manifestations of impaired emotional control are often associated with lesions of the cortico-bulbar tract and a dysfunction of the prefrontal and anterior temporal cerebral cortex.[55,56] The phenomenology of depression in stroke patients is basically the same as that of major depression and in accordance with DSM-IV. The clinical diagnosis of mood disorder may prove to be difficult however. This is partly due to admixture of neurological deficits including communication problems.

There are several possible explanations for increased vulnerability to affective disorders following stroke, such as the localization and severity of the brain lesion, the reduction of serotonin, dopamine and other transmitter levels, the patient's age, premorbid personality and socio-economic factors.[57,58] Robinson and associates analysed the relationship between depression and the localization of the cerebrovascular lesion, finding that the severity of depression was directly correlated to the closeness of the lesion to the frontal pole, irrespective of the aetiology of the brain injury. Forty-nine per cent of patients with left hemisphere lesions and 7% with right hemisphere lesions were affected initially and remained in this state for at least 6 months. The prevalence of depression in patients with brainstem lesions was 36%. Further studies have confirmed the strong association between depression and left hemisphere lesions.[59,60]

Thus great controversies concerning pathological correlates to depression in stroke patients still remain. The strong correlations between depression and anterior left hemisphere lesions and between symptoms of emotional indifference and euphoria related to right hemisphere lesions are supported by findings in other patient groups.[61,62] Depression might be considered a natural consequence of the patient's awareness of intellectual and physical disabilities. The production of a depressive syndrome probably depends on the degree of function in the better preserved cerebral structures. The relationship between mood and cognition in stroke is complex. Depression accentuates the cognitive dysfunction and the presence of cognitive deficits increases the likelihood of developing depression.

Robinson et al[63] also found that patients who suffered depression combined with cognitive impairment had smaller lesions than non-depressed patients with corresponding cognitive impairment. Eastwood et al,[64] after studying CT scans, reported depression in more than 50% of a group of patients with vascular lesions. The severity of depression was negatively correlated with the distance of the lesion from the frontal pole and with the amount of brain tissue involved in the left but not in the right hemisphere.[64] By contrast, Dam and co-workers,[65] using CT scans for the localization of vascular lesions, found a higher degree of depression in patients with right hemisphere lesions, especially when the frontal right region was involved. Sharpe and co-workers[66] found no evidence of correlation between the degree of depression and impaired physical function or proximity of the lesion to the anterior pole of the left cerebral hemisphere.

Morris and Robinson,[67] who studied 99 patients 2 months after they had suffered a stroke, diagnosed minor depression in 18% and major depression in 14%. Major depression was characterized by an average duration of 39 weeks and a mortality rate of 23% and was related to a positive family history of affective or anxiety disorder. In patients with left hemisphere lesions, major depression was combined with cognitive impairment. Minor depression had a shorter average duration. These two affective syndromes may define distinct subtypes of post-stroke depression. There was, however, no evidence of a significant link between gross hemispheric lesion localization and depression. The association between depression and left hemispheric lesions remains difficult to explain. However, a relation to hemispheric differences in cerebral biogenic amine function and a common factor linking cognitive dysfunction and depression to the left hemisphere have been suggested.

An additional affective syndrome of hypomanic type with symptoms such as elated mood, increased cheerfulness and hyperactivity has also been described in VAD.[60] This type of secondary or symptomatic mania was reported in a substantial number of cases following cerebral insults. Little is known about the pathological substrate, although MRI often shows white matter hyperintensities in the frontal lobes and the frontal/parietal junction, which are evenly divided between the two hemispheres in older patients with bipolar disorder.[68] These findings suggest mood disorders as possible subcortical disconnection syndromes.[69,70] White matter lesions are, however, common in healthy elderly people and the more specific association between depression and white matter lesions has yet to be clearly understood. In a meta-analysis of MRI findings[71] deep white matter lesions were found more frequently than expected in both unipolar and bipolar patients. Damage to deep white matter structures plays a role in the initiation, maintenance and outcome of major depression in the elderly.[72] Alexopoulos et al[73] view 'vascular depression' as a heterogeneous entity mediated by several mechanisms such as small vascular lesions in the left frontal pole and the left caudate head. A pathogenic mechanism may also be the accumulation of vascular lesions exceeding a threshold which predisposes into depression. Depression developing 3 months after stroke was predicted by impairment in activities in daily living, while depression occurring 12 months after stroke was predicted by social isolation.[74] Moreover the severity of white matter lesions predicted poor outcome in elderly patients with major depression.[72]

Mood disorder, changes of personality, psychotic reactions and cognitive impairment are all associated with cerebrovascular disease. The clinical picture and brain imaging findings, contribute to the diagnosis of type and location of the underlying vascular lesion.[14–16] In a recent study symptoms of depression and anxiety were studied in patients with postmortem verified pure forms of Binswanger's disease and MID. The age at onset was 68 years in Binswanger's disease and 60 years in MID and the mean duration of psychiatric symptoms was 12 and 15 years respectively. Depression and symptoms of anxiety were reported at an early stage of dementia in 23% and 15% of the Binswanger cases and in 38% and 23% respectively in MID cases. However, when the total clinical course was considered, depression was recorded in 70% of both Binswanger's disease and MID cases and symptoms of anxiety in 31% and 62% respectively.[75] The clinical importance of subcortical vascular involvement is indicated by findings that depression is more common in subcortical than in cortical VAD,[76] but the specificity of this association remains to be proved.

The clinical significance of white matter lesions for cognitive dysfunction in VAD is controversial. Positive correlations between the total volume of white matter lesions shown with MRI and the severity of dementia have been reported,[77–80] while other studies have failed to corroborate this.[81,82] These discrepancies may be partly explained by the heterogeneity of white matter lesions and different criteria for patient selection.

The individual case

A clear understanding of the complex relationship between symptoms and brain pathology is crucial for the clinical diagnosis and treatment of

VAD. This is illustrated by the medical report of a male patient who developed VAD which was confirmed post-mortem. The patient was a businessman living under good, stable socio-economic conditions. As a teenager he had experienced dizziness and faintness, probably due to low blood pressure. These complaints became more marked at the age of 56. Two years later this patient, with previously good physical and mental health, started to complain of general tiredness, lack of concentration and inertia. He was diagnosed as depressive and was treated with tricyclic antidepressants. There was no improvement in his depressed mood and he suffered repeated attacks of dizziness and falls. Later on he started complaining of memory failure and he displayed a general psychomotor retardation, a slow shuffling wide-based gait and hypomimia. Systolic blood pressure was low with a marked orthostatic blood pressure drop. Four years later, at the age of 64, he was still diagnosed as depressed. His systolic blood pressure in a supine position was 120 with a marked decrease to 70 mmHg in a standing position. A CT scan showed widespread leukoareosis. One year later a new CT scan showed progression of the white matter changes and a small right-sided frontal haematoma, probably due to repeated falls. His clinical state fluctuated with episodes of delirium, hallucinosis and delusions, and syncopal attacks associated with orthostatic hypotension of a postural type. The patient's performance on psychological tests was markedly better when he was tested in a supine position than in a standing position. Regional cerebral blood flow (rCBF) measured in a supine position showed a general reduction of cortical flow, most marked in the temporoparietal cortex. The rCBF level showed a further 25% reduction, most marked in frontal cortical areas, when the patient was re-examined in a standing position. A SPECT scan showed bilateral symmetrical temporoparietal and subcortical periventricular rCBF decreases. The dementia condition progressed and the patient became bedridden, disorientated and dysphasic. The patient died at the age of 67. The neuropathological examination performed by Arne Brun showed a general amyloid angiopathy with multiple minimal to small cortical infarctions, partly haemorrhagic, in addition to widespread incomplete white matter ischaemic lesions. The cingulate gyrus was involved bilaterally. There was also a mild Alzheimer encephalopathy and a severe degeneration with Lewy bodies in substantia nigra. No cortical Lewy bodies were found. Thus the progressive dementia with marked clinical fluctuations, psychotic features and extrapyramidal signs seemed to be caused by a cerebral amyloid angiopathy in combination with episodic orthostatic hypoperfusion and a mild Alzheimer encephalopathy. The structural and, especially, the functional brain imaging indicated the presence of vascular as well as degenerative brain disease.

Our knowledge of the broad spectrum of clinical manifestations of cerebrovascular disease and its underlying etiologies is still limited. The current concept of VAD covers a large variety of clinical and pathological entities and the understanding of the relationship between clinical and pathological findings has important implications for improved diagnostics, classification, prevention and treatment in this field.

References

1. Goldstein K, Functional disturbances in brain damage. In: Arieti S, ed, *American Handbook of Psychiatry*, vol I (Basic Books Inc: New York, 1959) 770–94.

2. Gustafson L, Hagberg B, Dementia with onset in the presenile period. A cross-sectional study, *Acta Psychiatr Scand* (1975) **257**:9–71.

3. Rotschild D, Neuropathologic changes in arteriosclerotic psychoses and their psychiatric significance, *Arch Neurol Psychiatr* (1942) **48**:417–36.

4. Yamamoto H, Bogousslavsky J, Mechanisms of second and further strokes, *Neurol Neurosurg Psychiatry* (1998) **64**:771–6.

5. Alvarez WC, The management of persons with little strokes, *Geriatrics* (1957) **12**:421–5.

6. Brun A, Gustafson L, Zerebrovaskuläre Erkrankungen. In: Kisker KP, Lauter H, Meyer J-E, Muller C, Strömgren E, eds, vol 6 *Psychiatrie der Gegenwart* (Springer-Verlag: Heidelberg, 1988) 253–95.

7. Snowden DA, Greiner LH, Mortimer JA et al, Brain infarction and the clinical expression of Alzheimer disease—the Nun study, *JAMA* (1997) **277**:813–17.

8. Brun A, Englund E, Gustafson L et al, Consensus statement—clinical and neuropathological criteria for frontotemporal dementia, *J Neurol Neurosurg Psychiatry* (1994) **57**:416–18.

9. Segarra JM, Cerebral vascular disease and behaviour, *Arch Neurol* (1970) **22**:408–18.

10. Poirier J, Barbizet J, Gaston A, Meyrignac C, Démence thalamique. Lacunes expansives du territoire thalamomésencéphalique paramédian. Hydrocéphalie par sténose de l'aqueduc de sylvius, *Rev Neurol (Paris)* (1983) **139**:349–58.

11. Brun A, Frontal lobe degeneration of non-Alzheimer type. I. Neuropathology, *Arch Gerontol Geriatr* (1987) **6**:193–208.

12. Pasquier F, Lebert F, Petit H, Dementia, apathy, and thalamic infarcts, *Neuropsychiatry Neuropsychol Behav Neurol* (1995) **8**:208–14.

13. Riechfield EK, Twyman R, Berent S, Neurological syndrome following bilateral damage to the head of the caudate nuclei, *Ann Neurol* (1987) **22**:767–71.

14. Jellinger K, Neumayer E, Progressive subcorticale vasculäre Encephalopathie Binswanger, *Arch Psychiatr Nervenkr* (1964) **205**:523–54.

15. Janota I, Dementia, deep white matter damage and hypertension: Binswanger's vascular dementia with lacunes? *Neurology* (1981) **11**:39–48.

16. Tomonaga M, Yamanouchi H, Tohgi H et al, Clinicopathologic study of progressive subcortical vascular encephalopathy (Binswanger type) in the elderly, *J Am Geriatr Soc* (1982) **30**:524–9.

17. Fredriksson K, Brun A, Gustafson L, Pure subcortical arteriosclerotic encephalopathy (Binswanger's disease): a clinicopathologic study.

Part 1: clinical features, *Cerebrovasc Disord* (1992) **2**:87–92.

18. Brun A, Gustafson L, Incomplete infarction is an important component in cerebrovascular dementia. In: Hartmann A, Kuschinsky W, Hoyer S, eds, *Cerebral Ischemia and Dementia* (Springer-Verlag: Berlin, Heidelberg, 1991) 54–9.

19. Andrew J, Nathan PW, Lesions of anterior frontal lobes and disturbances of micturition and defecation, *Brain* (1964) **87**:232–62.

20. Brun A, Gustafson L, Zerebrovaskuläre Erkrankungen. In: Kisker KP, Lauter H, Meyer JE, Muller C, Strömgren E, eds, vol 6, *Psychiatrie der Gegenwart. Organishe Psychosen* (Springer-Verlag: Heidelberg, 1988) 253–95.

21. Dejerine J, Roussy G, Le syndrome thalamique, *Rev Neurol* (1906) **12**:521–32.

22. Ladurner G, Iliff LD, Sager WD, Lechner H, A clinical approach to vascular multiinfarct dementia, *Exp Brain Res* (1982) **5**:243–50.

23. Critchley M, The enigma of Gerstmann's syndrome, *brain* (1966) **89**:183–98.

24. Gertsmann J, Fingeragnosie. Eine umschriebene Störung der Orientierung am eigenen Körper, *Wien Klin Wochenschr* (1927) **37**:152–77.

25. Benton AL, The fiction of the 'Gerstmann syndrome', *J Neurol Neurosurg Psychiatry* (1961) **24**:176–81.

26. Benson DF, Cummings JL, Tsai SY, Angular gyrus syndrome simulating Alzheimer's disease, *Arch Neurol* (1982) **39**:616–20.

27. Gustafson L, Hagberg B, Dementia with onset in the presenile period. A cross-sectional study, *Acta Psychiatr Scand* (1975) **65**:9–71.

28. Hachinski VC, Iliff LD, Zilkha E et al, Cerebral blood flow in dementia, *Arch Neurol* (1975) **32**:632–7.

29. Maroney JT, Bagiella E, Desmond VC et al, Meta-analysis of the Hachinski Ischemic Score in pathologically verified dementias, *Neurology* (1997) **49**:1096–105.

30. Roth M, The diagnosis of dementia in late and middle life. In: Mortimer JA, Schuman LM, eds, *The Epidemiology of Dementia* (Oxford University Press: New York, Oxford, 1981) 24–61.

31. Lassen NA, Incomplete cerebral infarction: focal incomplete ischemic tissue necrosis not leading to emollision, *Stroke* (1982) **13**:522–3.

32. Hossmann K-A, Neurological progress: viability thresholds and the penumbra of focal ischemia, *Ann Neurol* (1994) **36**:557–65.

33. Gustafson L, Nilsson L, Differential diagnosis of presenile dementia on clinical grounds, *Acta Psychiatr Scand* (1982) **65**:194–209.

34. Wagner O, Oesterreich K, Hoyer S, Validity of the ischemic score in degenerative and vascular dementia and depression in old age, *Arch Gerontol Geriatr* (1985) **4**:333–45.

35. Gustafson Y, Olsson T, Eriksson S et al, Acute confusional states (delirium) in stroke patients, *Cerebrovasc Dis* (1991) **1**:257–64.

36. Hénon H, Lebert F, Durieu I et al, Confusional state in stroke. Relation to preexisting dementia, patient characteristics, and outcome, *Stroke* (1999) **30**:773–9.

37. Mesulam M, Waxman SG, Geschwind N, Sabin TD, Acute confusional states with right middle cerebral territory infarctions, *J Neurol Neurosurg Psychiatry* (1976) **39**:84–9.

38. Santamaria J, Blesa R, Tolosa ES, Confusional syndrome in thalamic stroke, *Neurology* (1984) **34**:1618.

39. Koponen H, Hurri L, Stenbäck U et al, Acute confusional states in the elderly. A radiological evaluation,

Acta Psychiatr Scand (1987) **76**: 726–31.

40. Mori E, Yamadori A, Acute confusional state and acute agitated delirium, *Arch Neurol* (1987) **44**:1139–43.

41. Horenstein S, Chamberlain W, Conomy J, Infarction of the fusiform and calcarine regions: agitated delirium and hemianopia, *Trans Am Neurol Assoc* (1962) **92**:357–67.

42. Caplan LR, 'Top of the basilar' syndrome, *Neurology* (1980) **30**: 72–9.

43. Bogousslavsky J, Ferrazzini M, Regli F et al, Manic delirium and frontal-like syndrome with paramedian infarction of the right thalamus, *J Neurol Neurosurg Psychiatry* (1988) **51**:116–19.

44. Price J, Whitlock FA, Hall RT, The psychiatry of vertebro-basilar insufficiency with the report of a case, *Psychiatr Clin* (1983) **16**: 26–44.

45. Englund E, Brun A, Gustafson L, A white-matter disease in dementia of Alzheimer's type—clinical and neuropathological correlates, *Int J Geriatr Psychiatry* (1989) **4**: 87–102.

46. Londos E, Passant U, Brun A, Gustafson L, Clinical Lewy body dementia and the impact of vascular components, *Int J Geriatr Psychiatry* (1999) in press.

47. Williams D, Wilson TG, The diagnosis of the major and minor syndromes of basilar insufficiency, *Brain* (1962) **85**:741–74.

48. Sulkava R, Erkinjuntti T, Vascular dementia due to cardiac arrythmias and systemic hypotension, *Acta Neurol Scand* (1987) **76**: 123–8.

49. Benson DF, Marsden CD, Meadows JC, The amnestic syndrome of posterior cerebral artery occlusion, *Acta Neurol Scand* (1974) **50**:133–45.

50. Hochman MS, Sowers JJ, Bruce-Gregorios J, Syndrome of the mesencephalic artery: report of a case with CT and necropsy findings, *J Neurol Neurosurg Psychiatry* (1985) **48**:1179–81.

51. Trimble MR, Cummings JL, Neuropsychiatric disturbances following brainstem lesions, *Br J Psychiatry* (1981) **138**:56–9.

52. Kraeplin E, *Psychiatrie, ein Lehrbuch für Studierende und Ärtze* (Leipzig, 1904).

53. Post F, *The Significance of Affective Symptoms in Old Age. A Follow-up Study of One Hundred Patients* (Oxford University Press: London, 1962).

54. Fujikawa T, Yamawaki S, Touhouda Y, Incidence of silent cerebral infarction in patients with major depression, *Stroke* (1993) **24**:1631–4.

55. Luria AR, *The Working Brain. An Introduction to Neuropsychology* (The Penguin Press: New York, 1980).

56. Sackeim HA, Greenberg MS, Weiman AL et al, Hemispheric asymmetry in the expression of positive and negative emotions. Neurologic evidence, *Arch Neurol* (1982) **39**:210–18.

57. Gottfries CG, Blennow K, Karlsson I, Wallin A, The neurochemistry of vascular dementia, *Dementia* (1994) **5**:163–7.

58. Allard P, Englund E, Marcusson J, Reduced number of caudate nucleus dopamine uptake sites in vascular dementia, *Dementia Geriatr Cogn Disord* (1999) **10**: 77–80.

59. Lipsey JR, Robinson RG, Pearlson GD, Rao K et al, Dexamethasone suppression test and mood following stroke, *Am J Psychiatry* (1985) **142**:318–23.

60. Robinson RG, Kubos KL, Starr LB, Rao K et al, Mood changes in stroke patients. Relationship to

lesion location, *Compr Psychiatry* (1983) **24**:677–98.

61. Flor-Henry P, On certain aspects of the localization of the cerebral systems regulating and determining emotion, *Biol Psychiatry* (1979) **14**:677–98.

62. Gainotti G, Emotional behaviour and hemispheric side of the lesion, *Cortex* (1972) **81**:41–55.

63. Robinson RG, Bolla-Wilson K, Kaplan E et al, Depression influences intellectual impairment in stroke patients, *Br J Psychiatry* (1986) **148**:541–7.

64. Eastwood MR, Rifat SL, Nobbs H, Ruderman J, Mood disorder following cerebrovascular accident, *Br J Psychiatry* (1989) **154**:195–200.

65. Dam H, Pedersen HE, Ahlgren P, Depression among patients with stroke, *Acta Psychiatr Scand* (1989) **80**:118–24.

66. Sharpe M, Hawton K, House A et al, Mood disorders in long-term survivors of stroke: associations with brain lesion location and volume, *Psychol Med* (1990) **20**:815–28.

67. Morris PL, Robinson RG, Prevalence and course of depressive disorders in hospitalized stroke patients, *Int J Psychiatry Med* (1990) **20**:349–64.

68. Aylward EH, Robets-Twillie JV, Barata PE et al, Basal ganglia volumes and white matter hyperintensities in patients with bipolar disorder, *Am J Psychiatry* (1994) **151**:687–93.

69. Leuchter AF, Dunkin JJ, Lufkin RB et al, Effect of white matter disease on functional connections in the aging brain, *J Neurol Neurosurg Psychiatry* (1994) **57**:1347–54.

70. Tarvonen-Schröder S, Röyttär M, Räihä I et al, Clinical features of leuko-araiosis, *J Neurol Neurosurg Psychiatry* (1996) **60**:431–6.

71. Videbeck P, Review article: MRI findings in patients with affective disorder: a meta-analysis, *Acta Psychiatr Scand* (1997) **96**:157–68.

72. O'Brien J, Ames D, Chiu E et al, Severe deep white matter lesions and outcome in elderly patients with major depressive disorder: follow up study, *Br Med J* (1998) **317**:982–4.

73. Alexopoulos GS, Meyers BS, Young RC et al, 'Vascular depression' hypothesis, *Arch Gen Psychiatry* (1997) **54**:915–22.

74. Åström M, Adolfsson R, Asplund K, Major depression in stroke patients. A 3-year longitudinal study, *Stroke* (1993) **24**:976–82.

75. Gustafson L, Brun A, Johanson A, Vascular dementia—clinical and classification aspects. *IPA–Beijing Joint Meeting, Plenary Lectures* (1999) **9**:73–87.

76. Erkinjuntti R, Types of multi-infarct dementia, *Acta Neurol Scand* (1987) **75**:391–9.

77. Liu CK, Miller MD, Cummings JL et al, A quantitative MRI study of vascular dementia, *Neurology* (1992) **42**:138–43.

78. Miyao S, Takano A, Teramoto J, Tahahashi A, Leukoaraiosis in relation to prognosis for patients with lacunar infarctions, *Stroke* (1992) **23**:1434–8.

79. Breteler M, van Swieten J, Bots ML et al, Cerebral white matter lesions, vascular risk factors, and cognitive function in a population-based study: The Rotterdam study. *Neurology* (1994) **44**:1246–52.

80. Skoog I, Berg S, Johanson B, Palmertz B, Andreasson L. The influence of white matter lesions on neuropsychological functioning in demented and non-demented 85-year-olds. *Acta Neurol Scand* (1996) **93**(2–3):142–8.

81. Hunt A, Orrison W, Yeo R et al, Clinical significance of MRI white matter lesions in the elderly. *Neurology* (1989) **39**:1470–4.

82. Mirsen T, Lee D, Wong C et al, Clinical correlates of white-matter changes on magnetic resonance imaging in dementia. *Arch Neurol* (1991) **48**:1015–21.

11
Classification and criteria

Timo Erkinjuntti

Introduction

Vascular dementia (VAD) as a clinical syndrome relates to different vascular mechanisms and changes in the brain, and has different causes and clinical manifestations. VAD is not only the traditional multi-infarct dementia.[1,2] The pathophysiology of VAD incorporates interactions between vascular aetiologies (cerebrovascular disorders and vascular risk factors), changes in the brain (infarcts, white matter lesions, atrophy), host factors (age, education) and cognition.[3–7] Critical issues related to the classification and diagnosis of VAD include the cognitive syndrome (type, extent and combination of impairments in different cognitive domains) and the vascular causes (vascular aetiologies and changes in the brain).

As vascular causes of cognitive impairment are common, they may be preventable. These patients could benefit from therapy, early detection and accurate diagnosis of VAD.[8] Research in VAD, until recently overshadowed by that into Alzheimer's disease (AD), is now developing rapidly, as it is an area that holds great promise for intervention. Accordingly, developments in classification, diagnosis and treatment are on the horizon.

Pathophysiology

Different types of cerebrovascular disorders incorporate the main aetiologies of VAD. The prevalent types of *cerebrovascular disorders* include large artery disease (artery-to-artery embolism, occlusion of an extra- or intracranial artery), cardiac embolic events, small vessel disease (lacunar infarcts, ischaemic white matter lesions) and haemodynamic mechanisms (Table 11.1).[9–11] In most patients diagnosed with VAD, several factors are involved. However, the individual roles these factors play in causation have not been identified in detail, and which of these mechanisms are typical for VAD compared to non-demented patients with cerebrovascular disorders is not known precisely.[1–4,6,12]

Table 11.1   Approaches in classification of VADs.

1. **According to primary vascular aetiology**
    Large artery disease
        artery-to-artery embolism
        occlusion of an extra- or intracranial artery
    Cardiac embolic events
    Small vessel disease
        lacunar infarcts
        ischaemic white matter lesions
    Haemodynamic mechanisms
    Specific ateriopathies
    Haemorrhages
        intracranial
        subarachnoidal
    Haematological factors
    Venous diseases
    Hereditary entities
    Undiscovered cause(s)

2. **According to primary type of ischaemic brain lesion**
    Arterial territorial infarct
    Distal field (watershed) infarct
    Lacunar infarct
    Ischaemic white matter lesions
    Incomplete ischaemic injury

3. **According to primary location of brain lesions**
    Cortical
        focal lesions in distinct areas (ACA, MCA, PCA)
        combined cortical areas
        distal field areas
    Subcortical
        multiple deep lacunae
        extensive ischaemic white matter change
    Cortical and subcortical
    Strategic
        cortical
        deep

4. **According to primary clinical syndrome**
    Cortical
    Subcortical
    Defined behavioural network
        limbic-medial
        prefrontal-subcortical
        defined heteromodal brain areas

Different changes in the brain have been related to VAD.[3,4,9,10] The prevalent ischaemic lesions are listed in Table 11.1. Incomplete ischaemic injury incorporates laminar necrosis, focal gliosis, granular atrophy and incomplete white matter infarction.[13,14] Furthermore, both focal (around the ischaemic lesion) and remote (disconnection, diaschisis) functional ischaemic changes relate to VAD, and the volume of functionally inactive tissue exceeds that of focal ischaemic lesions in VAD.[15]

To what extent the given aetiologies and changes in the brain cause, compound or only coexist with VAD syndrome is still not known precisely. The vascular changes in the brain can be the main cause of cognitive impairment, as is assumed in VAD,[16,17] they can contribute to the risk and clinical picture of a dementia syndrome including that of AD,[6,18] but may only be coincidental.

The relationship between vascular lesions in the brain and cognitive impairment is an important question, but which type, extent, side, site and tempo of vascular lesions in the brain relate to different types of VAD is a matter of debate.[3-5,9] VAD has been related to the volume of brain infarcts (size reaching a critical threshold), the number of infarcts (additive, synergistic), the site of infarcts (bilateral, strategic cortical or subcortical sites), the ischaemic white matter lesions (extent, site, type, density), the other ischaemic factors (incomplete ischaemic injury, delayed neuronal death, functional changes), the atrophic changes (origin, location, extent) and finally to the additive effects of other pathologies (AD, Lewy body dementia, frontal lobe dementias).

Classification

Classification of VAD may be based according to:

1. the primary vascular aetiology
2. the primary type of ischaemic brain lesions
3. the primary location of brain lesions
4. the primary clinical syndrome (Table 11.1).

The currently proposed subtypes of VAD (Table 11.2) incorporate a variable combination of the given categories reflecting heterogeneity. However, subcortical VAD may be a more homogeneous subtype as it incorporates all the categories: small vessel disease as primary vascular aetiology, lacunar infarct and ischaemic white matter lesions as primary type of brain lesions, subcortical location as the primary location of lesions and subcorical syndrome as the primary clinical manifestation.

The subtypes of VAD included in current classifications are cortical

Table 11.2 Subtypes of VAD.

Cortical VAD or
   multi-infarct dementia
Subcortical VAD or
   small vessel dementia
Strategic infarct dementia
Hypoperfusion dementia
Haemorrhagic dementia
Hereditary VAD
Other VADs
AD with CVD (combined or mixed dementia)

VAD or mutli-infarct dementia, subcortical VAD or small vessel dementia and strategic infarct dementia (Table 11.2),[10,19–24] and many also include hypoperfusion dementia.[10,20,22,25] Further subtypes suggested include haemorrhagic dementia, hereditary VAD and combined or mixed dementia (AD with cerebrovascular disease) (Table 11.2).

A question of debate is whether these suggested subtypes are distinct disorders, having their own pathological and clinical features as well as response to therapy.[23] However, the goal is to identify homogeneous subtypes, which would facilitate comparison of independent studies and benefit multi-centre collaboration.[26]

Subtypes of VAD in current clinical criteria

The current clinical criteria for VAD differ in their classification of VAD into subtypes. None of these clinical criteria include detailed criteria for their subtypes.

The DSM-IV criteria do not specify subtypes.[27] The ICD-10[28] include six subtypes with rather superficial clinical descriptions (acute onset, mutli-infarct, subcortical, mixed cortical and subcortical, other and unspecified). The ADDTC criteria[26] do not specify detailed subtypes, but emphasize that classification of ischaemic VAD for research purposes should specify features of the infarcts that may differentiate the disorder, such as location (cortical, white matter, periventricular, basal ganglia, thalamus), size (volume), distribution (large, small or microvessel), severity (chronic ischaemia vs infarction) and aetiology (embolism, atherosclerosis, arteriosclerosis, cerebral amyloid angiopathy, hypoperfusion). The NINDS-AIREN criteria[20] include, without detailed description, cortical VAD, subcortical VAD, Binswanger's disease (BD) and thalamic dementia.

Main subtypes of VAD

Multi-infarct dementia or cortical VAD and small vessel dementia or sub-cortical VAD are the two common types, but the frequency of these varies in different series (Table 11.3).[10,21,22] In addition, strategic infarct dementia is widely cited as a subtype.

Cortical VAD relates to large vessel disease, cardiac embolic events and also hypoperfusion. It displays predominantly cortical and cortico-subcortical arterial territorial and distal field (watershed) infarcts. Typical clinical features are lateralized sensimotor changes and abrupt onset of cognitive impairment and aphasia.[21] In addition, some combination of different cortical neuropsychological syndromes has been suggested to be present in cortical VAD.[19]

Subcortical VAD, or small vessel dementia, incorporates the old entities 'lacunar state' and 'Binswanger's disease', relates to small vessel disease and hypoperfusion and shows predominantly lacunar infarcts, focal and diffuse ischaemic white matter lesions and incomplete ischaemic injury.[21,29,30] Clinically, small vessel dementia is characterized by pure motor hemiparesis, bulbar signs and dysarthria, depression and emotional lability, and especially deficits in executive functioning.[29-32]

In *strategic infarct dementia*, focal, often small, ischaemic lesions involving specific sites critical for higher cortical functions have been classified as causes of VAD. The angular gyrus is one example of the cortical site and the subcortical sites include the hippocampus, thalamus, cyrus cinguli, fornix, basal forebrain, caudate, globus pallidus and the genu of the anterior capsule.[1,3,9]

Table 11.3 Vascular mechanisms and changes in the brain related to the main subtypes of VAD.

Vascular mechanisms	Changes in the brain
Cortical VAD or multi-infarct dementia	
Large vessel disease	Arterial territorial infarct
Cardiac embolic events	Distal field (watershed) infarct
Subcortical VAD or small vessel dementia	
Small vessel disease	Lacunar infarct
Hypoperfusion	Focal and diffuse white matter lesions
	Incomplete ischaemic injury
Strategic infarct dementia	
Large vessel disease	Arterial territorial infarct
Cardiac embolic events	Distal field (watershed) infarct
Small vessel disease	Lacunar infarct
Hypoperfusion	Focal and diffuse white matter lesions

Clinical criteria

Since the 1970s several clinical criteria for VAD have been used.[33-35] The most widely used criteria for VAD include the DSM-IV,[27] the ICD-10,[28] the ADDTC[26] and the NINDS-AIREN criteria.[20]

The two cardinal elements implemented in the clinical criteria for VAD are the definition of the cognitive syndrome of dementia[36] and the definition of the vascular cause of the dementia.[34,35,37] All the clinical criteria used are consensus criteria, which are neither derived from prospective community-based studies on vascular factors affecting the cognition, nor based on detailed natural histories.[20,26,33,34,38] All the criteria cited are based on the ischaemic infarct concept and are designed to have high specificity, although they have been poorly implemented and validated.[33,38]

Variations in defining the dementia syndrome[36,39] and the vascular cause[35,40] have led to a critical consequence; different definitions give different point prevalence estimates, identify different groups of subjects and further identify different types and distribution of brain lesions.

The *DSM-IV* definition for VAD (Table 11.4) requires focal neurological signs and symptoms *or* laboratory evidence of focal neurological damage clinically judged to be related to the disturbance.[27] The course is specified by sudden cognitive and functional losses. The DSM-IV criteria do not detail brain imaging requirements. The DSM-IV definition for VAD is reasonably broad and lacks detailed clinical and radiological guidelines.

The *ICD-10* criteria[28] (Table 11.5) require unequal distribution of cognitive deficits, focal signs as evidence of focal brain damage and significant cerebrovascular disease judged to be aetiologically related to the

Table 11.4 The DSM-IV definition for VAD.

- Focal neurological signs and symptoms (for example, exaggeration of deep tendon reflexes, extensor plantar response, pseudobulbar palsy, gait abnormalities, weakness of an extremity, etc.)
  or
  laboratory evidence of focal neurological damage (for example, multiple infarctions involving cortex and underlying white matter)
- The cognitive deficits cause significant impairment in social or occupational functioning and represent a significant decline from a previously higher level of functioning
- The focal neurological signs, symptoms and laboratory evidence are judged to be aetiologically related to the disturbance
- The deficits do not occur exclusively during the course of delirium
- The course is characterized by sustained periods of clinical stability punctuated by sudden significant cognitive and functional losses

Table 11.5 The ICD-10 criteria for VAD.

- Unequal distribution of deficits in higher cognitive functions with some affected and others relatively spared. Thus memory may be quite markedly affected while thinking, reasoning and information processing may show only mild decline
- There is evidence for focal brain damage, manifest as at least one of the following: unilateral spastic weakness of the limbs, unilaterally increased tendon reflexes, an extensor plantar response, pseudobulbar palsy
- There is evidence from the history, examination or test of significant cerebrovascular disease, which may reasonably be judged to be aetiologically related to the dementia (history of stroke, evidence of cerebral infarction)

Table 11.6 Subtypes of VAD in the ICD-10 classification.

Acute onset (F01.0)
The dementia develops rapidly (i.e. usually within 1 month but within no longer than 3 months) after a succession of strokes or (rarely) after a single large infarction

Multi-infarct (F01.1)
The onset of the dementia is more gradual (i.e. within 3–6 months) following a number of minor ischaemic episodes. Comments: it is presumed that there is an accumulation of infarcts in the cerebral parenchyma. Between the ischaemic episodes there may be periods of actual clinical improvement

Subcortical (F01.2)
A history of hypertension and evidence from clinical examination and special investigations of vascular disease located in the deep white matter of the cerebral hemispheres, with preservation of the cerebral cortex

Mixed cortical and subcortical (F01.3)
Mixed cortical and subcortical components of the VAD may be suspected from the clinical features, the results of investigation or both

Other (F01.8)
Unspecified (F01.9)
In the ICD-10 criteria no specific diagnostic guidelines are given for these two VAD subtypes

dementia. The criteria do not detail brain imaging requirements. The ICD-10 criteria specify altogether six subtypes of VAD (Table 11.6). The ICD-10 criteria for VAD have been shown to be highly selective and only a subset of those fulfilling the general criteria for ICD-10 VAD can be classified into defined subtypes.[35,37] The shortcomings of these criteria include lack of detailed guidelines (for example, unequal cognitive deficits and neuroimaging), lack of aetiological cues and heterogeneity.[35,37]

106 Cerebrovascular Disease and Dementia

Table 11.7 The ADDTC criteria for probable ischaemic vascular dementia (IVD).

A The criteria for the clinical diagnosis of probable IVD include all of the following:
  1 Dementia
  2 Evidence of two or more ischaemic strokes by history, neurological signs and/or neuroimaging studies (CT or T1-weighted MRI), or
     Occurrence of a single stroke with a clearly documented temporal relationship to the onset of dementia
  3 Evidence of at least one infarct outside the cerebellum by CT or T1-weighted MRI

B The diagnosis of probable IVD is supported by
  1 Evidence of multiple infarcts in brain regions known to affect cognition
  2 A history of multiple transient ischaemic attacks
  3 History of vascular risk factors (for example, hypertension, heart disease, diabetes mellitus)
  4 Elevated Hachinski ischaemic scale (original or modified version)

C Clinical features that are thought to be associated with IVD, but await further research, include
  1 Relatively early appearance of gait disturbance and urinary incontinence
  2 Periventricular and deep white matter changes on T2-weighted MRI that are excessive for age
  3 Focal changes in electrophysiological studies (for example, EEG, evoked potentials) or physiological neuroimaging studies (for example, SPECT, PET, NMR spectroscopy)

D Other clinical features that do not constitute strong evidence either for or against a diagnosis of probable IVD include
  1 Periods of slowly progressive symptoms
  2 Illusions, psychosis, hallucinations, delusions
  3 Seizures

E Clinical features that cast doubt on a diagnosis of probable IVD include
  1 Transcortical sensory aphasia in the absence of corresponding focal lesions on neuroimaging studies
  2 Absence of central neurological symptoms/signs, other than cognitive disturbance

The *ADDTC* criteria are exclusively criteria for ischaemic VAD (IVD)[26] (Table 11.7). They require evidence of two or more ischaemic strokes by history, neurological signs or neuroimaging studies (CT or T1-weighted MRI) or, in the case of a single stroke, a clearly documented temporal relationship (not specified in detail), and always neuroradiological evidence of at least one infarct outside the cerebellum. Ischaemic white matter changes on CT or MRI do not qualify as brain imaging evidence of probable IVD, but may support a diagnosis of possible IVD. The criteria list features supporting the diagnosis, as well as a list of features casting doubt on a diagnosis of probable IVD.

Table 11.8 The NINDS-AIREN criteria for probable VAD.

I The criteria for the clinical diagnosis of probable VAD include *all* of the following:
1 *Dementia*
2 *Cerebrovascular disease*, defined by the presence of focal signs on neurological examination, such as hemispheres, lower facial weakness, Babinski sign, sensory deficit, hemianopsia, dysarthria etc., consistent with stroke (with or without history of stroke), and
evidence of relevant CVD by brain imaging (CT or MRI) including *multiple large-vessel strokes* or a *single strategically placed infarct* (angular gyrus, thalamus, basal forebrain, PCA or ACA territories), as well as *multiple basal ganglia and white matter lacunes* or *extensive periventricular white matter lesions*, or combinations thereof
3 *A relationship between the above two disorders*, manifested or inferred by the presence of one or more of the following:
   a Onset of dementia within 3 months following a recognized stroke
   b Abrupt deterioration in cognitive functions; or fluctuating, stepwise progression of cognitive deficits

II Clinical features consistent with the diagnosis of probable VAD include the following:
   a Early presence of a gait disturbance (small-step gait or *marche a petits-pas*, magnetic, apraxic-ataxic or Parkinsonian gait)
   b History of unsteadiness and frequent, unprovoked falls
   c Early urinary frequency, urgency and other urinary symptoms not explained by urological disease
   d Personality and mood changes, abulia, depression, emotional incontinence, other subcortical deficits including psychomotor retardation and abnormal executive function

III Features that make the diagnosis of VAD uncertain or unlikely include:
   a Early onset of memory deficit and progressive worsening of memory and other cognitive functions such as language (transcortical sensory aphasia), motor skills (apraxia) and perception (agnosia), in the absence of corresponding focal lesions on brain imaging
   b Absence of focal neurological signs, other than cognitive disturbance
   c Absence of cerebrovascular lesions on brain CT or MRI

The *NINDS-AIREN* research criteria for VAD[20] include dementia syndrome, cerebrovascular disease and a relationship between those (Table 11.8). Cerebrovascular disease is defined by the presence of focal neurological signs and detailed brain imaging evidence of ischaemic changes in the brain. A relationship between dementia and cerebrovascular disorder is based on the onset of dementia within 3 months following a recognized stroke, or an abrupt deterioration in cognitive functions or fluctuating, stepwise progression of cognitive deficits. The criteria include a list of features consistent with the diagnosis, as well as a list of features that make the diagnosis uncertain or unlikely. In addition different levels of certainty of the clinical diagnosis (probable, possible, definite) are included. The NINDS-AIREN criteria recognize heterogeneity of the syndrome[41] and variability of the clinical course in VAD, and highlight detection of ischaemic lesions and a relationship between lesion and cognition, as well as stroke and dementia onset.

The inter-rater reliability of the NINDS-AIREN criteria has been shown to be moderate to substantial (κ 0.46–0.72).[42]

Brain imaging requirements in clinical criteria for VAD

The DSM-IV[27] and the ICD-10[28] criteria for VAD do not specify brain imaging requirements.

The ADDTC criteria for IVD[26] require for the diagnosis of probably IVD 'evidence of two or more ischemic strokes by history, neurologic signs, and/or neuroimaging studies (CT or T1-weighted MRI), and evidence of at least one infarct outside the cerebellum by CT or T1-weighted MRI'. The diagnosis is further supported by 'evidence of multiple infarcts in brain regions known to affect cognition', but the sites are not detailed. Furthermore, features that are thought to be associated with IVD, but await further research, include 'periventricular and deep white matter changes on T2-weighted MRI that are excessive for age'. In the category of possible IVD the criteria include 'Binswanger's syndrome', with 'extensive white matter changes on neuroimaging', which are not specified.

The NINDS-AIREN criteria for probable VAD[20] require 'evidence of relevant cerebrovascular disorder by brain imaging (CT or MRI) including multiple large-vessel stroke or a single strategically placed infarct (angular gyrus, thalamus, basal forebrain, PCA or ACA territories), as well as multiple basal ganglia and white matter lacunes or extensive periventricular white matter lesions, or combinations thereof'. The criteria state that 'White matter lesions on CT/MRI alone may be considered evidence for cerebrovascular disease; however, to be significant, these changes must be diffuse and extensive, and characterized by irregular periventricular hyperintensities on T1 and T2 MRI extending to the deep white matter but sparing the areas thought to be protected from perfusion insufficiency (for example, subcortical U-fibres, external capsule-claustrum-extreme capsule). Changes observed only on T2 MRI may be insignificant', and 'it has been suggested that, in VAD, white matter changes involve at least one-fourth of the total white matter'. The criteria list features that make the diagnosis of VAD uncertain or unlikely include 'absence of cerebrovascular lesion on brain CT/MRI rules out probable VAD'. However, the class of possible VAD may include patients who have 'focal neurologic signs but in the absence of brain imaging confirmation of definite cerebrovascular disorder'.

Patients with subcortical VAD (small vessel dementia) often present with multiple lacunes and extensive white matter lesions on neuroimaging, but give only a clinical history of 'prolonged TIA' or 'multiple TIAs' (which mostly are minor strokes) without residual symptoms and only mild focal findings (for example, drift, reflex asymmetry, gait disturbance). This underlines the importance of neuroimaging criteria in the definitions of VAD.

In conclusion, the clinical criteria for VAD of older origin (DSM-IV and ICD-10) do not specify brain imaging requirements for the diagnosis in detail. The ADDTC requires one CT or T1 MRI infarct outside the cerebellum, but white matter lesions do not qualify for support of probable IVD. The NINDS-AIREN criteria require multiple infarcts (more than one cortico-subcortical or lacunar) or extensive white matter lesions (CT or T1 MRI), but also accept a clinically 'strategic' single infarct as evidence of 'relevant cerebrovascular disease'.

As evaluated neuropathologically the ADDTC criteria seem to be more sensitive and the NINDS-AIREN criteria more specific, neither are perfect.[43]

Comparison of clinical criteria for VAD

The current criteria for VAD are not interchangeable; they identify different numbers and clusters of patients diagnosed with VAD. The DSM-IV criteria are less restrictive compared to the ICD-10, the ADDTC and the NINDS-AIREN criteria (Table 11.9).[35,44]

The NINDS-AIREN criteria are currently most widely used in clinical drug trails on VAD, despite their limitations. In a neuropathological series sensitivity of the NINDS-AIREN criteria was 58% and specificity was 80%.[43] The criteria successfully excluded AD in 91% of cases, and the proportion of combined cases misclassified as probably VAD was 29%.[43] Compared to the ADDTC criteria the NINDS-AIREN criteria were more specific and they better excluded combined cases (54% vs 29%).[43]

Perspective

There is a vital need for international agreement on clinical criteria for VAD. The constructs should be based on homogeneity in the aetiologies and changes in the brain, and should show a predictable natural history and outcomes. A proposal for a more homogeneous subtype with a more predictable outcome is the subcortical VAD. Meanwhile, a modular approach has been proposed for clinical studies and drug trials, defining in detail the elements in the cognitive syndrome (type, extent and combination of impairments in different cognitive domains) and the vascular causes.

Table 11.9 Comparison of clinical criteria for VAD.

	DSM-IV	ICD-10	ADDTC	NINDS-AIREN
Ischaemic stroke	+	+	+	+
Haemorrhage	+	+	–	+
Focal signs	+	+	NS	+
Focal symptoms	+	–	NS	–
Causal relation	+	+	+	+
List of supporting and non-supporting features	–	–	+	+
Different levels of certainty	–	–	+	+
Structural neuroimaging	–	–	One infarct outside cerebellum	Multiple large vessel or single strategically placed or multiple lacunes or extensive WMLs

References

1. Erkinjuntti T, Hachinski VC, eds, Rethinking vascular dementia, *Cerebrovasc Dis* (1993) **3**:3–23.
2. Chui HC, Rethinking vascular dementia: moving from myth to mechanism. In: Growdon JH, Rossor MN, eds, *The Dementias* (Butterworth-Heinemann: Boston) 377–401.
3. Tatemichi TK, How acute brain failure becomes chronic. A view of the mechanisms and syndromes of dementia related to stroke, *Neurology* (1990) **40**:1652–9.
4. Chui HC, Dementia: a review emphasizing clinicopatholgic correlation and brain–behaviour relationships, *Arch Neurol* (1989) **46**:806–14.
5. Desmond DW, Vascular dementia: a construct in evolution, *Cerebrovasc Brain Metab Rev* (1996) **8**:296–325.
6. Pasquier F, Leys D, Why are stroke patients prone to develop dementia? *J Neurol* (1997) **244**:135–42.
7. Skoog I, Status of risk factors for vascular dementia, *Neuroepidemiology* (1998) **17**:2–9.
8. Bowler JV, Hachinski V, Vascular cognitive impairment: a new approach to vascular dementia, *Baillières Clin Neurol* (1995) **4**:357–76.
9. Erkinjuntti T, Clinicopatholgical study of vascular dementia. In: Prohovnik I, Wade J, Knezevic S, Tatemichi TK, Erkinjuntti T, eds, *Vascular Dementia. Current concepts* (John Wiley & Sons: Chichester, 1996) 73–112.
10. Brun A, Pathology and pathophysiology of cerebrovascular dementia: pure subgroups of obstructive and hypoperfusive etiology, *Dementia* (1994) **5**:145–7.
11. Amar K, Wilcock G, Vascular dementia, *Br Med J* (1996) **312**:227–31.
12. Pantoni L, Garcia JH, The significance of cerebral white matter abnormalities 100 years after Binswanger's report. A review, *Stroke* (1995) **26**:1293–301.
13. Pantoni L, Garcia JH, Pathogenesis of leukoaraiosis: a review, *Stroke* (1997) **28**:652–9.
14. Englund E, Brun A, Alling C, White matter changes in dementia of Alzheimer's type. Biochemical and neuropathological correlates, *Brain* (1988) **111**:1425–39.
15. Mielke R, Herholz K, Grond M, Kessler J, Heiss WD, Severity of vascular dementia is related to volume of metabolically impaired tissue, *Arch Neurol* (1992) **49**:909–13.
16. Tatemichi TK, Paik M, Bagiella E, Risk of dementia after stroke in a hospitalized cohort: results of a longitudinal study, *Neurology* (1994) **44**:1885–91.
17. Erkinjuntti T, Haltia M, Palo J, Sulkava R, Paetau A, Accuracy of the clinical diagnosis of vascular dementia: a retrospective clinical and post-mortem neuropathological study, *J Neurol Neurosurg Psychiatry* (1988) **51**:1037–44.
18. Snowdon DA, Greiner KH, Mortimer JA et al, Brain infarction and the clinical expression of Alzheimer disease. The Nun Study [see comments]. *JAMA* (1997) **277**:813–17.
19. Konno S, Meyer JS, Terayama Y, Margishvili GM, Mortel KF, Classification, diagnosis and treatment of vascular dementia, *Drugs Aging* (1997) **11**:361–73.
20. Roman GC, Tatemichi TK, Erkinjuntti T et al, Vascular dementia: diagnostic criteria for research studies. Report of the NINDS-

AIREN International Work Group, *Neurology* (1993) **43**:250–60.

21. Erkinjuntti T, Types of multi-infarct dementia, *Acta Neurol Scand* (1987) **75**:391–9.

22. Cummings JL, Vascular subcortical dementias: clinical aspects, *Dementia* (1994) **5**:177–80.

23. Wallin A, Blennow K. The clinical diagnosis of vascular dementia, *Dementia* (1994) **5**:181–4.

24. Loeb C, Meyer JS, Vascular dementia: still a debatable entity? *J Neurol Sci* (1996) **143**: 31–40.

25. Sulkava R, Erkinjuntti T, Vascular dementia due to cardiac arrhythmias and systemic hypotension, *Acta Neurol Scand* (1987) **76**: 123–8.

26. Chui HC, Victoroff JI, Margolin D et al, criteria for the diagnosis of ischemic vascular dementia proposed by the State of California Alzheimer's Disease Diagnostic and Treatment Centers [see comments], *Neurology* (1992) **42**: 473–80.

27. American Psychiatric Association, *Diagnostic and Statistical Manual of Mental Disorders*, 4th edn (American Psychiatric Association: Washington, DC, 1994).

28. World Health Organization, *ICD-10 Classification of Mental and Behavioural Disorders: Diagnostic Criteria for Research* (WHO: Geneva, 1993).

29. Mahler ME, Cummings JL, The behavioural neurology of multi-infarct dementia, *Alzheimer Dis Assoc Disord* (1991) **5**:122–30.

30. Roman GC, Senile dementia of the Binswanger type. A vascular form of dementia in the elderly, *JAMA* (1987) **258**:1782–8.

31. Babikian V, Ropper AH, Binswanger's disease: a review, *Stroke* (1987) **18**:2–12.

32. Ishii N, Nishihara Y, Imamura T, Why do frontal lobe symptoms predominate in vascular dementia with lacunes? *Neurology* (1986) **36**:340–5.

33. Rockwood K, Parhad I, Hachinski V et al, Diagnosis of vascular dementia: Consortium of Canadian Centres for Clinical Cognitive Research consensus statement, *Cand J Neurol Sci* (1994) **21**:358–64.

34. Erkinjuntti T, Clinical criteria for vascular dementia: the NINDS-AIREN criteria, *Dementia* (1994) **5**:189–92.

35. Wetterling T, Kanitz RD, Borgis KJ, Comparison of different diagnostic criteria for vascular dementia (ADDTC, DSM-IV, ICD-10, NINDS-AIREN), *Stroke* (1996) **27**:30–6.

36. Erkinjuntti T, Ostbye T, Steenhuis R, Hachinski V, The effect of different diagnostic criteria on the prevalence of dementia, *N Engl J Med* (1997) **337**:1667–74.

37. Wetterling T, Kanitz RD, Borgis KJ. The ICD-10 criteria for vascular dementia, *Dementia* (1994) **5**:185–8.

38. Erkinjuntti T, Vascular dementia: challenge of clinical diagnosis, *Int Psychogeriatr* (1997) **9**(Suppl 1):51–8.

39. Pohjasvaara T, Erkinjuntti T, Vataja R, Kaste M, Dementia three months after stroke. Baseline frequency and effect of different definitions of dementia in the Helsinki Stroke Aging Memory Study (SAM) cohort, *Stroke* (1997) **28**:785–92.

40. Skoog I, Nilsson L, Palmertz B, Andreasson LA, Svanborg A, A population-based study of dementia in 85-year-olds [see comments], *N Engl J Med* (1993) **328**:153–8.

41. Erkinjuntti T, Clinical criteria for vascular dementia: the NINDS-AIREN criteria, *Dementia* (1994) **5**:189–92.

42. Lopez OL, Larumbe MR, Becker JT et al, Reliability of NINDS-AIREN clinical criteria for the diagnosis of vascular dementia [see comments], *Neurology* (1994) **44**:1240–5.
43. Gold G, Giannakopoulos P, Montes-Paixao JC et al, Sensitivity and specificity of newly proposed clinical criteria for possible vascular dementia, *Neurology* (1997) **49**:690–4.
44. Verhey FR, Lodder J, Rozendaal N, Jolles J, Comparison of seven sets of criteria used for the diagnosis of vascular dementia, *Neuroepidemiology* (1996) **15**:166–72.

12
Behavioural neurology of vascular dementia

Kjell Martin Moksnes and Anders Wallin

Introduction

Vascular dementia (VAD) is a heterogeneous syndrome, encompassing a wide variety of symptoms. The reason is at least partly the heterogeneity of the pathophysiological processes and of the size, number and locations of the various tissue lesions. The current description of vascular dementia VAD symptomatology was outlined by Roth[1] and by Mayer-Gross et al[2] in the textbook *Clinical Psychiatry*. The main characteristics of VAD were stated as 'dementia associated with focal signs and symptoms indicative of cerebrovascular disease' and 'a remittent or markedly fluctuating course at some stage of dementing process'. Interest in VAD has been increasing recently. Special attention has been paid to the subtypes and the preliminary stages of VAD.

Clinical features of VAD—general description

The clinical picture of VAD varies. Some patients with VAD show signs of advanced vascular disease with hypertension, diabetes, angina pectoris and intermittent claudication with complications. Cerebral ischaemic attacks may occur but are not compulsory events. Other patients with VAD show no signs of vascular disease but have a history with signs of a single transient ischaemic attack (TIA).

Important features of VAD include relatively abrupt onset (days to weeks) of cognitive impairment. The course may be stepwise progressive, fluctuating or in some cases (20–40%) more insidious and continuously progressive.[3,4] When the progression is continuous, the differential diagnosis from Alzheimer's disease (AD) may be difficult. Examination of the neurological status may reveal multiple focal neurological symptoms, indicating that, due to several infarcts, the brain is affected in patches. There may, however, be no focal neurological signs at all. Mental slowing, along with a slow gait and stiffness of extremities, is common and predominates in many patients. In some cases, perceptual disturbances like those seen in AD also occur in VAD, and epileptic seizures may occur. In other cases behavioural psychiatric symptoms predominate.

Identifying VAD – history and status examination

Every patient suspected of a dementia disorder requires comprehensive evaluation. A careful history is essential. The clinical picture will often remain incomplete, and an interview with a relative or caregiver is absolutely necessary. Time spent in obtaining a detailed history is always rewarded and may give more important clues to the correct diagnosis than a multitude of investigations. Statements derived from the patient alone frequently prove misleading, both with regard to the severity of the symptoms and the time course of their evolution. This is clear when the patient is confused or suffers from obvious memory impairment. In some cases there will be a genuine loss of insight. Such matters require information from someone who has known the patient intimately throughout the evolution of the disorder. Particular attention must always be paid to the mode of onset of the disorder, the duration of symptoms and the way they have progressed.

It is important that the investigation of the patient's symptomatology is comprehensive and well structured. This makes the work easier for the clinician and facilitates the documentation of silent symptoms in various phases of the disease process. It also facilitates the identification of various VAD subtypes (see below). Destruction of even a minor part of the brain causes changes in a number of functions that are difficult to study objectively.[5] A comprehensive investigation enables the clinician to identify symptoms or groups of symptoms that frequently occur in the various dementing illnesses and to follow the intensities of the symptoms over time. A tool for identification of regional brain syndromes in dementia is the Stepwise Comparative Status Analysis (STEP). It is adapted to the physician's way of working and may be used by both specialists and relatively inexperienced physicians.[6]

Vascular cognitive impairment

The cognitive syndrome of VAD differs from that of AD. VAD is characterized by predominant executive, subcortical and frontal lobe dysfunction rather than deficits in memory and language function. By requiring impairment in activities of daily living (ADL) for a diagnosis of dementia, many vascular dementia cases are detected only when the brain damage has reached a degree when successful treatment is no longer possible. Thus, it was suggested that the old concept should be substituted with a broader category including the whole spectrum of cognitive impairment related to cerebrovascular disease.[7] In vascular cognitive impairment (VCI), the term 'vascular' refers to all causes of ischaemic cerebrovascular disease, while cognitive impairment encompasses all levels of cognitive decline, including the earlier stages.

Subtypes of VAD

Different forms of VAD produce clinical pictures that differ to some extent. One part of the clinical presentation consists of symptoms and behaviour patterns directly related to the site of the brain damage. These are referred to as primary or deficit symptoms. The other part of the clinical presentation consists of what is called secondary symptoms. These may be connected to the disease process, the patient's personality, his efforts to compensate for his difficulties, side-effects of drugs or an unfavourable psychosocial situation.[8] Primary symptoms reflect disturbances in different parts of the brain (Table 12.1). They include impaired practical abilities, a lowered ability to interpret sensory impressions, reduced mental speed and motor activity, a reduced ability to take initiatives and personality changes. Primary symptoms also encompass a reduction of memory and abstract thinking.

Thirty-one consecutive patients with the clinical diagnosis of VAD, defined as dementia with pronounced vascular disease, were examined with regard to symptoms reflecting disturbances in various brain regions. Frontal (77%) and subcortical (68%) disturbances were the most common clinical patterns.[9] Ninety-one per cent of the VAD patients were characterized by dominance of frontal and/or subcortical symptomatology.[10] Slowness in the rate of information processing is described as a cardinal symptom in the subcortical symptom complex. This complex also includes behavioural disturbances similar to those seen in patients with frontal damage. Although the patients were defined as VAD in general, most of them appeared to fit into the subcortical white matter dementia (SWMD) category (see below).

Multi-infarct dementia

Multiple large complete infarcts, usually from large-vessel occlusions involving cortical and subcortical areas, may result in a clinical syndrome of dementia.[11] Multi-infarct dementia (MID) is characterized by TIAs or stroke episodes in close time relation to the development of dementia. Stepwise deterioration is considered a hallmark of MID, but is sometimes difficult to identify. The history of illness usually comprises various types of vascular disease. Clinical examination reveals asymmetric neurologi-

Table 12.1 Symptoms and signs in some regional brain syndromes.

Regional brain syndromes	Symptoms and signs
Parietal brain syndrome	• Sensory aphasia (fluent aphasia, impaired ability to understand spoken language) • Visual agnosia (impaired ability to interpret primary visual acuity or field deficits; for instance difficulty in identifying a knife) • Visuospatial dysfunction (perceptual spatial dysfunction) • Body agnosia (inability to orient the body spatially) • Apraxia (impaired ability to perform purposeful movements)
Frontal brain syndrome	• Emotional bluntness (apathy, indifference, stereotypy, aspontaneity, lack of initiative) • Impaired control and modulation of emotions (disinhibition, tearfulness, inadequate smiling, indolent euphoria) • Lack of insight and judgment (loss of tact) • Change of oral/dietary/sexual behaviour • Perseveration • Poverty of language
Subcortical brain syndrome	• Mental slowness • Psychomotor retardation • Bilateral pyramidal signs (spasticity, increased tendon reflexes, Babinski's sign, subclonus, paraparetic gait, marche à petits pas) • Bilateral extrapyramidal signs (limb rigidity, cogwheel phenomenon, limb tremor, hypokinesia) • Pseudobulbar symptoms (positive masseter reflex, compulsive crying, dysarthria, dysphagia)
Global brain syndrome	• Memory impairment • Disorientation • Reduced problem-solving ability • Anomia • Concentration difficulties • Visuospatial disturbances

cal signs, such as field of vision deficits, hemiparesis and reflex abnormalities. Erkinkuntti[12] found the four most common symptoms after stroke in patients with cortical MID to be motor-sensory hemiparesis (22.6%), aphasia (19.5%), vertigo and dysequilibrium (12.3%) and apractic-atactic gait (9.9%). In subcortical MID, they were dysarthria (27.9%), pure motor hemiparesis (24.5%), vertigo and dysequilibrium (14.8%) and apractic-atactic gait (14.8%). Erkinjuntti also found that patients with cortical MID more often tended to have abrupt onset of cognitive failure, nocturnal confusion and atrial fibrillation than those with subcortical MID. The latter tended to be depressed and show emotional incontinence more frequently than those with cortical MID.

Strategic infarct dementia

The symptomatology of strategic infarct dementia (SID)[13] varies with the infarct location. Bilateral hippocampal infarcts are mainly characterized by amnesia. Bilateral thalamic lesions are characterized by attention deficits, slowing of thought processes, apathy, aphasia, agnosia and apraxia. Paramedian mesencephalic-diencephalic infarcts (PMDI) often cause impairments of ocular motility, co-ordination and gait, attention and mental control. There is a dramatic slowness of response, whether verbal or motor, and the patients are apathetic and lacking motivation. They often fall asleep when left alone, but always awake easily.[14]

Subcortical white matter disease

SWMD, which is also called subcortical small-vessel dementia or subcortical vascular dementia, is an underdiagnosed type of VAD.[10] TIAs or stroke episodes may appear in SWMD but are not always present. Hypertension, as well as hypotension, is associated with SWMD, and the presence of diabetes mellitus and ischaemic heart disease is the rule. In most cases, these multiple vascular disorders are pronounced and have peripheral complications. The course is seldom stepwise but usually continuous and slowly progressive.[4] Typical symptoms of SWMD are mental slowness, extrapyramidal deficits (rigidity, hypokinesia) and bilateral pyramidal deficits (short-step gait, increased reflexes in legs). Positive masseter reflex may occur. There may be focal neurological symptoms in the form of inability to distinguish between the left and right sides, but this finding is not as common as in MID. Emotional bluntness, which may be difficult to separate from mental slowness, is common. When emotional bluntness occurs with subcortical mental deficits, a frontosubcortical symptom pattern is present. Reduced power of initiative, emotional lability and loss of insight are very common additional symptoms. Memory disturbances are present in all patients but do not predominate. There is absence of instrumental symptoms, such as agnosia, aphasia and apraxia, that is those included in the parietal lobe syndrome. Lacunar dementia, which belongs to the SWMD spectrum, may initially produce symptoms such as pure motor hemiparesis or pure sensory stroke or dysarthria-clumsy hand syndrome, homolateral ataxia or other clinical syndromes.[15] Recovery from each event is the rule, but the neurological defects gradually accumulate to a state of dementia, combined with pyramidal, extrapyramidal, cerebellar or pseudobulbar symptoms.

Binswanger's disease, another variant in the spectrum of SWMD, is either acute, with evidence of stroke (33%), or insidious (66%), without clear-cut cerebral ischaemic attacks. The subsequent course follows one of three patterns:

1. gradual progression without acute deficits (43%)
2. stroke without progression (14%), and
3. gradual progression of symptoms exacerbated by acute focal deficits (43%).

Periods of relative improvement or stability are unusual. Amnesia dominates in the early phase of the illness in many patients. Alterations in mood, judgment and behaviour are prominent. Pyramidal (reflex asymmetries or hemiparesis), extrapyramidal (rigidity), or cerebellar (limb or gait ataxia) features are present in 89% of patients. Pseudobulbar symptoms (that is dysarthria) are frequent. Lateralizing signs appear to be less prominent in the early phase of the disease, when mental changes dominate.[16] Lacunar and Binswanger's disease produce a dementia syndrome including slowing of information processing, poor sustained attention, poor word list generation and verbal fluency, impaired motor programming with perseveration and impersistence and difficulty with set shifting. Memory loss is characterized by poor retrieval and intact recognition.[17]

Familial vascular encephalopathies

Cerebral autosomal dominant arteriopathy with subcortical infarcts and leukoencephalopathy (CADASIL) may be considered a new disease predominantly affecting the small vessels of the brain with an autosomal dominant transmission linked to chromosome 19. The disease has a progressive or stepwise course with age at onset in the forties. CADASIL causes subcortical lacunar infarction and dementia in over 80% of cases.[18] The clinical features include migraine, stroke or ischaemic episodes, mood disorders and dementia. Migraine with aura occurs in approximately one-third of families and is often one of the initial symptoms. Depression occurs in 30 to 50%.[19]

Other primary symptoms and signs in VAD

The coexistence of apathy with subcortical pathology and cognitive impairment is seen in patients with multiple vascular insults to paramedian diencephalic structures.[20] Some patients may show akinesia and mutism, a state of aspontaneity. They may say 'my mind is empty' or 'I have nothing to say'. Robinson et al[21] found apathy more strongly associated with lesions in the anterior part of the right hemisphere. Patients with VAD often became less energetic and more unreasonable. Typical early signs of dementia are loss of interest and initiative and inability to perform up to the usual standard. Despite full alertness and the preservation of normal levels of consciousness, the patient fatigues readily on mental effort.

Emotionalism is a heightened tendency to cry (or rarely to laugh), so that crying occurs more frequently, more easily, more vigorously or in circumstances that previously would have been out of character.[22] The prevalence in a community sample of stroke patients was found to be 15% at 1 month, 21% at 5 months and 11% at 1 year.[23] Emotionalism is found especially in patients with left frontal and temporal lesions. The most common precipitants have been found to be thoughts, kind gestures or expression of sympathy and visitors arriving or departing. Some patients show signs of euphoria or elation. Secondary mania is rare but seems to be associated with damage to structures functionally connected to the orbitofrontal cortex, mainly in the right hemisphere.[24] The right hemisphere plays an important role in mood regulation, and disruption of these functions may contribute to manic behaviour.

Personality change is the cardinal symptom of the frontal brain syndrome. Brain damage often results in a change of temperament or an alteration in the patient's habitual attitudes and patterns of behaviour, so that his reactions to events and people are different from what they were before. Areas typically affected include the control of emotions and impulses and aspects of motivation and social judgment.[25]

The frontal lobe syndrome is characterized by reduced initiative, emotional blunting, reduced control of emotions, impaired judgment, lack of awareness of one's illness, lack of insight, poor language skills, disorientation, perseveration, general disinhibition, loss of volition, disturbance of incentive, gross defects of integrative processes and changed oral and sexual behaviour. This may lead to antisocial conduct and conflicts with the law. Disinhibition, which is often marked, is seen in social interactions and in some cases in sexual behaviour. In some patients, the basic personality may be well preserved until late in the disease. The capacity for judgment may also persist, and a remarkable degree of insight is sometimes retained. In one study, patients with VAD showed a relatively more severe dysfunction of frontal lobes, as expressed in specific psychiatric and neuropsychological changes, than AD patients matched for age, sex and severity of dementia. They had more severe anosognosia, emotional lability and more severe deficits in tests of planning, sequencing and verbal fluency.[26] Verhey et al[27] concluded however, that depression, lack of insight and personality changes do not favour an aetiology of VAD over that of AD.

Difficulty with visual recognition combined with impaired reasoning and memory sometimes produce false recognitions and faulty orientation in place. Unfamiliar things and people tend to be mistaken for familiar things and people or may be interpreted as hostile or persecutory. Thus, the patient may misidentify a doctor as an old friend or enemy or a nurse as a relative. The hospital ward may be mistaken for home. Table 12.2 gives an overview of different perceptual deficiency-related syndromes.

Body image disturbances will often be revealed by the patient's subjective complaints or his own behaviour, but sometimes special tests or questions will be required to elicit them. A rough drawing of a man made by the patient will sometimes give the first indication of body image disorder. There is sometimes evidence of unilateral unawareness or neglect of the body, usually involving the left side. This side of the body may be relatively neglected in washing or dressing. The patient has unusual subjective sensations or beliefs about the limbs of one half of his body. Disordered auditory perception makes verbal communication difficult. A chance noise may be misinterpreted and contribute to the formation of delusions. The perceptual disorder is often reinforced by affects of fear and suspiciousness.

Stereotypical, repetitive, ritualistic behaviour can be marked. Picking, scratching and other purposeless activities frequently complicate VAD with frontal lobe syndrome. Episodes of weirdly inappropriate behaviour may occur.

Secondary psychiatric symptoms of VAD

Secondary symptoms can sometimes be difficult to differentiate from more specific brain damage symptoms. The psychological symptoms

Table 12.2 Syndromes of misidentification.

Capgras syndrome	The delusion that significant people have been replaced by identical-appearing imposters
Fregoli syndrome	The patient identifies his persecutor in several persons, the persecutor being accused of changing faces, like an actor
Intermetamorphosis syndrome	The delusion that people have taken on the physical appearance of others
De Clerambault syndrome	Erotomania or the delusional belief that one is secretly loved by another person

and behavioural disturbances in dementia are primarily a manifestation of the brain disease and a consequence of the demented patient's inability to cope with an environment that does not adapt to his needs (Tables 12.3 and 12.4). The patient's mental symptoms are also affected by his premorbid personality and his past experiences.

Skoog[28] found anxiety syndromes slightly more common in VAD than in AD (26% versus 20%). Anxiety and fear are especially common and tormenting in patients with VAD, delirium and other psychotic syndromes. In VAD, anxiety sometimes increases to terror and panic. The symptoms are often accompanied by various vegetative symptoms, such as palpitations, tremor, sweating, dizziness, dry mouth, epigastric discomfort and urgency of micturition. These symptoms are often misinterpreted and are considered to be due to somatic disease. The power of concentration is

Table 12.3 Psychological symptoms and signs of vascular dementia.

Intellect	Impairment of intellect, concentration and memory, distractibility, disorientation
Insight	Impaired early insight, impaired judgment, lack of awareness of one's illness, denial of illness, unreasonableness
Sleep disturbances	Insomnia, delayed sleep, early awakening, nocturnal arousals, sleeplessness, sleep during daytime
Anxiety	Anxiety, intense feeling of discomfort, worry, fear, anxiousness, perplexity, catastrophic reaction
Affective disturbances	• Blunted affect, emotional withdrawal, emotional lability, pathological crying and laughing • Depression, worrying, brooding, morning depression, crying, somatic concerns, hypochondria, loss of interest and appetite, lack of initiative, hopelessness, feelings of helplessness, feelings of worthlessness, lack of self-confidence, self-neglect, self-depreciation, guilt feelings, loss of libido, suicidal plans and attempts • Mania, euphoria, inappropriate cheerfulness
Personality changes	Changes of character, general disinhibition, loss of volition, disturbance of incentive, gross defects of integrative processes, rigid adherance to routines
Misidentification	Distortion of body image, disordered perception of internal body sensation
Psychosis	Suspiciousness, paranoid attitudes, delusions, persecutory ideas, hallucinations

Table 12.4 Behavioural psychiatric symptoms and signs of vascular dementia.

Apathy	Indifference reaction, lack of emotional concern, reduced energy, fatigability, reduced vitality, subjective anergia, loss of libido, low motivation, poor hygiene, aspontaneity, semi-mutism
Agitation	Wandering, pacing, shadowing, meaningless repetition of questions, folding pages in a book, stereotypical, repetitive, ritualistic behaviour, screaming, episodes of noisy crying or laughing
Aggressiveness	Irritability, inappropriate anger, cursing, explosive emotional outbursts, outbursts of rage, aggressive and violent behaviour, hostility
Psychomotor activity	Motor retardation, profound slowing, diminished drive, restlessness, perseveration, inability to perform up to usual standard, purposeless overactivity, stereotyped organization of behaviour
Language	Reduced speech, poor language skills, expressive deficits, articulation defects
Social functioning	Low motivation, inappropriate dressing and undressing, social withdrawal
Eating problems	Impaired eating abilities, eating flowers or other inappropriate things
Disinhibition	A tendency to indulge in foolish jokes, episodes of tactless behaviour, intrusiveness, grossly insensitive behaviour, sexual disinhibition
Delirium	Acute confusional state, disturbance of consciousness, fluctuating cognitive disturbances, sleep-wake disturbances, nocturnal delirium

impaired. When taxed beyond his ability, the patient may become evasive or sullen or react abruptly with an explosion of primitive affect, such as anger, anxiety or tears (catastrophic reaction).

Depression affects 40–50% of stroke patients[29] and poses one of the most critical challenges to the physician. Skoog et al[30] suggested that cerebrovascular disease may be the leading cause of dementia at age 85 and older and they found depression in 29% of these patients. The frequency and severity of depression are significantly increased during the period from 6 months to 2 years after the stroke.[31] Clinicians working with patients suffering from vascular brain lesions need to maintain a high sensitivity to concomitant depression. '… subtle cerebral changes may make aging persons increasingly liable to affective disturbances'. This statement by Post[32] has been pursued with some vigour over the past decades. Patients with a history of psychiatric disorder have been found to have high rates of post-stroke depression.[29] Usual symptoms are worrying, brooding, loss of interest, hopelessness, suicidal plans, social withdrawal, self-depreciation, lack of self-confidence, pathological guilt, irritability, anxiety, anxious foreboding, morning depression, weight loss, delayed sleep, subjective anergia, early awakening and loss of libido.

Several factors increase the difficulty of accurately assessing mood in demented patients. These patients are unable to introspect or adequately report their mood states. Anosognosia or poor insight may prevent patients from recognizing their cognitive losses and possibly their mood states. Sultzer et al[33] found that patients with VAD had more severe behavioural disturbing depression and anxiety than those with AD at similar levels of cognitive impairment. Other investigators found that patients with VAD were more likely to have depression in all stages of dementia.[34]

Major depressive disorder after brain injury may itself produce intellectual impairment. Starkstein et al[35] showed that when patients with and without major depression were matched for size and location of lesion, the Mini-Mental State scores were significantly lower for depressed than for non-depressed patients. Some studies suggest that lesion location is related to severity of post-stroke depression, although this relationship may be more complex than previously suggested. In patients with left hemisphere lesions, the severity of depression tended to be greater with increasing proximity of the lesion to the frontal pole, whereas posterior lesions of the right hemisphere were separately associated with higher depression scores.[36] Other studies conclude that lesion location is not an important factor in determining the emergence of depression after stroke.[37,38]

Difficulty in falling asleep, fragmentation of sleep, nocturnal arousals, sleep during daytime and sleep apnoea are disturbances commonly reported in demented patients. Many demented patients need to be fed, some refuse food although they are capable of swallowing, and binge eating occurs occasionally. Impaired eating abilitiy increases the risk of social isolation.

Motor agitation in the form of restless pacing behaviour and difficulty in sitting still may be an expression of a disinhibition due to frontal lobe lesions, but is also seen in patients with extrapyramidal syndromes and subcortical brain damage. Restlessness and wandering are also common and correlate with executive and visuospatial dysfunction. Wandering is more common in the later stages of VAD, but is more likely in AD patients in all stages of disease.[34] Screaming behaviour may be a vocal variant of motor agitation. Difficulty in communication may prevent a patient from conveying the underlying cause, such as somatic pain or anxiety. Confusion is often present, and a frontal lobe syndrome is common among 'screamers'.

Delusions are false beliefs not alterable by evidence or reason. Delusional complications are not as common in VAD as in AD. The prevalence of delusions varies from 27% to 60% in MID.[39,40] Simple persecutory delusions seen in VAD often consist of elementary, loosely structured, usually transient beliefs, such as believing that possessions or money have been stolen or that one's spouse has been unfaithful. Suspiciousness against own family members and staff may be linked to difficulties of recognition. Troublesome, aggressive and violent behaviours and hallucinations are more likely to appear in delusional than in non-delusional patients.[41]

The denial of illness is a delusional syndrome in which the patient will not admit to physical deficits despite obvious dysfunction. Denial of blindness (Anton's syndrome) and denial of hemiparesis are the most well established delusional syndromes.[42] Delusions may also be associated with neurological deficits, such as reduplication of body, reduplicative paramnesia (a state in which the patient believes that he is simultaneously in two geographical locations). This last delusion is usually transient, occurs during recovery from an acute cerebral lesion and has been associated with right parietal or combined right parietal and bilateral frontal dysfunction.[43,44]

The frequency of hallucinations is higher in VAD than in AD. Hallucinations occur in approximately one-tenth of all VAD patients. Visual hallucinations are more frequent than auditory hallucinations, followed by gustatory, olfactory and haptic hallucinations.[40] Hallucinations typically co-occur with delusions, unless they are produced by an age-related comorbid process, such as blindness or deafness. It is important to differentiate delusions and hallucinations from misinterpretations and loss of the ability to interpret sensory impressions. The patients probably experience failure to distinguish inner images from outer percepts, and from vivid dreams carried over into the waking state. Simple visual hallucinations consist of flashes of light, geometrical patterns or colours. Some patients with visual hallucinations have homonymous visual field abnormalities associated with geniculocalcarine lesions and experience formed hallucinatory images within the field defect.[45]

Delirium or confusional states are characterized by disturbances of consciousness, inability to focus attention, fluctuating cognitive disturbances, variations of the condition, sleep and wake disturbances and potentiation of other symptoms of dementia. Delirium seems to be more common in brain disorders such as late onset AD (LAD) and VAD, in which the damage to the brain is more widespread.[46] The highest prevalence of delirium has been found among the most severely demented patients.[47]

Restlessness, irritability and aggressiveness are often parts of a more general condition, such as somatic disorders, pain, urinary retention and obstipation. Easily aroused aggression is encountered in 35–50% of patients with VAD. Aggressiveness is often linked to feelings of helplessness, despair, anxiety and delusions. The symptoms are often related to inability to understand, interact and to communicate with the surroundings. Underlying problems in the form of stress and setting limits are common. Some patients show impaired control of aggressive behaviour and in its extreme form this may be manifest as outbursts of uncontrollable violence.

Conclusion

The variety of symptoms in patients with VAD may reflect the heterogeneity of the pathophysiological processes, as well as of the size, number and locations of the various tissue lesions in these patients. This appears to be true for the infarct-related dementia subtypes (MID and SID), but in SWMD a more homogeneous symptom pattern, with emotional reduction, mental slowness and gait deficits, seems to predominate. The difference may be explained by the variety of locations of brain lesions in the infarct-related dementias, whereas the subcortical region is the primary site of vascular damage in SWMD.

The pronounced variety of symptoms in patients with VAD may also indicate that the phenomenological manifestations of VAD have not yet been clarified. In the view of the authors, an increased interest in the methodology of assessment and analysis of symptoms may contribute to a clearer description of the phenomenology of VAD and consequently to a better understanding of VAD, including its subtypes and preliminary stages.

References

1. Roth M, The natural history of mental disorders arising in the senium. *J Ment Sci* (1955) **101**:281–301.
2. Mayer-Gross W, Slater E, Roth M, *Clinical Psychiatry*, 3rd edn (Ballière, Tindall & Cassell: London, 1969) 593–7.
3. Erkinjuntti T, Vascular dementia: challenge of clinical diagnosis. *Int Psychogeriatr* (1997) **9** (Suppl 1):51–8.
4. Pantoni L, Garcia JH, Brown GG, Vascular pathology in three cases of progressive cognitive deterioration. *J Neurol Sci* (1996) **135**: 131–9.
5. Brodal A, Self-observations and neuro-anatomical considerations after a stroke. *Brain* (1973) **96**: 675–94.
6. Wallin A, Edman Å, Blennow K et al, Stepwise Comparative Status Analysis (STEP): a tool for identification of regional brain syndromes in dementia. *J Geriatr Psychiatry Neurol* (1996) **9**:185–99.
7. Bowler JV, Hachinski V, Vascular cognitive impairment: a new

approach to vascular dementia. *Baillieres Clin Neurol* (1995) **4**: 357–76.

8. Gustafson L, Hagberg B, Dementia with onset in the presenile period. A cross-sectional study. *Acta Psychiatr Scand* (1975) (Suppl) **257**:3–71.

9. Wallin A, Blennow K, Gottfires CG, Subcortical symptoms predominate in vascular dementia. *Int J Geriatr Psychiatry* (1991) **6**: 137–45.

10. Wallin A, Blennow K, Clinical subgroups of the Alzheimer syndrome. *Acta Neurol Scand* (1996) (Suppl) **165**:51–7.

11. Roman GC, Tatemichi TK, Erkinjuntii T et al, Vascular dementia: diagnostic criteria for research studies. Report of the NINDS-AIREN International Workshop. *Neurology* (1993) **43**:250–60.

12. Erkinjuntti T, Types of multi-infarct dementia. *Acta Neurol Scand* (1987); **75**:391–9.

13. Brun A, Gustafson L, Zerebrovaskuläre Erkrankungen. In: Kisker KP, Lauter H, Meyer J-E, Muller C, Strömgren E, eds, *Psychiatrie der Gegenwart, Band 6, Organische Psychosen*. (Springer-Verlag: Heidelberg 1988) 253–95.

14. Katz DI, Alexander MP, Mandell A, Dementia following strokes in the mesencephalon and diencephalon. *Arch Neurol* (1987) **44**:1127–33.

15. Fisher CM, Lacunar strokes and infarcts: a review. *Neurology* (1982) **32**:871–6.

16. Babikian V, Ropper AH, Binswanger's disease: a review. *Stroke* (1987) **229**:69–77.

17. Cummings JL, Vascular subcortical dementias: clinical aspects. *Dementia* (1994) **5**:177–80.

18. Chabriat H, Vahedi K, Iba-Zizen MT et al, Clinical spectrum of CADASIL: a study of 7 families. *Lancet* (1995) **346**:934–9.

19. Salloway S, Hong J, CADASIL syndrome: a genetic form of vascular dementia. *J Geriatr Psychiatry Neurol* (1998) **11**:71–7.

20. Marin RS, Differential diagnosis and classification of apathy. *Am J Psychiatry* (1990) **147**:22–30.

21. Robinson RG, Kubos KL, Starr LB et al, Mood disorders in stroke patients. *Brain* (1984) **107**:81–93.

22. Allman P, Emotionalism following brain damage. *Behav Neurol* (1991) **4**:57–62.

23. House A, Dennis M, Molyneux A et al, Emotionalism after stroke. *Br Med J* (1989) **298**:991–4.

24. Starkstein SE, Boston JD, Robinson RG, Mechanism of mania after brain injury. *J Nerv Ment Dis* (1988) **176**:87–100.

25. Lipowski ZJ, A new look at organic brain syndromes. *Am J Psychiatry* (1980) **137**:674–8.

26. Starkstein SE, Sabe L, Vazquez S et al, Neuropsychological, psychiatric, and cerebral blood flow findings in vascular dementia and Alzheimer's disease. *Stroke* (1996) **27**:408–14.

27. Verhey FR, Ponds RW, Rozendaal N et al, Depression, insight, and personality changes in Alzheimer's disease and vascular dementia. *J Geriatr Psychiatry Neurol* (1995) **8**:23–7.

28. Skoog I, The prevalence of psychotic, depressive and anxiety syndromes in demented and non-demented 85-year-olds. *Int J Geriatr Psychiatry* (1993) **8**:247–53.

29. Eastwood MR, Rifat SL, Nobbs H, Mood disorder following cerebrovascular accident. *Br J Psychiatry* (1989) **154**:95–200.

30. Skoog I, Nilsson L, Palmertz B et al, A population-based study of dementia in 85-year-olds. *N Engl J Med* (1993) **328**:153–8.

31. Robinson RG, Price TR, Poststroke depressive disorders: a follow-up study of 103 patients. *Stroke* (1982) **13**:635–41.
32. Post F, The factor of ageing in affective illness. In: Coppen A, Walk A, eds, *Recent Developments in Affective Disorders* Headley Bros: Kent (1968) 105–16.
33. Sultzer DL, Harvey SL, Mahler ME, A comparison of psychiatric symptoms in vascular dementia and Alzheimer's disease. *Am J Psychiatry* (1993) **150**:1806–12.
34. Cooper JK, Mungas D, Risk factor and behavioral differences between vascular and Alzheimer's dementias: the pathway to end-stage disease. *J Geriatr Psychiatry Neurol* (1993) **6**:29–33.
35. Starkstein SE, Robinson RG, Price TR, Comparison of patients with and without poststroke major depression matched for size and location of lesion. *Arch Gen Psychiatry* (1988) **45**:247–52.
36. Sinyor D, Jacques P, Kaloupek DG et al, Poststroke depression and lesion location. *Brain* (1986) **109**:537–46.
37. House A, Dennis M, Warlow C et al, Mood disorders after stroke and their relation to lesion location. *Brain* (1990) **113**:1113–29.
38. Sharpe M, Hawton K, House A, Mood disorders in long-term survivors of stroke: associations with brain lesion location and volume. *Psychol Med* (1990) **20**:815–28.
39. Flint AJ, Delusions in dementia: a review. *J Neuropsychiatr Clin Neurosci* (1991) **3**:121–30.
40. Wragg RE, Jeste DV, Overview of depression and psychosis in Alzheimer's disease. *Am J Psychiatry* (1989) **146**:577–87.
41. Flynn FG, Cummings JL, Gornbein J, Delusions in dementia syndromes: investigation of behavioral and neuropsychological correlates. *J Neuropsychiatry Clin Neurosci* (1991) **3**:364–70.
42. Cummings JL, Organic delusions: phenomenology, anatomical correlations and review. *Br J Psychiatry* (1985) **146**:184–97.
43. Benson DF, Gardner H, Meadows JC, Reduplicative paramnesia. *Neurology* (1976) **26**:47–151.
44. Fisher CM, Disorientation for place. *Arch Neurol* (1982) **39**:33–6.
45. Cummings JL, Miller B, Hill MA et al, Neuropsychiatric aspects of multi-infarct dementia and dementia of the Alzheimer type. *Arch Neurol* (1987) **44**:389–93.
46. Sjögren M, Wallin A, Edman Å, Symptomatological characteristics distinguish between frontotemporal dementia and vascular dementia with a dominant frontal lobe syndrome. *Int J Geriatr Psychiatry* (1997) **12**:656–61.
47. Robertsson B, Blennow K, Gottfries CG, Wallin A, Delirium in dementia. *Int J Geriatr Psychiatry* (1998) **13**:49–56.

13
Cognition and neuropsychology

Tammy M Scott and Marshal F Folstein

Vascular dementia (VAD) is the second most common form of dementia in the USA and Europe, and is the most common form in Asia.[1-3] Until recently, research on VAD has been impeded by a lack of standards in diagnosis, classification, methodology, and terminology, which created inconsistencies throughout the literature. During the 1990s, however, attempts have been made to create diagnostic criteria which will allow international comparison.[2,4,5]

In 1991, a joint committee of the Neuroepidemiology Branch of the National Institute of Neurological Disorders and Stroke (NINDS) and the Association Internationale pour la Recherche et l'Enseignement en Neurosciences (AIREN) worked to develop a definition of VAD and to develop diagnostic criteria for VAD for neuroepidemiologic studies. According to the criteria established by the NINDS–AIREN workshop, a neuropathologic classification of VAD includes cases of dementia resulting from ischemic and hemorrhagic brain lesions, as well as from cerebral ischemic hypoxic lesions such as those due to cardiac arrest; it excludes cases due to pure asphyxia or respiratory failure.[2] The definition of *dementia* adopted by the NINDS–AIREN committee is that of the ICD-10,[6] and specifies that cognitive decline should be demonstrated by loss of memory and deficits in *at least two other domains*. The criteria specify that the decline in memory and intellectual abilities must cause impairment in functioning in daily living.[2] The definition excludes cases of delirium, altered states of consciousness, other etiologic causes of dementia, as well as patients with conditions that interfere with assessment of intellectual functions. For better or worse, this last criterion requires that patients with severe aphasia and significant sensori-motor deficits precluding testing be excluded. Undoubtedly this stringent criterion will result in the false exclusion of many cases of VAD following stroke.

The report of the NINDS-AIREN workshop stresses the importance of a neuropsychological evaluation for the assessment of VAD. It suggests the following tests as being useful for screening for VAD[2]: a four-word memory test with 10-minute delayed recall; a cube-drawing test for copy; a verbal fluency test (i.e. number of animals named in 1 minute); Luria's alternating hand sequence or finger rings; a letter cancellation tests for neglect; a reaction-time test and; the grooved pegboard test.

While the report also suggests the use of the Mini-Mental Status Exam (MMSE)[7] as a screening tool for VAD, other studies suggest that a supplemental mental alternation test to be added to increase the sensitivity to subcortical dysfunction.[8] Following the screening phase, the NINDS-AIREN committee recommends that suspected cases should be evaluated by a neuropsychologist, and that tests used should cover each major cognitive domain in order to evaluate fully the spectrum of neuropsychological abnormalities. In addition, they recommend that the neuropsychological tests selected should have sensitivity in detecting subcortical lesions and in evaluating language and motor functioning since subcortical structure are commonly affected in VAD.[2]

Expanding on the neuropathological classifications outlined by the NINDS-AIREN report, Meyer and colleagues[9] have proposed the following eight subtypes of VAD:

1. multi-infarct dementias
2. strategically placed infarctions causing dementia
3. multiple subcortical lacunar lesions
4. Binswanger's disease (BD) (arteriosclerotic subcortical leukoencephalopathy)
5. mixtures of two or more of the above VAD subtypes
6. hemorrhagic lesions causing dementia
7. subcortical dementias due to cerebral autosomally dominant arteriolopathy with subcortical infarcts and leukoencephalopathy (CADASIL), or to familial amyloid angiopathies and coagulopathies
8. mixtures of DAT and VAD.

Neuropsychological or cognitive patterns of impairments have been published for six of the right subtypes. Findings of these studies are described below.

Subtypes of VAD

Multi-infarct dementia

The neuropathology of multi-infarct dementia (MID) includes multiple, large, cerebral infarcts caused by emboli or arising from occlusion by atherosclerotic plaques. The NINDS–AIREN criteria for MID specify that the cerebrovascular lesions associated with MID are multiple, large, *complete* infarcts that can involve cortical and subcortical areas. There have been a number of neuropsychological studies that have used clinical criteria consistent with the NINDS–AIREN criteria for MID.

The cognitive impairments associated with MID necessarily are dependent on the cortical or subcortical areas supplied by the affected blood vessels. For example, middle cerebral artery occlusions affecting the left hemisphere typically result in aphasia and apraxia;[10-12] infarctions anterior to the Rolandic fissure result in non-fluent aphasias and lesions posterior to the central fissure are associated with fluent aphasia.[13] Right middle cerebral artery infarctions are usually associated with abnormalities in prosody, the ability to dress, and problems with visuospatial orientation and visuomotor performance.[14,15] Since the definition of *dementia* specifies that multiple areas of cognition are impaired, pathology restricted to cortical areas usually requires multiple bilateral infarcts in order to meet the diagnostic criteria.[13] In studies of the psychiatric sequelae of stroke, Starkstein et al[16] found that those patients with left anterior lesions, either cortical or subcortical, had significantly greater frequency and severity of depression than patients with any other lesion location. In contrast, right hemisphere lesions were associated with a significantly higher incidence of excessive cheerfulness.

Strategically placed infarcts

Recent studies making use of advances in neuroimaging have shown that small infarctions which are strategically located are capable of creating deficits in multiple areas of cognitive functioning. While most of these regions are subcortical, infarcts to the angular gyrus have also been shown to result in multiple cognitive impairments. The subcortical areas which have been shown to result in a full dementia syndrome when infarcted include the basal ganglia, thalamus, and genu of the internal capsule. These latter sites have been shown to have pathways that project to the frontal or temporal lobes,[17-19] and it is thought that the cognitive and behavioral changes resulting from infarcts to these areas are a result of interruptions of the circuits connecting subcortical and cortical regions.[20,21]

Angular gyrus
The clinical syndrome associated with infarct to the left angular gyrus includes aphasia (with paraphasic errors), alexia with agraphia, Gerstmann syndrome (acalculia, right–left disorientation, dysgraphia, and finger agnosia), and constructional disturbance.[13] Patients with angular gyrus syndrome typically recognize their impairments and are frustrated by them. It is important to note that focal motor and/or sensory signs may be absent in these patients, and that their lesions are not always detectable by CT; this often makes the syndrome difficult to distinguish from other types of dementia including Alzheimer's disease (AD).[21]

Genu of the internal capsule
Small infarcts to the genu of the internal capsule have been shown to result in significant impairments in cognition. The main clinical features of

this syndrome have been described as acute confusional state soon after the stroke with fluctuating alertness, inattention, memory loss, apathy, abulia, and psychomotor retardation.[20] Contralateral weakness appears to be mild or absent, with the severity of weakness correlated to the extent of the infarct in the posterior limb. The chronic phase of this syndrome in patients with dominant hemisphere lesions include significant verbal memory loss—along with other neuropsychological impairments such as naming and verbal fluency—despite an improved level of consciousness.[20,22,23] Persistence of symptoms as a result of non-dominant hemisphere lesions appears to be more equivocal, with moderate impairment in visuospatial memory recovering within weeks in one patient.[20]

Thalamus
The consequences of thalamic infarction include fluctuating consciousness, apathy, lack of spontaneity, perseveration, and disorientation. Dominant-side lesions result in visuo-verbal memory impairment accompanied by a variable degree of dysphasic disturbances with sparing of repetition. Non-dominant lesions usually result in hemispatial neglect and visuospatial processing deficits.[20,24] Patients with bilateral paramedian thalamic infarctions have cognitive deficits which include memory impairment, reduced verbal fluency, and decreased mental control,[20,21,25-27] but with relatively intact language.[25] Not uncommonly, the blood supply for thalamic para-median structures can arise from one pedicle, which when occluded can produce a generalized or bilateral, i.e. non-material specific, amnestic syndrome. There is some evidence that amnesia due to thalamic infarction may differ in form from that due to hippocampal compromise, as occurs with posterior cerebral artery infarction, with better recognition skills and responsiveness to cueing found with the former.[28] Other studies have shown that anterior thalamic nuclei damage results in more consistent memory loss than does dorsomedial nuclear damage.[18]

Caudate and globus pallidus
Patients with bilateral and unilateral caudate hemorrhage have been reported in the literature to have executive functioning impairment (e.g. problem solving, set switching), recent and remote memory deficits (e.g. list learning and recall of a complex drawing), attention deficits, abulia, and verbal fluency impairments (with relatively spared naming abilities). Acute visual and auditory hallucinations, apraxia, motor impersistence, and anosognosia have also been reported in these patients.[20,29] Behaviorally, infarction of the dorsolateral portion of the caudate nucleus has been shown to result in apathy and hypokinesia, while infarction of the ventromedial caudate has resulted in disinhibition and impulsiveness.[29]

Studies of focal damage to the globus palidus are rare and are limited to case reports. There is some evidence, however, of bilateral globus pallidus hemorrhages resulting in impairments of memory and set shifting.[21,30]

Multiple subcortical lacunar infarcts

Neuropathological studies have shown that multiple subcortical lacunar infarcts occur following occlusion of penetrating arterioles and lenticulostriate arteries in the basal ganglia, pons, and white matter of the centrum ovale. These small vessels are susceptible to arteriosclerotic injuries, and it has been shown that multiple occlusions can produce a full dementia syndrome. In a study utilizing magnetic resonance imaging, Boone et al[31] found that large white matter lesions (> 10 cm^2) were associated with deficits in basic attention and impairments in frontal lobe functioning, but did not find consistent cognitive impairments in patients with lesions totalling less than 10 cm^2. This finding led them to hypothesize that a 'threshold' of white matter lesion area must be present before cognitive deficits are observed.

Few studies of lacunar infarcts have included neuropsychological assessments; those that do, however, agree that the syndrome includes deficits in executive functioning. Wolfe et al[32] found deficits including difficulties in set shifting, decreased verbal fluency, and apathy in their sample of 11 patients with multiple subcortical lacunar infarcts. Corbet et al[33] showed that the number of lacunes and extent of periventricular lucency, as well as the extent of ventricular enlargement, were related to deficits in phonemic and semantic fluency, simple attention, and abstraction. A CT study performed by Meyer et al[34] showed that in patients with multiple small strokes, cognitive performance was correlated with measures of ischaemia but not with measures of brain atrophy. It is hypothesized that like strategic infarcts in these areas, lacunes, in the basal ganglia and deep white matter disrupt subcortico-frontal pathways resulting in the above executive impairments.[21,35]

Binswanger's subcortical arteriosclerotic leukoencephalopathy

Binswanger's disease is a result of multiple and cumulative occlusions of deep penetrating arterioles supplying white matter, resulting in more severe patterns of the subcortical dementia described above, with the addition of abulia, incontinence, and limb rigidity.[21,36,37] It is a gradually progressive disorder. Patients usually have a history of repeated small strokes with discrete neurological impairments.[3,21,38,39] Binswanger's dementia is characterized by pseudobulbar palsy, emotional incontinence, lateralized motor signs, corticospinal or corticobulbar tract dysfunction, and gait disturbance. Changes in mood and behavior may include personality change, loss of incentive, impaired insight, mutism, and apathy. Motor disturbances can include bradykinesia, rigidity, and dysarthria. Incontinence and primitive reflexes are also often present.[21,38-40] Neuropsychologcial evaluations have revealed impairments in simple and divided attention, perseverativeness and difficulty shifting set on a card sorting task,[31] as well as impairments on task of motor performance and sequential reasoning and analysis.[41] Similar to lacunar state, BD has been hypothesized to create a disconnection of subcortical and cortical structures resulting in dementia.[21,37,42]

Subcortical dementias caused by genetically determined arteriolopathies

A number of studies have documented a syndrome of cerebral autosomal dominant arteriopathy with subcortical infarcts and leukoencephalopathy (CADASIL), which maps to chromosome 19 and potentially leads to cognitive decline and dementia.[3,43-45] Features of the syndrome of recurrent subcortical ischemic events can include progressive subcortical dementia with pseudobulbar features to those seen in BD, migraine with aura, and mood disorders with severe depressive episodes. Other studies on VAD have emphasized the role of apolipoprotein E polymorphism, which has been examined as a potential marker for AD. There has been some equivocal evidence that the ε4 allele may be associated with a predisposition toward atherosclerosis and ischemic CVD and that the frequency of the ε4 allele may be greater in MID relative to control subjects.[46-48] This has not been a consistent finding, however.[49]

Combined DAT and VAD

The coincidence of AD and vascular disorders is becoming increasingly recognized as common, especially in older patients. Mirsen and Hachinski[50] have estimated that patients with mixed dementia make up approximately 15-19% of all dementia cases. The report of the NINDS-AIREN International Workshop[2] discourages the use of the term *mixed dementia*, and proposes that when the NINCDS-ADRDA clinical criteria and typical radiological features of AD are present, the diagnosis of AD should take precedence over the diagnosis of VAD. They do concede, however, that CVD may be a confounder in AD since radiological evidence of stroke is commonly found, and that clear-cut differentiation of AD and VAD may be extremely difficult. Other investigators have also found it difficult to differentiate AD with CVD from MID, as well as AD from the dementia associated with lacunar infarcts.[51] The Hachinski Ischemic Scale (HIS)[52] has been widely used for these purposes with varying success (Table 13.1). For pure forms of AD and MID there appears to be a 70-80% sensitivity and specificity.[5] The HIS, however, appears to be relatively less sensitive in detecting cases of degenerative dementia plus stroke.[2] A neuropathological study for validating the HIS found that 21% of patients with primary degenerative dementia may have been incorrectly labeled by the HIS as having VAD.[53] Review of the HIS has progressively found that many of the original scale's 13 items were not particularly discriminating.[54,55]

Table 13.1 Clinical features of the Hachinski Ischemic Scale.[52]

Feature	Score*
Abrupt onset	2
Stepwise deterioration	1
Fluctuating course	2
Nocturnal confusion	1
Relative preservation of personality	1
Depression	1
Somatic complaints	1
Emotional incontinence	1
History of hypertension	1
History of strokes	2
Evidence of associated atherosclerosis	1
Focal neurologic symptoms	2
Focal neurologic signs	2

*A total score of 4 or less indicates Alzheimer's disease; a total of 7 or more indicates multi-infarct dementia.

Neuropsychological differentiation of VAD from dementias of other etiologies

A number of neuropsychological studies have attempted to show differences in the cognitive deficits found in the VADs and AD. Most of these studies have grouped all of the VADs into one syndrome. The results of the studies showed that relative to AD, patients with VAD perform more poorly on tests influenced by frontal and subcortical mechanisms—particularly in executive functioning (e.g. self-regulation, planning), attention, verbal fluency, and motor performance/fine motor coordination.[41,56,57] In addition, patients with VAD have been shown to have more severe behavioral retardation, depression, and anxiety than those with AD.[58] In contrast, patients with AD perform more poorly on tests of recent memory and story recall,[41,57,59] language repetition,[41] naming,[56,57] and orientation to time and place.[57] Directly comparing MID and AD patients, Erker et al[60] found that Alzheimer patients appear to have greater impairment with recent memory function compared with general intellectual ability, while MID patients exhibit the converse pattern. In studies comparing patients with MID to AD, a similar pattern of impairments was discovered with MID patients performing less well on tests of verbal fluency,[61,62] prosody,[63] and with a greater number of perseverations and intrusions.[64] Relying on language measures only, Kontiola et al[65] were able to discriminate mildly to moderately demented patients from healthy controls, and with 97% accuracy discriminate Alzheimer's patients from those independently classified as suffering MID, even after controlling for general severity of the dementia. The factor structure of discriminant functions produced by their research suggested that MID patients suffer relatively more disturbance to elementary linguistic functions, such as word or phoneme repetition, and colour naming, while Alzheimer's patients' difficulties were at the level of understanding and constructing complex grammatical structures. Although given the heterogeneity present in MID cognitive impairment, the generalizability of these results to the clinical situation when attempting to assign individual patients diagnostic groups is likely to be limited. Bennet et al[66] compared patients with BD to those with AD and found that Binswanger's patients had relatively less profound impairments in episodic memory, more depressive symptomatology, and a more variable rate of cognitive decline.

In a study comparing AD, VAD, and senile dementia of Lewy body type (SDLT), Ballard et al[59] found that patients with SDLT had significantly greater deterioration in verbal fluency than patients with AD or VAD, as well as a trend toward greater overall cognitive decline in the course of a year (as measured by the CAMCOG). Cherrier et al[67] compared patients with frontotemporal dementia (FTD) with those with VAD, and found that FTD patients performed significantly better than the VAD patients on tests of digit span and constructions, while there was a trend that the VAD patients performed relatively less well on tests of verbal fluency and abstractions. While there does not appear to be a neuropsychological literature on differentiating VAD from the dementias related to Parkinsons' disease, Pick's disease, Creutzfeldt–Jakob disease, progressive supranuclear palsy, and Huntington's disease, it is recommended that these etiologies can be ruled out by detailed clinical history, neuroimaging studies, and microscopic evaluation of adequately selected samples of brain parenchyma.[2]

Treatment and prevention

The early detection of VAD is important because there is some evidence in the literature for the treatment and prevention of the disorder.[68–70] A number of studies[68] have suggested that modification of risk factors for cerebrovascular disease (such as hypertension, diabetes, cholesterol, and smoking) may be useful as preventative measures against VAD. There has also been some research on the secondary pharmacological treatment of VAD. In a study of the effects of propentofylline on patients with VAD (propentofylline is a xanthine derivative that blocks reuptake of adenosine by neurons and glia cells, and which purportedly reduced ischemic nerve cells' deaths in the brain[71]), Mielke et al[70] found that visual information processing was improved in the treatment group, and that there was also a trend towards the slowing of the progression of cognitive deterioration as measured by the MMSE and digit symbol subtest. Parnetti et al[69] looked at the usefulness of posatirelin (a synthetic peptide having modulatory activity on the monoaminergic and cholinergic systems and neurotrophic effects) in the treatment of VAD. Their results showed a significant improvement in intellectual performance, orientation, motivation, and memory as compared to placebo. In addition to the above treatments, both aspirin and ticlopidine (antiplatelet agents) have been found to be useful in preventing strokes and worsening dementia in patients with VAD.[21,68]

Cognitive rehabilitation of dementia patients in general has had limited success, although there have been some exceptions. The majority of the techniques, however, have been geared to patients with AD, and make use of cognitive functions which are relatively spared.[68,72,73] These programs rely heavily on spared motor learning or implicit memory. One approach includes *spaced retrieval* which involves the patient repeatedly recalling information at increasingly longer intervals of time. This technique is often used to teach adult day-care attendees the names and faces of staff members.[68] A second technique which has shown some success involves activities of daily living (ADL) training in which the training concentrates on the motor aspects of the activity (such as tooth brushing and table setting) in order to reduce the demands on other forms of memory. Unfortunately the cognitive areas utilized in these techniques are often affected in VAD. Little or no literature exists on the cognitive rehabilitation of VAD since it is difficult to arrive at general principles because the pattern of neuropsychological deficits depends on the site of the lesions.[68]

More successful approaches to facilitating the lives of dementia patients involve designing the environment so that it makes the best use of the patient's remaining skills. Examples include camouflaging exits in order to decrease wandering, marking doorways to bathrooms with bright colors and symbols, and increasing the use of open plan design to decrease spatial disorientation.[68,74,75] A behavioral approach can also be used to modify behavioral disturbances commonly found in dementia patients such as agitation, aggression, screaming, and apathy. Increasing the rate of pleasant activities, reinforcing desirable responses, and ignoring or gently redirecting undesirable responses can be extremely useful.[63,75–78]

Summary

Neuropsychological testing is an invaluable tool for clinical assessment and research on the cognitive impairments associated with VAD. While there are a number of subcategories of VAD resulting from ischemic and hemorrhagic brain lesions, most variations are thought to create interruptions of subcortico-frontal pathways resulting in executive functioning impairments. Relative to AD, patients with VAD perform more poorly on tests influenced by frontal and subcortical mechanisms—particularly in self-regulation, planning, attention, verbal fluency, and motor performance/fine motor coordination. In addition, patients with VAD have been shown to have more severe behavioral retardation, depression, and anxiety than those with AD. The early detection of VAD is important because there is some evidence for successful treatment and prevention of the disorder.

References

1. Roman GC, The epidemiology of vascular dementia. In: Hartmann A, Kuschinsky W, Hoyer S, eds, *Cerebral Ischemia and Dementia* (Springer-Verlag: Berlin, 1991) 9–15.
2. Roman GC, Tatemichi TK, Erkinjuntti T et al, Vascular dementia: diagnostic criteria for research studies—Report of the NINDS-AIREN International Workshop, *Neurology* (1993) **43**: 250–60.
3. Desmond DW, Vascular dementia: a construct in evolution, *Cerebr Brain Metab Rev* (1996) **8**: 296–325.
4. Graham JE, Rockwood K, Beattie BL et al, Standardization of the diagnosis of dementia in the Canadian study of health and aging, *Neuroepidemiology* (1996) **15**:246–56.
5. Chui HC, Victoroff JI, Margolin D et al, Criteria for the diagnosis of ischemic vascular dementia proposed by the State of California Alzheimer's Disease Diagnostic and Treatment Centers, *Neurology* (1992) **42**:473–80.
6. WHO, The neurological adaptation of the International Classification of Diseases (ICD-10NA) (draft) (World Health Organization: Geneva, 1991).
7. Folstein M, Folstein S, McHugh PR, Mini-Mental State: a practical method for grading the cognitive state of patients for the clinician, *J Psychiatr Res* (1975) **12**:189–98.
8. Jones BN, Teng EL, Folstein MF, Harrison KS, A new bedside test of cognition for patients with HIV infection, *Ann Intern Med* (1993) **119**:1001–4.
9. Meyer JS, Shirai T, Akiyama H, Neuroimaging for differentiating vascular from Alzheimer's dementias, *Cerebr Brain Metab Rev* (1996) **8**:1–10.
10. Benson DF, Geschwind N, Psychiatric conditions associated with focal lesions of the central nervous system. In: Arieti S, Reiser M, eds, *American Handbook of Psychiatry* (Basic Books: New York, 1975), vol 4.
11. Benson DF, Aphasia, alexia, and agraphia (Churchill Livingstone: New York, 1979).

12. Geschwind N, The apraxias: neural mechanisms of disorders of learned movement, *Am Sci* (1975) **63**:188–95.
13. Cummings JL, Benson DF, Dementia: a clinical approach (Butterworth-Heinemann: Boston, 1992).
14. Hemphill RE, Klein R, Contribution to the dressing disability as a focal sign and to the imperception phenomena, *J Ment Sci* (1948) **94**:611–22.
15. Ross ED, The aprosodias, *Arch Neurol* (1981) **38**:561–9.
16. Starkstein SE, Robinson RG, Price TR, Comparison of cortical and subcortical lesions in the production of poststroke mood disorders, *Brain* (1987) **110**:1045–59.
17. Alexander GE, Crutcher MD, DeLong MR, Basal ganglia-thalamocortical circuits: parallel substrates for motor, oculomotor, 'prefrontal' and 'limbic' functions. In: Uylings HBM, Eden CGV, Bruin JPCD, Corner MA, Feenstra MGP, eds, *Progress in Brain Research*, vol 85 (Elsevier Science Publishers: New York, 1990) 119–46.
18. Tatemichi TK, Desmond DW, Mayeux R, Dementia after stroke: baseline frequency, risks, and clinical features in a hospitalized cohort, *Neurology* (1992) **42**:1185–93.
19. Cummings JL, Frontal-subcortical circuits and human behavior, *Arch Neurol* (1993) **50**:873–80.
20. Tatemichi TK, Desmond DW, Prohovnik I, Strategic infarcts in vascular dementia—a clinical and brain imaging experience, *Arzneim-Forsch/Drug Res* (1995) **45**:371–85.
21. McPherson SE, Summings JL, Neuropsychological aspects of vascular dementia, *Brain Cogn* (1996) **31**:269–82.
22. Kooistra CA, Heilman KM, Memory loss from a subcortical white matter infarct, *J Neurol Neurosurg Psychiatry* (1988) **51**:866–9.
23. Markowitsch HJ, Cramon DY, Hormann E, Sick CD, Kinsler P, Verbal memory deterioration after unilateral infarct of the internal capsule in an adolescent, *Cortex* (1990) **26**:597–609.
24. Bogousslavsky J, Ferrazzini M, Regli F, Assal G, Tanabe H, Manic delirium and frontal lobe syndrome with paramedian infarction of the right thalamus, *J Neurol Neurosurgery Psychiatry* (1988) **51**:116–19.
25. Eslinger PJ, Warner GC, Grattan LM, Easton JD, 'Frontal lobe' utilization behavior associated with paramedian thalamic infarction, *Neurology* (1991) **41**:450–2.
26. Gentilini M, Renzi ED, Crisi G, Bilateral paramedian thalamic artery infarcts: report of eight cases, *J Neurol Neurosurg Psychiatry* (1987) **50**:900–9.
27. Stuss DT, Guberman A, Nelson R, Larochelle S, The neuropsychology of paramedian thalamic infarction, *Brain Cogn* (1988) **8**:348–78.
28. Mattis S, Kovner R, Goldmeier E, Different patterns of amnestic syndromes, *Brain Lang* (1978) **6**:170–91.
29. Mendez MF, Adams NL, Lewandowski KS, Neurobehavioral changes associated with caudate lesions, *Neurology* (1989) **39**:349–54.
30. Strub RL, Frontal lobe syndrome in a patient with bilateral globus pallidus lesions, *Arch Neurol* (1989) **46**:1024–7.
31. Boone KB, Miller BL, Lesser IM et al, Neuropsychological correlates of white-matter lesions in healthy elderly subjects–a threshold effect, *Arch neurol* (1992) **49**:549–54.
32. Wolfe N, Linn R, Babikian VL, Albert ML, Frontal systems impair-

ment following multiple lacunar infarcts, *Arch Neurol* (1990) **47**: 129–32.
33. Corbett AJ, Bennett H, Kos S, Cognitive dysfunction following subcortical infarction, *Arch Neurol* (1994) **51**: 999–1007.
34. Meyer JS, Obara K, Muramatsu K, Mortel KF, Shirai T, Cognitive performance after small strokes correlates with ischemia, not atrophy of the brain, *Dementia* (1995) **6**: 312–22.
35. Sultzer DL, Mahler ME, Cummings JL et al, Cortical abnormalities associated with subcortical lesions in vascular dementia, *Arch Neurol* (1995) **52**:773–80.
36. Fisher CM, Binswanger's encephalopathy: a review *J Neurol* (1989) **236**:65–69.
37. Roman GC, Senile dementia of the Binswanger type—a vascular form of dementia in the elderly, *JAMA* (1987) **258**:1782–8.
38. Babikian V, Ropper AH, Binswanger's disease: a review, *Stroke* (1987) **18**:2–12.
39. Nichols FT, Mohr JP, Binswanger's subacute arteriosclerotic encephalopathy. In: Barnett HJM, Mohr JP, Stein VM, eds, *Stroke: Pathophysiology, Diagnosis, and Management* (Churchill Livingstone: New York, 1986).
40. Lotz PR, Ballinger J, Quisling RG, Subcortical arteriosclerotic encephalopathy: CT spectrum and pathologic correlation, *Am J Roentgenol* (1986) **147**:1209–14.
41. Kertesz A, Clydesdale S, Neuropsychological deficits in vascular dementia vs Alzheimer's disease, *Arch Neurol* (1994) **51**: 1226–31.
42. Loeb C, Meyer JS, Vascular dementia: still a debatable entity, *J Neurol Sci* (1996) **143**:31–40.
43. Baudrimont M, Dubas F, Joutel A, Tournier-Lasserve E, Bousser MG, Autosomal dominant leukoencephalopathy and subcortical ischemic stroke: a clinicopathological study, *Stroke* (1993) **24**: 122–5.
44. Sabbadini G, Francia A, Calandriello L, Cerebral autosomal dominant arteriopathy with subcortical infarcts and leucoencephalopathy (CADASIL). Clinical, neuroimaging, pathological and genetic study of a large Italian family, *Brain* (1995) **118**:207–15.
45. Tournier-Lasserve E, Joutel A, Melki J, Cerebral autosomal dominant arteriopathy with subcortical infarcts and leukoencephalopathy maps to chromosome 19q12, *Nat Genet* (1993) **3**:256–9.
46. Pedro-Botet J, Senti M, Nogues X, Lipoprotein and apolipoprotein profile in men with ischemic stroke. Role of lipoprotein 9a, triglyceride-rich lipoproteins, and apolipoprotein E polymorphism, *Stroke* (1992) **23**:1556–62.
47. Frisoni GB, Bianchetti A, Govoni S et al, Association of apolipoprotein E E4 with vascular dementia, *JAMA* (1994) **271**:1317.
48. Shimano H, Ishibashi S, Murase T, Plasma apolipoproteins in patients with multi-infarct dementia, *Atherosclerosis* (1989) **79**:257–60.
49. Kawamata J, Tanaka S, Shimohama S, Ueda K, Kimura J, Apolipoprotein E polymorphism in Japanese patients with Alzheimer's disease or vascular dementia, *J Neurol Neurosurg Psychiatry* (1994) **57**:1414–16.
50. Mirsen T, Hachinski V, Epidemiology and classification of vascular and multi-infarct dementia. In: Meyer JS, Lechner H, Marshall J, Toole JF, eds, *Vascular and Multi-infarct Dementia* (Future Publishing: New York, 1988).
51. Skoog I, Risk factors for vascular dementia: a review, *Dementia* (1994) **5**:137–44.

52. Hachinski V, Multi-infarct dementia, *Neurol Clin* (1983) **1**:27–36.
53. Fischer P, Jellinger K, Gatterer G, Danielczyk W, Prospective neuropathological validation of Hischinski's ischemic score in dementias, *J Neurol Neurosurg Psychiatry* (1991) **54**:580–3.
54. Loeb C, Gandolfo C, Diagnostic evaluation of degenerative and vascular dementia, *Stroke* (1983) **14**:399–401.
55. Rosen W, Terry R, Fuld P, Katzman R, Peck A, Pathological verification of ischemic score in differentiation of dementias, *Ann Neurol* (1980) **7**:486–8.
56. Almkvist O, Neuropsychological deficits in vascular dementia in relation to Alzheimer's disease: reviewing evidence for functional similarity or divergence, *Dementia* (1994) **5**:203–9.
57. Villardita C, Alzheimer's disease compared with cerebrovascular dementia. Neuropsychological similarities and differences, *Acta Neurol Scand* (1993) **87**:299–308.
58. Sultzer DL, Levin HS, Mahler ME, High WM, Cummings JL, A comparison of psychiatric symptoms in vascular dementia and Alzheimer's disease, *Am J Psychiatry* (1993) **150**:1806–12.
59. Ballard C, Patel A, Oyebode F, Wilcock G, Cognitive decline in patients with Alzheimer's disease, vascular dementia and senile dementia of Lewy body type, *Age Ageing* (1996) **25**:209–13.
60. Erker G, Searight H, Peterson P, Patterns of neuropsychological functioning amongst patients with multi-infarct and Alzheimer's dementia: a comparative analysis, *Int J Psychogeriatr* (1995) **7**:393–406.
61. Hier DB, Hagenlocker K, Schindler AG, Language disintegration in dementia: effects of etiology and severity, *Brain Lang* (1985) **25**:117–33.
62. Gainotti G, Galtagirone C, Masullo C, Miceli G, Patterns of neuropsychologic impairment in various diagnostic groups of dementia. In: Amaducci L, Davidson AN, Antuono P, eds, *Aging of the Brain and Dementia: Aging*, vol 13 (Raven Press: New York, 1980).
63. Powell AL, Cummings JL, Hill MA, Benson DF, Speech and language alterations in multi-infarcy dementia, *Neurology* (1988) **38**:717–19.
64. Schindler AG, Caplan LR, Hier DB, Intrusions and perseverations, *Brain Lang* (1984) **23**:148–58.
65. Kontiola P, Laaksonen R, Erkinjuntti T, Pattern of language impairment is different in Alzheimer's disease and multi-infarct dementia, *Brain Lang* (1990) **38**:364–83.
66. Bennett DA, Gilley DW, Lee S, Cochran EJ, White matter changes: neurobehavioral manifestations of Binswanger's disease and clinical correlates in Alzheimer's disease, *Dementia* (1994) **5**:148–52.
67. Cherrier MM, Mendez MF, Perryman KM et al, Frontotemporal dementia versus vascular dementia: differential features on mental status examination, *J Am Geriatr Soc* (1997) **45**:579–83.
68. Jorm AF, Disability in dementia: assessment, prevention, and rehabilitation, *Disabil Rehabil* (1994) **16**:98–109.
69. Parnetti L, Ambrosoli L, Agliati G et al, Posatirelin in the treatment of vascular dementia: a double-blind multicentre study vs placebo, *Acta Neurol Scand* (1996) **93**:456–63.
70. Mielke R, Kittner B, Ghaemi M et al, Propentofylline improves regional cerebral glucose metabolism and neuropsychologic performance in vascular dementia, *J Neurol Sci* (1996) **141**:59–64.
71. Parkinson FE, Rudolphi KA, Fredholm BB, HWA 285: a nucleoside

transport inhibitor with neuroprotective effects in cerebral ischemia, *Gen Pharmac* (1994) **25**:1053–8.

72. Kotik-Harper D, Harper RG, Techniques for enhancing memory, orientation, and communication in the Alzheimer patient. In: Dippel RL, Hutton JT, eds, *Caring for the Alzheimer Patient: A Practical Guide*, 2nd edn (Prometheus Books: New York, 1991) 93–109.

73. Backman L, Memory training and memory improvement in Alzheimer's disease: rules and exceptions, *Acta Neurol Scand* (1992) **139**(Suppl):84–9.

74. Shroyer JAL, Hutton JT, Optimal living environments for Alzheimer patients. In: Dippel RL, Hutton JT, eds, *Caring for the Alzheimer Patient: A Practical Guide*, 2nd edn (Prometheus Books: New York, 1991) 44–50.

75. Matteson MA, Linton AD, Cleary BL, Barnes SJ, Lichtenstein MJ, Management of problematic behavioral symptoms associated with dementia: a cognitive developmental approach, *Aging Clin Exp Res* (1997) **9**:342–55.

76. Dyck G, Management of geriatric behavior problems, *Geriatr Psychiatry* (1997) **20**:165–80.

77. Green GR, Linsk NL, Pinkston EM, Modification of verbal behavior of the mentally impaired elderly by their spouses, *J Appl Behav Anal* (1986) **19**:329–36.

78. Teri L, Uomoto JM, Reducing excess disability in dementia patients: training caregivers to manage patient depression, *Clin Gerontol* (1991) **10**:49–63.

14
Neuroimaging in vascular dementia

John T O'Brien

Introduction

Neuroimaging may be useful in patients suspected of having vascular dementia (VAD) to exclude any other intracranial lesion that may be responsible for dementia, to add support and confirmation to the clinical diagnosis, to help determine the subtype of VAD and to correlate brain changes with clinical symptoms and neuropsychology to inform clinical understanding and management. As a number of different vascular pathologies can cause dementia, including haemorrhage, infarction (both single large and multiple small infarction) and diffuse white matter change,[1] it is not surprising that there is no pathognomonic neuroimaging feature of VAD. However, all these vascular changes can be visualized using structural imaging techniques [computed tomography (CT) and magnetic resonance imaging (MRI)] and the use of neuroimaging is increasingly becoming an essential requirement for an accurate clinical diagnosis of VAD.[2] It should, however, be emphasized that the role of imaging is to provide confirmatory support for a diagnosis of VAD which has been formulated on clinical grounds. A diagnosis of VAD can never be made on the basis of scan appearances alone.

There are still many important areas which remain controversial, including the degree of vascular change on scanning needed to support a diagnosis of VAD, the relative significance of different types of vascular lesions and the contribution of functional as opposed to structural imaging. This chapter will review structural and functional brain imaging changes in VAD and summarize the neuroimaging evidence required to fulfil different sets of current diagnostic criteria for VAD.

Structural imaging in VAD

This consists of CT or MRI scanning. A detailed description of imaging modalities is outside the scope of this text but excellent summaries are contained elsewhere.[3] CT scanning involves the use of traditional radiography and a detector system which rotates around the head with reconstruction of the brain image, based on electron density, performed by back projection. Although recent haemorrhage (fresh blood) shows us areas of high attenuation (bright), after a few days both haemorrhage and infarction appear as areas of low attenuation (dark). CT scanning is cheap, widely available, quick (30 seconds per scan on modern scanners), well tolerated and an effective way of showing cortical and subcortical infarcts as well as white matter changes.

In contrast to CT, MRI builds an image based on proton density and the physical properties of protons using a strong magnetic field (typically 1.5 Tesla) and a series of brief pulses of electromagnetic radiation. The image produced depends on three main properties, proton density and T1 and T2 relaxation times. Proton density, as the name implies, reflects actual density of protons in the tissue. T1 is essentially the relaxation time (time taken for protons excited by a radiofrequency pulse to lose energy and return to normal) in three-dimensional space whilst T2 is the relaxation time reflecting loss of spin phase or coherence between adjacent protons (which initially spin in phase after a radiofrequency pulse). Both T1 and T2 depend on the physical and chemical environment of the protons, not just on their density. No image relies purely on a single of these properties, although scans weighted towards one parameter rather than another have different appearances and uses. Good anatomical resolution is provided by heavily T1-weighted images (for example, inversion recovery sequences) while proton density and T2-weighted images (for example, spin-echo sequences) are sensitive to changes in water content and provide good visualization of white matter lesions and smaller infarcts.

MRI is less widely (though increasingly) available, more expensive (about twice the cost of CT), is unsuitable for patients with pacemakers or metallic implants in the head and can be claustrophobic. It does not visualize bone but provides superior resolution to CT, particularly in the white matter. MRI, particularly T2-weighted sequences, has been criticized as being too sensitive to detecting pathological changes which may not always be of clinical significance (see below). Although MRI would be preferred to CT if both were equally available, in practice CT will usually be performed first in most clinical services, with MRI reserved for cases where the CT is equivocal or uninformative or when better visualization of particular lesions (such as in the white matter or in subcortical areas) is required.

On structural imaging VAD, like Alzheimer's disease (AD), is associated with relatively non-specific changes such as generalized cerebral atrophy and ventricular dilatation.[4-8] There may sometimes be focal atrophy, either cortical or ventricular, corresponding to focal infarction and subsequent local atrophy (see Figure 14.1). A wide variety of other brain lesions can be seen including cortical infarcts, infarcts in strategic brain areas (basal ganglia and thalamus), multiple lacunes, extensive white matter change (or 'leuokoaraiosis') or combinations thereof.

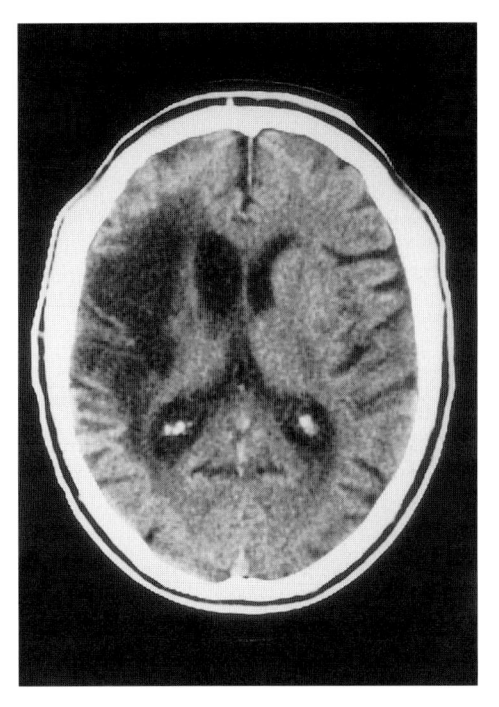

Figure 14.1
Axial CT scan showing large areas of cortical and subcortical infarction in the right hemisphere. Note classic appearances of infarcts and the associated dilatation of the right ventricle.

A major difficulty is in interpreting the clinical significance of infarcts and, in particular, white matter changes seen on CT and MRI. Large infarcts, in keeping with the clinical symptoms and neuropsychological profile, may pose little problem. However, smaller infarcts, infarcts in 'silent' areas and more subtle white matter changes may be difficult to interpret (see 'leukoaraiosis' below). The opposite difficulty is that many stroke patients have extensive scanning evidence of cerebrovascular disease yet do not develop cognitive impairment. The essential question, therefore, in interpreting scanning changes is in terms of the extent to which these are known to be robustly associated with VAD. This can be determined by considering (a) studies which have compared patients with VAD to other groups of patients and (b) studies which have compared stroke patients who subsequently develop dementia to those who remain cognitively intact

VAD compared to other disorders

Several studies have compared structural imaging changes between patients with VAD and AD. Degree of cortical atrophy or ventricular enlargement does not seem to separate groups,[4,5] although VAD is invariably associated with an increased prevalence of infarcts and more extensive white matter change.[4,5,9] In contrast, focal atrophy of the frontal lobes occurs in approximately 50% of cases of frontal lobe dementia while focal atrophy of the medial temporal lobes on CT or MRI, especially with serial scanning, is associated with AD[10–12] (see Figure 14.2). In a comparison of CT and MRI in distinguishing between VAD and AD, Erkinjuntti et al[4] found MRI more sensitive but CT more specific. Reed et al[13] compared MRI changes in 25 patients with AD and 25 with multi-infarct dementia. Although there was overlap between groups, six MRI variables provided 84% correct diagnostic classification, these were ventricular to brain ratio, presence of subcortical infarcts, bifrontal ventricular ratio, bicaudate ventricular ratio, third ventricular ratio and the presence of diffuse periventricular high intensity white matter lesions. Other studies also show overlap between diagnostic groups, for example, VAD can be associated with temporal lobe atrophy on CT or MRI,[10,14,15] while AD may be associated with an increased prevalence of white matter changes.[16,17]

In summary, structural imaging studies which have compared VAD with AD generally confirm a higher prevalence of vascular lesions (particularly white matter change and infarction) in vascular compared with Alzheimer patients, although some degree of overlap appears to exist. These studies indicate that there are no pathognomonic imaging features characteristic of VAD and again emphasize the role of imaging in terms of providing confirmatory support rather than absolute diagnosis.

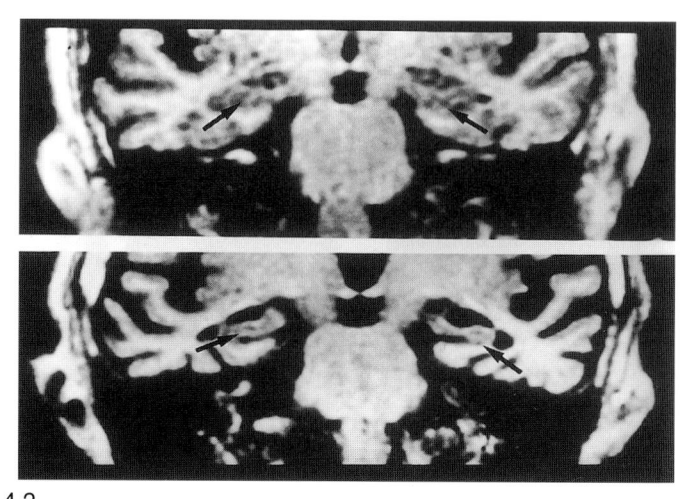

Figure 14.2
Coronal T1-weighted MRI scan of subject with relatively normal temporal lobes and hippocampus (top) compared below to a subject with AD (bottom). Note the marked atrophy of the hippocampus (arrows), temporal horn and temporal lobe in the subject with AD.

The extent of vascular change necessary for dementia

There are two ways of approaching this, one is to consider the site of the lesion, the other the extent of damage, although ultimately a combination of the two will undoubtedly be the variable of interest. The classic neuropathological study of Tomlinson et al[18] found that a volume of infarction of at least 50 ml, and usually 100 ml, was necessary for VAD. However, patients with presumed VAD clinically but with smaller volumes of infarction are well recognized. Erkinjuntti et al[19] studied 27 patients with VAD and found the mean volume of infarction was only 40 ml (range 1–229 ml) with an average of 3.4 infarctions (range 2–7) microscopically evident on neuropathological examination. Del Ser et al[20] divided patients with evidence of cerebrovascular disease at post mortem into 28 who were demented during life and 12 who were not. Demented subjects had three times the infarct volume of non-demented subjects, although a volume of infarction of only 1% was sufficient to produce dementia. Such neuropathological studies have great relevance for understanding neuroimaging changes in VAD. If very small vascular changes can be associated with VAD in some cases then very small and subtle vascular changes on imaging may sometimes be sufficient to support a clinical diagnosis of VAD.

Charletta et al[21] compared 66 patients with VAD, 56 subjects who had had a stroke but who were not demented and 56 subjects with AD. Patients with VAD and stroke without dementia had a similar extent of white matter lesions, but differed from each other by the size of the third ventricle. Gorelick et al[7] compared CT findings in 58 patients with multi-infarct dementia and 74 patients who had had multiple infarcts without evidence of cognitive impairment. Dementia after stroke was associated with stroke severity, left cortical infarction, left ventricular enlargement and also level of education. In subjects with cerebrovascular disease, a number of studies have related both the extent of white matter change and cerebral atrophy to the presence of dementia.[7,22,23] The total number of infarcts also appears to be important,[7,23] as may left-sided or bilateral lesion location[7,23] or location in strategic areas such as thalamus and anterior capsule.[23]

Imaging changes in post-stroke dementia

Several studies have investigated lesion size and location in patients after stroke in relation to whether they subsequently develop dementia. In a large series of 972 subjects who had undergone CT, dementia was associated with advancing age, number of infarcts, location of infarcts in temporo-parietal areas and extent of white matter lesions.[8] No relationship was found between volume of infarct and dementia, consistent with some other reports,[24,25] although at variance with others.[23,26,27] Most authors agree that location of lesions is important, with lesions in the thalamus,[24] temporo-parietal and temporo-occipital areas,[8] temporal lobes,[25] frontal lobe and medial cerebral artery infarct location[26] and left cortical and parietal infarcts[27] all shown to be important. Several studies report an association between post-stroke dementia and generalized measures such as cortical and central atrophy.[8,23,25–28]

Pohjasvaara et al[29] examined 337 patients aged 55–85 who, 3 months after ischaemic stroke, had a comprehensive neuropsychological examination and MRI scan. Frequency of post-stroke dementia at 3 months was 32% and was associated with advancing age, low level of education, past history of stroke and left hemisphere location. Left-sided location associated with dementia after stroke has also been shown by others.[26,30] In a prospective study, Meyer et al[31] compared repeat CT changes in 24 patients with VAD and 24 subjects with AD. Many VAD patients were treated with anti-platelet therapy and risk factor control. Cognitive decline amongst patients with a VAD was associated with recurrent 'silent' strokes and perfusion changes (measured using Xenon CT) in frontal white matter, and thalamic and internal capsule. Progressive cerebral atrophy and ventricular enlargement were much greater in the group with AD.

In summary, evidence from studies of patients with established VAD and post-stroke dementia suggests that associations of VAD include cortical and central atrophy and indicate that both volume of lesion and location are important. In particular, bilaterality, left-sided lesions, diffuse white matter change and small infarcts in strategic areas may all be important. However, in addition to a 'lesion based' view of VAD, clinical features such as age and level of education may play an important role. Progressive cognitive decline in VAD may be associated with an increase in 'silent' cerebral infarction.

Leukoaraiosis

This term, meaning 'rarefaction of the white matter', was introduced by Hachinski et al[32] as a descriptive term for white matter changes seen on imaging which are not invariably associated with subcortical VAD or 'Binswanger's disease' (BD). The nature and significance of such changes remains an area of uncertainty and controversy and leukoaraiosis is one of the neuroimaging changes most widely misunderstood and misinterpreted. While BD is likely to be associated with leukoaraiosis on scan, the converse does not apply. Leukoaraiosis, or white matter changes, can be associated with a number of different disorders including other types of VAD, AD, multiple sclerosis, hydrocephalus, various leukodystrophies, cerebral oedema, neurosarcoid and conditions such as late life depression.[2,17] On CT, leukoaraiosis is seen as diffuse low density areas in the

Neuroimaging in vascular dementia 151

white matter surrounding the cerebral ventricles (see Figure 14.3). MRI, because it builds an image based on proton, rather than electron, density has greater sensitivity for demonstrating white matter lesions (Figures 14.4a,b).

Although previously felt to be entirely non-specific, it is now recognized that at least two types of white matter change can be demonstrated: periventricular and deep white matter lesions (Figure 14.5). Periventricular lesions consist of, in milder forms, caps around the frontal and occipital horns of the lateral ventricles. More advanced periventricular change can be seen as a smooth halo surrounding the lateral ventricles which extends a variable distance into the white matter. Pathological studies have indicated that the pathogenesis of this periventricular type of lesion is essentially non-vascular.[33-36] Periventricular changes are associated with loss of the ependymal lining of the ventricles, increased interstitial fluid and gliosis. Such lesions are not only common in the healthy elderly (where there are seen in up to 90% of cases, depending on age) but are common in all types of dementia. For example, we have recently shown[15] that periventricular lesions occur with high but equal frequency in VAD, AD and dementia with Lewy bodies.

In contrast, deep white matter lesions are separate from the ventricles (Figure 14.5) and appear to have a different pathogenesis.[33-35] A number

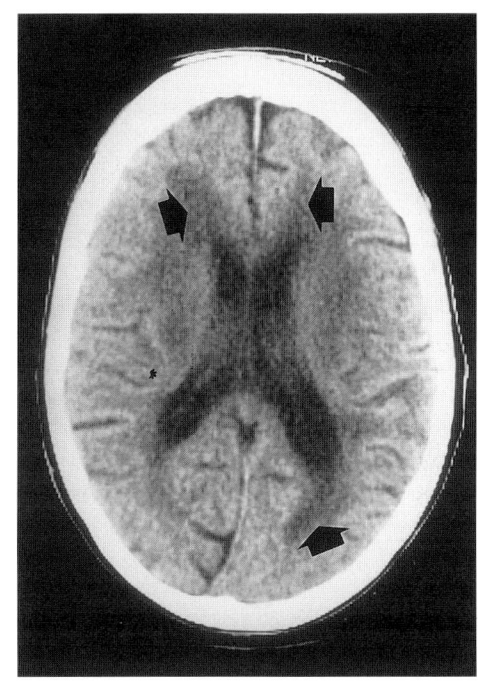

Figure 14.3

Axial CT scan showing severe leuokoaraiosis extending into most of the white matter, particularly around the frontal and occipital horns of the ventricles (arrows).

152   Cerebrovascular Disease and Dementia

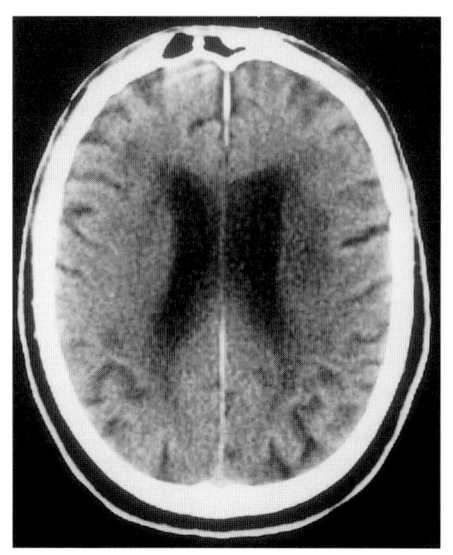

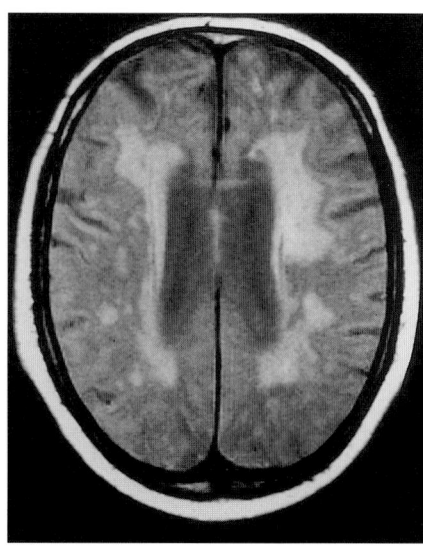

Figure 14.4
(a) Axial CT scan showing white matter change in a 73-year-old man with a clinical diagnosis of VAD.
(b) Proton density MRI scan of the same subject. Note the superior visualization of white matter change on the MRI scan compared to the CT scan.

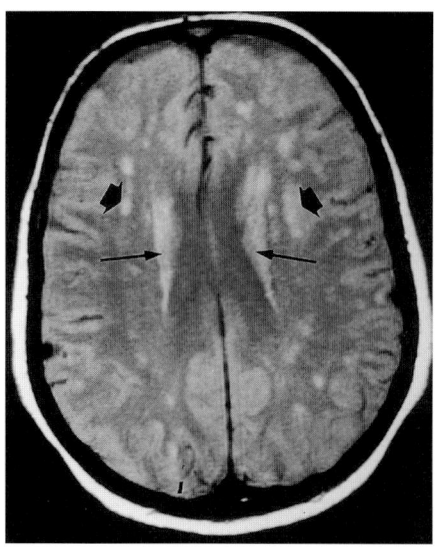

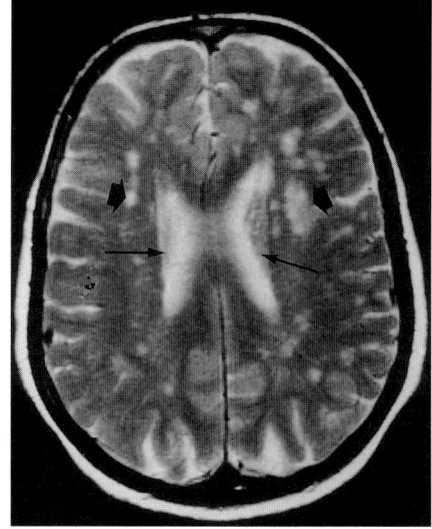

Figure 14.5
(a) Proton density and (b) T2-weighted axial MRI scans showing moderate white matter changes in a female subject with late-onset depression. Note the two discrete types of white matter change: periventricular lesions adjacent to the lateral ventricles (thin arrows) and deep white matter lesions which are clearly distinct from the natural ventricles (thick arrows). These two types of lesions have a different pathogenesis (see text for details).

of different pathologies have been related to deep white matter changes which is, perhaps, not surprising as these changes have been described in a number of different conditions including normal ageing and dementia. Very small punctate white matter lesions can be associated with small areas of demyelination or the pathological change of etat crible, where dilatation of perivascular spaces and increased tortuousity of vessels is seen, not necessarily associated with atherosclerosis. Other possible causes of white matter change include focal cerebral oedema, hypoxia and acidosis as well as chronic perfusion changes. More severe types of deep white matter change, however, can be associated with atherosclerotic disease.

Given the variety of pathologies known to underlie white matter change, it is extremely important not to overinterpret imaging changes (particularly on proton density and T2-weighted MRI) with regard to vascular contribution to dementia. For example, in Figure 14.5 the prominent white matter changes in this elderly depressed patient were not associated with any demonstrable cognitive decline. However, in non-demented populations, including the healthy elderly[37-39] and those with depression,[40-42] minor degrees of white matter lesion may be associated with more subtle neuropsychological deficits. It should be emphasized that although these fall well short of dementia, a proportion of such subjects may show cognitive decline over time.[43]

Imaging requirements for the application of current diagnostic systems for VAD

These are summarized in Table 14.1. The Hachinski ischaemic index[44] is composed of a number of clinical features and does not require any imaging information for its application. Requirements for ICD-10[45] are open to interpretation. It is clear that structural neuroimaging is not mandatory for the diagnosis, although the criteria do indicate that in some cases it will be needed. DSM-IV criteria[46] require 'laboratory evidence of cerebrovascular disease', which may include laboratory evidence such as imaging. They state that structural imaging 'usually' demonstrates multiple vascular lesions, but this implies that diagnosis can still be made when scanning is normal or shows a single lesion. The California criteria for probable ischaemic VAD (IVD)[47] require at least one infarct outside the cerebellum. A diagnosis of possible IVD does not require neuroimaging evidence of infarction. The NINDS-AIREN criteria[2] are the most rigorous with regard to the need for neuroimaging confirmation. The criteria for probable VAD include multiple infarcts or strategic single infarcts as well as multiple subcortical or white matter lesions. The criteria specifically state that the absence of cerebrovascular lesions on brain CT or MRI make the diagnosis of VAD uncertain. In the accompanying paper[2] it is stated that 'absence of cerebrovascular lesions CT or MRI is strong evidence against vascular aetiology and constitutes the most important brain imaging element to distinguish AD from VAD. There are no pathognomonic brain CT or MRI images of VAD'. The criteria adopt what seems to be, on the basis of previous work discussed above, a sensible approach which requires radiological findings to fulfil minimum standards for both severity and topography.

One difference between the NINDS-AIREN criteria and the California criteria is that the former criteria recognize that a single lesion may cause VAD. They also accept that radiological lesions regardless of location may be taken as evidence of cerebrovascular disease. However, the criteria do exclude 'trivial' infarcts, for example, frontal horn capping or one or two lacunes. The brain imaging changes required for the NINDS-AIREN criteria are shown in Table 14.2. Perhaps one of the more difficult areas is the role of white matter change alone. The criteria deal with this by stating that white matter lesions on CT or MRI may be considered as evidence for cerebrovascular disease, but for this to be the case they must be diffuse and extensive, extending to deep white matter. Changes observed only on T2 MRI are felt to be of doubtful significance. Importantly, the guide has suggested that the changes should involve at least one quarter of the total white matter, on the basis of previous studies.[4,19] The discussion emphasizes the need to correlate radiological images with clinical and neuropsychological changes combined with neuropathology in patients with VAD.

However, the NINDS-AIREN criteria have also been criticized as being too dependent on the presence of changes on brain imaging for diagnosis.[48] Frisoni et al[49] examined 77 patients with AD and 17 with

Table 14.1 Neuroimaging requirements for the application of current diagnostic systems.

Diagnostic criteria	Vascular brain changes required on structural imaging
Hachinski ischaemic scale (Hachinski et al[44])	No requirement for brain imaging
ICD-10 (World Health Organization[45])	In some cases, confirmation can be provided only by computerized axial tomography or, ultimately, neuropathological examination In addition, the ICD-10 research diagnostic criteria require evidence from the history, examination or tests of significant cerebrovascular disease, which may reasonably be judged to be aetiologically related to the dementia (for example, a history of stroke; evidence of cerebral infarction)

Diagnostic criteria	Vascular brain changes required on structural imaging
DSM-IV (American Psychiatric Association[46])	There must be evidence of cerebrovascular disease (that is, focal neurological signs and symptoms or laboratory evidence) that is judged to be aetiologically related to the dementia. CT of the head and MRI usually demonstrate multiple vascular lesions of the cerebral cortex and subcortical structures. The extent of central nervous system lesions detected by CT and MRI in VAD typically exceeds the extent of changes detected in the brains of healthy elderly persons (for example, periventricular and white matter hyperintensities noted on MRI scans). Lesions often appear in both white matter and grey matter structures, including subcortical regions and nuclei. Evidence of old infarctions (for example, focal atrophy) may be detected, as well as findings of more recent disease
California criteria (Chui et al[47])	The criteria for the clinical diagnosis of probable ischaemic VAD (IVD) include evidence of two or more ischaemic strokes by history, neurological signs and/or neuroimaging studies (CT or T1-weighted MRI) and evidence of at least one infarct outside the cerebellum on CT or T1-weighted MRI The diagnosis of probable IVD is supported by evidence of multiple infarcts in brain regions known to affect cognition. Features that are thought to be associated with IVD, but await further research, include periventricular and deep white matter changes on T2-weighted MRI that are excessive for age. A clinical diagnosis of possible IVD may be made when there is dementia and Binswanger's syndrome (without multiple strokes) that includes extensive white matter changes on neuroimaging
NINDS/AIREN criteria (Roman et al[2])	The criteria for the clinical diagnosis of probable VAD require the presence of cerebrovascular disease (CVD), defined by the presence of focal signs on neurological examination and evidence of relevant CVD by brain imaging (CT or MRI) including multiple large-vessel infarcts (angular gyrus, thalamus, basal forebrain or PCA or ACA territories), as well as multiple basal ganglia and white matter lesions, or combinations thereof. Features that make the diagnosis of VAD uncertain or unlikely include absence of cerebrovascular lesions on brain CT or MRI

Table 14.2 Brain imaging lesions associated with VAD (NINDS/AIREN criteria).

I Topography

Radiological lesions associated with dementia include *any* of the following or combinations thereof:

1. Large-vessel strokes in the following territories:
   Bilateral anterior cerebral artery
   Posterior cerebral artery, including paramedian thalamic infarctions, inferior medial temporal lobe lesions
   Association areas: parietotemporal, temporo-occipital territories (including angular gyrus)
   Watershed carotid territories: superior frontal, parietal regions
2. Small-vessel disease:
   Basal ganglia and frontal white matter lacunes
   Extensive periventricular white matter lesions
   Bilateral thalamic lesions

II Severity

In addition to the above, relevant radiological lesions associated with dementia include:

- Large-vessel lesions of the dominant hemisphere
- Bilateral large-vessel hemispheric strokes
- Leukoencephalopathy involving at least one quarter of the total white matter

Although the volume of the lesion is weakly related to dementia, an additive effect may be present. White matter changes observed only on T2 MRI but not on T1 MRI or CT may not be significant. The absence of vascular lesions on brain CT/MRI rules out probable VAD.

multi-infarct dementia (MID) according to DSM-III-R criteria. Seven (41%) of patients clinically diagnosed as having MID either had no lesion or insufficient lesions for diagnosis of probable VAD according to the NINDS/AIREN criteria. MID patients with CT evidence of cerebral vascular disease sufficient to meet probable VAD criteria were six times more likely to have a history of stroke than those without such lesions. Without large prospective studies to determine diagnostic accuracy it is difficult to assess whether the requirement for neuroimaging changes is sensible or not. It seems likely the NINDS-AIREN criteria will have high specificity but, if neuropoathological work is correct in suggesting less than 1% infarction may be associated with dementia, sensitivity may be low.

Functional brain imaging in VAD

Functional brain imaging techniques include single photon emission tomography (SPET) which can use a number of tracers, most commonly a perfusion tracer like Technetium 99-HMPAO. Positron emission tomography (PET) is primarily a research tool which can use a variety of ligands to look at cerebral metabolism and receptor changes. Other functional imaging techniques include magnetic resonance spectroscopy and EEG brain mapping. The latter technique can demonstrate areas of power change, particularly slowing, which correspond to areas of ischaemic damage. Changes with MRI spectroscopy are less clear. Several groups have demonstrated that neuronal loss occurring in AD is associated with reduced levels of *N*-acetyl aspartate (NAA), a putative neuronal marker.[50-52] More controversial is an increase in myoinositol (MI), although Shonk et al[50] have suggested that the MI/NAA ratio can assist in differential diagnosis of AD from normal ageing and frontal lobe dementia. The role spectroscopy will play in the recognition of VAD is unclear, although preliminary evidence suggests that white matter lesions, irrespective of cause, may have similar spectroscopic appearances.[53]

Studies using PET show that both blood flow and metabolic rate for oxygen decrease in parallel. Glucose metabolism in VAD generally shows asymmetric patterns deflecting regional abnormalities, particularly decreased metabolism in the transitional zone of temporal, parietal and occipital lobes.[54,55] In addition, diaschisis (a decrease in metabolism owing to distance effect) commonly occurs contralaterally in the cerebellum or cerebral hemisphere, thus complicating interpretation of changes.

For the foreseeable future SPET will remain the functional imaging technique accessible to clinicians in their assessment of patients with VAD. Although structural imaging is undoubtedly the investigation of first choice to perform in the assessment of patients with vascular lesions, both to exclude some other intracranial cause for the cognitive impairment and to confirm the presence of vascular change, SPET can have a useful role in some cases. Numerous studies now demonstrate that SPET has high sensitivity and specificity (over 80%) in the distinction of patients with AD from age-matched controls.[10,56] Classically, bilateral temporo-parietal patterns of hypoperfusion are seen (Figure 14.6), and with frontal perfusion in some cases, particularly with more severe disease. SPET is often considered the investigation of choice in supporting a diagnosis of dementia of frontal lobe type, where prominent hypoperfusion of frontal lobes is seen, with relative preservation (in most cases) of posterior perfusion. In VAD a variable pattern of perfusion is seen. Classically, a 'patchy' multifocal pattern, corresponding to perfusion deficits, but that will depend on the actual site of vascular lesions (Figure 14.7). Large cortical infarcts are represented by areas of absent blood flow. More diffuse white matter change can be associated with more generalized cortical reduction in blood flow, with some regional variations which depend both on the site of lesion and the projection pathways. For example, infarcts in the basal ganglia can result in reduced cortical blood flow to frontal lobes, consistent with main projection pathways. As with PET, cerebellar and cerebral diaschisis can commonly be observed, especially after large infarcts.

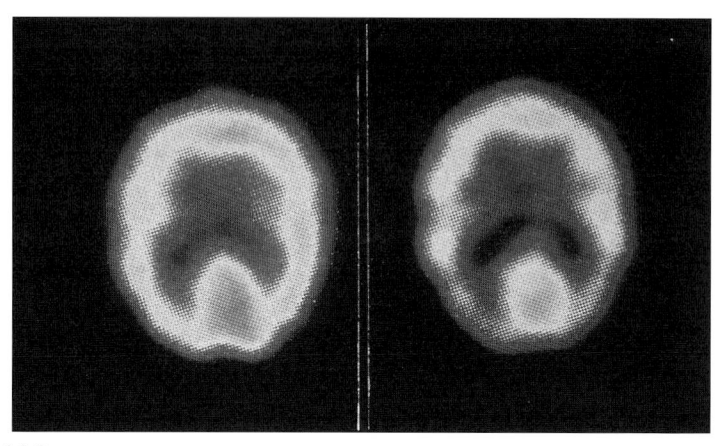

Figure 14.6
Axial ^{99}Tc-HMPAO perfusion SPET scan showing normal control subject (left) and subject with mild AD (right). Note the classic appearance of bilateral temporo-parietal hypoperfusion in the subject with AD.

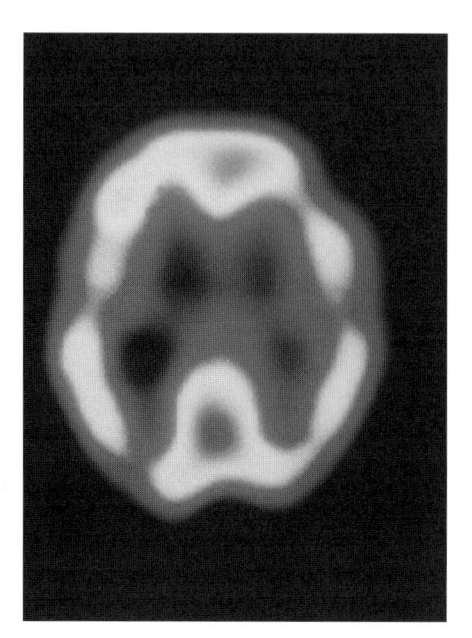

Figure 14.7
Axial perfusion SPET scan of subject with VAD. Note the patchy mottled appearance which is characteristic of multi-infarct disease, particularly when compared with the classic appearances in AD (Figure 14.6).

Read et al[57] compared results from SPET scanning against neuropathological diagnosis and found SPET could demonstrate abnormalities due to ischaemic lesions not seen on structural imaging. Interestingly, two patients with a clinical diagnosis of multi-infarct dementia were found to have AD at post mortem; both had in vivo SPET changes more consistent with AD. Other studies report similar findings,[10,58] although the extent to which SPET is useful in routine clinical practice remains unclear[59] as most clinicopathological studies investigating the accuracy of SPET scanning in terms of diagnosis have been limited to a small number of subjects primarily with a diagnosis of AD. No large samples of patients with VAD have been reported. At the present time, it is probably sensible to reserve SPET as an investigation to use when information from structural imaging is not definitive enough to confirm or refute a diagnosis of VAD.

Mixed dementias

One difficulty with current classification systems is that they do not take account of mixed dementias, which are known to occur for 10–20% of cases. The importance of mixed pathology was demonstrated by Snowdon et al[60] who found that, among 61 subjects who met neuropathological criteria for AD, those with brain infarcts (particularly lacunar infarcts in the basal ganglia, thalamus or deep white matter) had poorer cognitive function and a higher prevalence of dementia than those without infarcts. Neuroimaging offers great potential to tease out mixed pathology as the vascular component to cognitive impairment can be demonstrated by structural imaging, with the necessary caveats regarding issues such as deep white matter change. The component of degenerative change to cognitive impairment is, perhaps, more difficult to quantify. However, it has been demonstrated that atrophy of the temporal lobe and hippocampus appears to be related to the presence of Alzheimer change, particularly tangle count in the medial temporal lobe.[61,62] Further prospective studies are needed to confirm this, but it remains possible that selective volume change in medial temporal lobe areas may primarily reflect in current Alzheimer type pathology, whereas ischaemic and other change would reflect vascular pathology. As such, imaging could prove a useful tool to help distinguish the contribution of different underlying pathologies to the clinical picture.

New avenues of research would involve the use of longitudinal imaging to measure serial change.[12] New ligands, increasingly becoming available, are still primarily research tools. Kuhl et al[63] have shown profound loss of the choline transporter system (a putative presynaptic marker for cholinergic systems) in patients with AD and in patients with Parkinson's disease and dementia. The advent of such chemical imaging techniques offers the opportunity to investigate individual neurotransmitter systems by studying either receptor changes or presynaptic markers (or both) and, ultimately, offers great potential to investigate neurochemical correlates of ischaemic lesions on scanning.

References

1. Amar K, Wilcock G, Vascular dementia, *BMJ* (1996) **312**: 227–31.
2. Roman GC, Tatemichi T, Erkinjuntti T et al, Vascular dementia: diagnostic criteria for research studies. Report of the NINCDS AIRENS International Workshop, *Neurology* (1993) **43**:250–60.
3. Ames D, Chiu E, *Neuroimaging and the Psychiatry of Late Life* (Cambridge University Press: Cambridge, 1997).
4. Erkinjuntti T, Ketonen L, Sulkava R et al, CT in the differential diagnosis between Alzheimer's disease and vascular dementia, *Acta Neurol Scand* (1987) **75**:262–70.
5. Aharon-Peretz J, Cummings JL, Hill MA, Vascular dementia and dementia of the Alzheimer type. Cognition, ventricular size, and leukoaraiosis, *Arch Neurol* (1988) **47**:719–21.
6. Loeb C, Gandolfo C, Bino G, Intellectual impairment and cerebral lesions in multiple cerebral infarcts. A clinical-computed tomography study, *Stroke* (1988) **19**:560–5.
7. Gorelick P, Chatterjeea A, Pateld C et al, Cranial computed tomographic observations in multi-infarct dementia. A controlled study, *Stroke* (1992) **23**:801–11.
8. Tatemichi TK, Foulkes MA, Mohr JP et al, Dementia in stroke survivors in the stroke data bank cohort, relevance, incidence, risk factors, and computed tomographic indings, *Stroke* (1990) **21**:858–66.
9. Pullicino P, Benedict RH, Capruso DX et al, Neuroimaging criteria for vascular dementia, *Arch Neurol* (1996) **53**:723–8.
10. Jobst KA, Barnetson LP, Shepstone BJ, Accurate prediction of histologically confirmed Alzheimer's disease and the differential diagnosis of dementia, *Int Psychogeriatr* (1997) **9**(Suppl 1):191–222.
11. O'Brien JT, Desmond P, Ames D et al, Temporal lobe magnetic resonance imaging can differentiate Alzheimer's disease from normal ageing, depression, vascular dementia and other causes of cognitive impairment, *Psych Med* (1997) **27**:1267–75.
12. Fox NC, Freeborough PA, Rossor MN, Visualisation and quantification of rates of atrophy in Alzheimer's disease, *Lancet* (1996) **348**:94–7.
13. Reed K, Rogers R, Myer J, Cerebral magnetic resonance imaging compared in Alzheimer's and multi-infarct dementia, *J Neuropsychiatry Clin Neurosci* (1991) **3**:51–7.
14. Laakso MP, Partanen K, Riekkinen P et al, Hippocampal volumes in Alzheimer's disease, Parkinson's disease with and without dementia, and in vascular dementia: an MRI study, *Neurology* (1996) **46**: 678–81.
15. Barber R, Gholkar A, Scheltens et al, Medial temporal lobe atrophy on MRI in dementia with Lewy bodies. *Neurology* (1999) **52**: 1153–8.
16. Scheltens PH, Barkhof F, Valk J et al, White matter lesions of magnetic

resonance imaging in Alzheimer's disease. Evidence for heterogeneity, *Brain* (1992) **115**:735–43.
17. O'Brien JT, Desmond P, Ames D et al, A magnetic resonance imaging study of white matter lesions in depression and Alzheimer's disease, *Br J Psychiatry* (1996) **168**:477–85.
18. Tomlinson BE, Blessed G, Roth M, Observations on the brains of demented old people, *Neurol Sci* (1970) **11**:205–42.
19. Erkinjuntti T, Heltia M, Palo J et al, Accuracy of the clinical diagnosis of vascular dementia: a prospective clinical and post-mortem neuropathological study, *J Neurol Neurosurg Psychiatry* (1988) **51**:1037–44.
20. Del Ser T, Bermejof B, Porteraa C et al, Vascular dementia: a clinical pathological study, *J Neurol Sci* (1990) **96**:1–17.
21. Charletta D, Gorelick PB, Dollear TJ et al, CT and MRI findings among African-Americans with Alzheimer's disease, vascular dementia, and stroke without dementia, *Neurology* (1995) **45**:1456–61.
22. Tanaka Y, Tanaka O, Mizuno Y et al, A radiologic study of dynamic processes in lacunar dementia, *Stroke* (1989) **20**:1488–93.
23. Figueroa M, Tatemichi TK, Cross DT et al, CT correlates of dementia after stroke, *Neurology* (1992) **42**:176.
24. Ladurner G, Illiff LD, Lechner H, Clinical factors associated with dementia in ischaemic stroke, *J Neurol Neurosurg Psychiatry* (1982) **45**:97–101.
25. Schmidt R, Mechtler L, Kinkel PR et al, Cognitive impairment after hemispheric stroke: a clinical and computed tomographic study, *Neurology* (1992) **42**(Suppl 3):176.
26. Censori B, Manara O, Agostinis C et al, Dementia after first stroke, *Stroke* (1996) **27**:1205–10.
27. Liu CK, Miller BL, Cummings JL et al, A quantitative MRI study of vascular dementia, *Neurology* (1992) **42**:138–43.
28. Hershey LA, Modic MT, Greenough PG et al, Magnetic resonance imaging in vascular dementia, *Neurology* (1987) **37**:29–36.
29. Pohjasvaara T, Erkinjuntti T, Ylikoskir C et al, Clinical determinance of post-stroke dementia, *Stroke* (1998) **29**:75–81.
30. Tatemichi T, Desmond D, Paik M, Clinical determinance of dementia related to stroke, *Ann Neurol* (1993) **33**:568–75.
31. Meyer JS, Muramatsu K, Mortel KF et al, Prospective CT confirms differences between vascular and Alzheimer's dementia, *Stroke* (1995) **26**:735–42.
32. Hachinski VC, Potter P, Merskey H, Leukoaraiosis: an ancient term for a new problem, *Arch Neurol* (1987) **44**:21–3.
33. Awad IA, Johnson PC, Spetzler RE et al, Incidental subcortical lesions identified on magnetic resonance imaging in the elderly, II, Post-mortem pathological correlations, *Stroke* (1986) **17**:1090–7.
34. Fazekas F, Kleinert R, Offenbacher H et al, The morphologic correlates of incidental punctate white matter hyperintensities on MR images, *Am J Neuroradiol* (1991) **12**:915–21.
35. Fazekas F, Kleinert R, Offenbacher H et al, Pathologic correlates of incidental MRI white matter signal hyperintensities, *Neurology* (1993) **43**:1683–9.
36. Scheltens PH, Kamphorst W, Barkhof F et al, Histopathological correlates of white matter changes on MRI in Alzheimer's disease and normal ageing, *Neurology* (1995) **45**:883–8.

37. Schmidt R, Fazekas F, Offenbacher H et al, Neuropsychologic correlates of MRI white matter hyperintensities: a study of 150 normal volunteers, *Neurology* (1993) **43**:2490–4.

38. Boone KB, Miller BL, Lesser JM et al, Neuropsychological correlates of white matter lesions in healthy elderly subjects. A threshold effect, *Arch Neurol* (1992) **49**:549–54.

39. Breteler MMB, van Amerongen NM, van Swieten JC et al, Cognitive correlates of ventricular enlargement and cerebral white matter lesions on magnetic resonance imaging, *Stroke* (1994) **25**:1109–15.

40. Jenkins M, Malloy P, Salloway S et al, Memory processes in depressed geriatric patients with and without subcortical hyperintensities on MRI, *J Neuroimaging* (1998) **8**:20–6.

41. Salloway S, Malloy P, Kohn R et al, MRI and neuropsychological differences in early- and late-life-onset geriatric depression, *Neurology* (1996) **46**:1567–74.

42. Simpson S, Jackson A, Baldwin RC et al, Subcortical hyperintensities in late-life depression; acute response to treatment and neuropsychological impairment, *Int Psychogeriatr* (1997) **3**:257–75.

43. Hickie I, Scott E, Wilhelm K et al, Subcortical hyperintensities on magnetic resonance imaging in patients with severe depression—a longitudinal evaluation, *Biol Psychiatry* (1996) **42**:367–74.

44. Hachinski VC, Iliff LD, Zilhka E et al, Cerebral blood flow in dementia, *Arch Neurol* (1975) **32**:632–7.

45. World Health Organization, *International Classification of Diseases and Health Related Problems*, 10th revn (World Health Organization: Geneva, 1992).

46. American Psychiatric Association, *Diagnostic and Statistical Manual of Mental Disorders*, 4th edn (American Psychiatric Association: Washington DC, 1994).

47. Chui HC, Victoroff JI, Margolin D et al, Criteria for the diagnosis of ischaemic vascular dementia proposed by the state of California Alzheimer's disease diagnostic and treatment centres, *Neurology* (1992) **42**:473–80.

48. Amar KA, Wilcock GK, Vascular dementia, *Neurology* (1995) **45**:1423–4.

49. Frisoni G, Beltramolloa, Binetti G et al, Computed tomography in the detection of the vascular component in dementia, *Gerontology* (1995) **41**:121–8.

50. Shonk TK, Moats RA, Gifford P et al, Probable Alzheimer's disease: diagnosis with proton MR spectroscopy, *Radiology* (1995) **195**:65–72.

51. Ernest T, Chang C, Melchor R et al, Frontotemporal dementia and early Alzheimer's disease: differentiation with frontal lobe H-1 MR spectroscopy, *Radiology* (1997) **203**:829–36.

52. Schuff N, Amend D, Ezekiel F et al, Changes of hippocampal N-acetyl aspartate and volume in Alzheimer's disease: a proton MR spectroscopic imaging and MRI study, *Neurology* (1997) **49**:1513–21.

53. MacKay S, Ezekiel F, Di Sclafani V et al, Alzheimer's disease and subcortical ischemic vascular dementia: evaluation by combining MR imaging segmentation and H-I MR spectroscopic imaging, *Radiology* (1996) **198**:537–45.

54. Duara R, Barker W, Loewenstein D et al, Sensitivity and specificity of positron emission tomography and magnetic resonance imaging studies in Alzheimer's disease and multiinfarct dementia, *Eur Neurol* (1989) **29**(Suppl 3):9–15.

55. Meguro K, Doi C, Ueda M et al, Deceased cerebral glucose

metabolism associated with mental deterioration in multiinfarct dementia, *Neuroradiology* (1991) **33**:305–9.

56. O'Brien JT, Eagger S, Syed GMS et al, A study of regional cerebral blood flow and cognitive performance in Alzheimer's disease, *J Neurol Neurosurg Psychiatry* (1992) **55**:1182–7.

57. Read SL, Miller BL, Mena I et al, SPECT in dementia: clinical and pathological correlation, *J Am Geriatr Soc* (1995) **43**:1243–7.

58. Bonte FJ, Weiner MF, Bigio EH et al, Brain blood flow in dementias: SPECT with histopathologic correlation in 54 patients, *Radiology* (1997) **202**:793–7.

59. Pasquier F, Lavenue I, Lebert F et al, The use of SPECT in a multidisciplinary memory clinic, *Dementia Geriatric Cog Disord* (1997) **8**:85–91.

60. Snowdon DA, Greiner LH, Mortimer JA et al, Brain infraction and the clinical expression of Alzheimer's disease, *JAMA* (1997) **277**:813–17.

61. Huesgen CT, Burger PC, Crain BJ et al, In vitro MR microscopy of the hippocampus in Alzheimer's disease, *Neurology* (1993) **43**:145–52.

62. Harvey GT, O'Brien JT, Hughes J et al, Magnetic resonance imaging differences between dementia with Lewy bodies and Alzheimer's disease, *Psychol Med* (1999) **29**:181–7.

63. Kuhl DE, Minoshima S, Fessler JA et al, In vivo mapping of cholinergic terminals in normal ageing, Alzheimer's disease, and Parkinson's disease, *Ann Neurol* (1996) **40**:399–410.

15
qEEG and dementia with special reference to vascular dementia

Ingmar Rosén

EEG—basic features

The electroencephalogram (EEG) is a recording of cerebral electrical potentials by electrodes on the scalp. It is a spatiotemporal average of synchronous postsynaptic potentials arising in radially oriented cortical pyramidal cells. Synchronous neuronal activity arises by various mechanisms. Specific pacemakers exist in the thalamocortical neuronal circuitry that produce rhythmic synchronous activity. These are under the influence of afferents from the brain stem reticular formation, which stimulate individual neurons into independent asynchronous activity. These effects are mediated by cholinergic and noradrenergic neuronal systems. Thus, synchrony is reduced by arousal and increased by reduced vigilance.[1,2] The rhythmic activity of the normal adult awake EEG is dominated by frequencies in the 8–13 Hz (alpha) range and is generated by several independent generators in the cerebral cortex and thalamus.[3] Slow waves between 0.5 and 4 Hz (delta) prevail during the deep stage of normal synchronized sleep but are scarce in the normal waking condition. Both metabolic and structural pathology can give rise to diffusely distributed polymorphic delta activity. Cholinergic deafferentation may play a role in the production of cortical delta activity[4-6]. Localized delta activity is usually attributed to a lesion with some destruction of cerebral tissue. The pathophysiological mechanisms of slow waves in the 4–8 Hz range (theta) is not well known. Often, theta activity represents a slowing down of the alpha activity and then representing the dominant background activity. There is a relationship between the dominant or mean EEG frequency and the rate of cerebral blood flow and oxygen uptake in cortical grey matter.[7,8] Such slowing of the background activity is seen in mild to moderate hypoxia, cerebrovascular disease, dementias and in mild degrees of metabolic encephalopathies.[2,9] An increased number of theta waves in combination with alpha activity of normal frequency may represent the mildest form of polymorphic delta activity (see above).[1] EEG waves with frequencies above 13 Hz (beta) are normally present with a symmetric frontocentral predominance. Excessive prominent beta activity is usually the result of a medication effect, most frequently produced by benzodiazepines or barbiturates. Otherwise, excessive generalized beta activity is of little diagnostic significance.[10]

Interpretation and quantification of the EEG

Interpretation of the EEG record is still, 60 years after the initiation of clinical electroencephalography, made by visual inspection of recordings from a large number of electrodes distributed over the scalp. Over the years, several attempts have been made to quantify the EEG signal, making it available for statistical analysis and various display techniques.[11] Recent developments in computer technology have facilitated the application of such techniques in clinical practice. The most commonly used method of quantified frequency analysis of EEG is based on the fast Fourier transform (FFT). Features commonly extracted from the amplitude or power spectrum are:

(a) absolute band amplitude or power: the area under the curve between the two frequencies defining the bandwidth, usually delta (0.5–4 Hz), theta (4–8 Hz), alpha (8–13 Hz) and beta (>13 Hz);
(b) relative band values: one absolute band value divided by another, usually one band value divided by the absolute value of the whole spectrum;
(c) absolute peak frequency: the peak value in a selected band of the spectrum, usually the alpha band;
(d) mean frequency within a selected band.

By the application of quantitative techniques and the collection of normal age-matched control data it has been possible to substantiate the visual interpretation of the EEG. It has also become possible to estimate the degree of deviation from normality, usually expressed as Z scores for each band. Discriminant analysis and artificial neural networks are appearing as useful methods for separating dementia patients from controls and in the classification of subgroups of dementia.[12,13]

Spatial display of the scalp distribution of recorded activity is referred to as topographic or brain mapping, which has been applied in studies of dementia.[14-16] Maps can be constructed from statistical values derived from quantitative comparisons. Interpolation between the points of real measurements makes these maps appear very detailed. Artefacts from extracranial sources and electrodes are much more difficult to reveal as compared with the routine EEG display. Short transients in the EEG, that is epileptiform discharges or episodes of slow waves, which might be highly relevant clinically, do not usually appear in the frequency analysis of 1 to 2 minutes of EEG. Therefore it is mandatory that these new techniques of quantification and mapping be combined with careful inspection of the original EEG recording in a professional clinical neurophysiological setting.[17–20] One topographical technique which overcomes mass significance problems is dipole source estimations of different frequency components of the EEG; it has been applied in Alzheimer dementia studies.[21,22]

Scalp-recorded EEG coherence is a measure of the functional interrelation between pairs of neocortical regions. It is a function of distance between recording electrodes, due to volume conduction and density of cortico-cortical neuronal connections. It is not homogenous over the cortex, due to special long cortico-cortical tracts. Diffusely projecting thalamocortical systems add to the coherence measured. The coherence measures are highly dependent upon the mode of recording and are correlated with cognitive or behavioural measures, and are often specific for certain frequency components of the EEG.[23] Coherence as an adjunct to conventional frequency analysis has recently been used in dementia research.[24–27]

Non-linear EEG analysis can provide information about the functional state of neural networks that cannot be obtained with linear analysis. The correlation dimension (D2) is considered to be a reflection of the complexity of the cortical dynamics. Quantification can be obtained by comparison of D2 from original EEG data with phase randomized surrogate data. Recent reports show decreased D2 values in dementia.[28–30]

Whatever the method used for quantitative evaluation of EEG, a prerequisite is that a sufficiently long sequence of artefact-free EEG (or added multiple sequences) is sampled at a well-defined level of alertness, usually awake with eyes closed. Critical evaluations of the reproducibility of qEEG in senile dementia are scarce.[31,32] Available results indicate that this is worse in dementia patients than in healthy controls, due to large fluctuations of the background activity.[33] In a few studies, attempts have been made to stabilize the vigilance level during EEG recording by various activation procedures.[34,35] As a possibly better alternative to EEG in wakefulness, qEEG during REM sleep, which provides full muscle relaxation, has been shown to discriminate between patients with dementia of Alzheimer type (DAT) and normal controls.[36,37] The EEG alpha reactivity to opening of the eyes can be quantified (EC/EO ratio), and has been shown to correlate with several neuropsychological variables in VAD.[38]

EEG and normal aging

Once the adult EEG is established around the age of 15 years, this pattern is very stable over the years into healthy senescence.[39,10] The change of EEG most commonly reported in elderly subjects is slowing of alpha frequency. Although this slowing is statistically significant, most healthy elderly individuals will maintain alpha activity within the range 9.5–10 Hz.[33,40–42] A frequent abnormality observed with advancing age is episodic local slowing over temporal regions.[10,42–44] Focal, left-sided, anterior temporal EEG abnormality in normal elderly subjects has been reported to be correlated with deterioration of language function.[45] In a group of elderly healthy women, 75–95 years of age, theta activity increased with age without correlation with psychometric features.[46] Increase of delta activity with age has been correlated with impairment of memory function and with reduced acetylcholinesterase activity of the CSF.[47] Beta activity has been reported to increase with age, particularly in women,[48] and has shown a positive correlation with cognitive performance.[49] In a group of normal elderly women beta activity carries a negative risk for cognitive impairment 5 years later.[50] The spatial distribution of EEG activity seems to change with normal aging, with increasing uniformity across the brain associated with an increased coupling of activity between areas.[51]

EEG in non-VADs

A pathological EEG in a histologically verified case of Alzheimer dementia and a correlation between EEG slowing and the degree of senile dementia was observed by Berger.[52,53] Since then a large number of reports have been published on the subject of EEG and dementia, particularly verified or probable DAT. EEG, visually interpreted, shows a high percentage of abnormalities in DAT.[54–58] Most of these studies also showed a correlation between the degree of EEG abnormality and the severity of dementia. Systematized blind interpretation of EEG[59] in a large group of patients with DAT showed abnormal findings in 87.2% at the initial examination, and in 92% at follow-up (negative predictive value: 0.825 with respect to the diagnosis of DAT). A group of patients with probable DAT and depression was found to have abnormal EEG, whereas patients with depression or depressive pseudodementia had normal EEG or only mild abnormality.[60] This was later confirmed with quantified EEG techniques.[61–63]

A large number of studies have been reported, comparing different quantitative EEG variables in patients with DAT with healthy control subjects. The criteria for the clinical diagnoses as well as the degree of dementia vary to a large extent and are not always well defined. In only a fraction of the patients have the diagnoses been verified by post-mortem histological examinations. In mild DAT relative theta power[64,65] seems to provide the highest sensitivity. Alpha and theta relative power together with temporoparietal alpha coherence discriminated between Alzheimer's disease (AD) patients of mild and moderate degree and controls at

77.8% sensitivity and 100% specificity.[26] With principal component analysis with age as a moderator 95.5% correct classifications were reached.[13] In the study of Penttilä et al,[65] where one single channel was used for quantification, slowing of the occipital peak frequency and distinct accentuation of relative delta power only occurred in cases of advanced DAT.

In a longitudinal study[66,67] over 2.5 years relative delta and theta power increased and alpha and beta power as well as mean frequency decreased in correlation with the disease progress. Again, relative theta power most effectively distinguished between four stages of dementia. Another longitudinal study over 2 years failed to demonstrate EEG progression.[68] In a third longitudinal study,[69-71] the degree of EEG abnormality was demonstrated to carry prognostic information about the rate and type of clinical progression.[72,73] Patients with the most marked slowing of the dominant occipital rhythm were found to have the lowest concentrations of noradrenaline in the thalamus[74] and the lowest levels of choline acetyltranferase activity in the frontal cortex at post-mortem examination.[75] The heterogeneity of DAT was further illustrated with multi-channel brain mapping applied to two groups of DAT patients, one with predominant memory deficit and one group with progressive spatial impairment,[76] with differences located to the parietal region. Patients with DAT with relative intactness of parietal lobe function as measured by psychometric testing and FDG-PET (fluorodeoxyglucose positive emission tomography) showed preservation of the EEG alpha background.[77,78] Also parietal rCBF (regional cortical blood flow) measured with 99mTc-HMPAO-SPECT correlated with qEEG.[79] Marked differences in EEG power spectra between AD patients of early and late onset were found in a recent study by Pucci et al.[80] Late onset AD patients showed a preserved although slowed dominant activity in contrast to the early onset patients, indicating differences in the underlying pathophysiology. A PET study by Kuhl et al[81] demonstrated a more widespread reduction of cholinergic terminals in early onset as compared with late onset DAT. DAT patients have also been shown to vary considerably in terms of degree of subcortical white matter abnormalities.[82,83]

EEG in patients with histologically verified frontotemporal cortical atrophy was found to be normal or moderately abnormal despite prolonged dementia of increasing severity.[56,84] Quantified EEG showed a moderate and diffuse increase in relative theta activity in a group of FTD (frontotemporal dementia) patients, identified by their clinical features and rCBF.[85]

In Parkinson's disease (PD) without dementia the EEG has been reported to be abnormal in 30–50% of cases, with an abnormal diffuse increase in low-frequency activity and slowing of the occipital alpha frequency. The degree of abnormality could be correlated with the degree of motor disability.[86-88] PD patients with dementia differed from those without dementia with more advanced diffuse EEG slowing, particularly with more delta activity. In practice, it would not be possible to differentiate PD with dementia from DAT on the basis of conventional EEG features.

The characteristic feature in Creutzfeldt–Jakob disease (CJD) is diffuse or focal slowing developing into periodic sharp wave complexes (PSWC). The PSWC pattern appears within 12 weeks of disease in 88% of the cases, usually correlated with a marked worsening of the clinical picture.[89–91] Focal or asymmetric PSWC are common at onset (about 50%) with correspondence with focal clinical signs. A subgroup of patients (10%) had unusually long courses, and showed PSWC in only 55%. The EEG pattern is not pathognomonic for CJD and has been reported in cases of severe post-anoxic encephalopathy,[92] AIDS dementia complex,[93] herpes encephalitis,[94] lithium toxic encephalopathy,[95,96] Binswanger's disease[97] and severe DAT.[98]

EEG in VAD

Studies of conventional and quantified EEG in VAD are difficult to summarize, due to the fact that the pathophysiological processes are presumably even more heterogeneous than for DAT, including patients with few or multiple cortical lesions as well as patients with ischaemic white matter disease, which would affect the electrocortical activity differently. Early studies are focused on MID as verified by CT and clinically by ischaemic scoring,[99] whereas more recent studies are based on NINDS-AIREN criteria,[100] often supplemented by additional neuroimaging techniques such as MRI, SPECT or PET. Many studies have addressed the question whether EEG may help in the differentiation of VAD from DAT at an early stage. Conventional visual interpretation of EEG[57,101–104] showed similar diffuse EEG abnormalities in both groups. The MID groups showed a higher rate of regional or asymmetric abnormalities.[57,103] Quantified spectral analysis of EEG in a subsample of patients showed a similar deterioration of mean frequency with severity of dementia in VAD and DAT groups. An EEG brain mapping study comprising 54 DAT and 57 MID patients also failed to demonstrate group differences regarding global spectral parameters. Both groups showed extensive increase of delta/theta and slowing of dominant frequency. However, a better differentiation was obtained using differences between the maximum and the minimum and interhemispheric asymmetries, reaching a level of 63.1% correctly classified patients.[16]

A multi-channel qEEG study of 49 DAT, 29 MID (multi-infarct dementia) of mild to moderate degree and 38 elderly controls using several spectral power and spectral ratio measurements and discriminant analysis revealed that none of the qEEG parameters detected large differences between the two dementia groups. In the MID group associations between cognitive status and qEEG were less robust than in the DAT group.[105] The same patients were subjected to an exploration of the cortical connectivity by coherence analysis using complex combinations of multiple bipolar leads in order to contrast long-distance frontoparietal connections to short-distance broad connective networks within the frontal and occipitoparietal areas, respectively.[24] Long-distance coherence was decreased in subjects with DAT but not significantly in MID patients. Short-distance coherence showed the largest decreases among MID patients. A ratio of coherence from short- and long-distance coherence correctly classified 76% of subjects into DAT and MID categories. In contrast to previous spectral power studies, a number of later studies have reported quantitative differences between DAT and MID groups.[69,85,106,107] In these studies the alpha activity was less affected and the delta and theta power less increased in MID than in DAT patients. In a further analysis by Sloan et al,[108] clinical and rCBF-SPECT data were combined into coherent subsets of patients with typical findings of temporoparietal defects (DAT), multiple low perfusion areas (MID) and functionally ill patients with normal SPECT. The AD group differed from the MID group in having significantly less alpha and more delta power. With the use of a more straightforward design than Leuchter et al,[24] the two dementia groups did not differ in terms of intrahemispheric or interhemispheric coherence spectra, but showed less coherence than the normal group. This study again emphasizes the importance of the parietal cortex for alpha activity production.

The value of combining qEEG and functional neuroimaging is illustrated by the study of Szelies et al.[109] FDG-PET was compared to qEEG in 24 patients with DAT, 19 patients with VAD and 15 controls. The metabolic ratio between typically affected and non-affected regions differentiated between DAT and VAD. The occipito/frontal alpha ratio also differentiated between groups. Relative theta power was the most sensitive EEG parameter distinguishing demented patients from controls. Optimal classification into three groups was obtained by combining the three parameters. EEG power changes in VAD were also related to regional changes in glucose metabolism.[110] Alpha power correlated directly with metabolism in the occipital lobe. Delta power was negatively correlated to local metabolism. Theta power correlated negatively with thalamic metabolism. This study emphasizes the impression reached in several previous EEG studies in dementia that activities in different EEG frequency bands represent functionally different aspects of brain function.

In addition to qEEG analysis of spontaneous activity during resting wakefulness with eyes closed, the alpha reactivity measured as the eyes closed/eyes open ratio has been shown to provide an improved assessment of brain dysfunction in VAD than background EEG variables.[38] Barbiturate-induced beta activity has been shown to be preserved in VAD as opposed to DAT.[111] Non-linear analysis of EEG may improve the differentiation between VAD and DAT.

Conclusions

Clinical electroencephalography is a relatively simple and inexpensive diagnostic tool with a high sensitivity for diffuse organic encephalopathy of various aetiology, but with a rather low specificity for the type of diagnosis. The highest sensitivity is shown in DAT and Parkinson dementia, and in these conditions the degree of EEG abnormality is correlated with the disease severity. Quantification of EEG makes these correlations more reliable and provides a method for monitoring therapeutic effects. VAD causes EEG changes similar to those in Alzheimer dementia, usually with more preserved posterior alpha activity. Additional analysis of cortical connectivities with coherence analysis, analysis of non-linear EEG properties, and functional or pharmacological provocations may add to the discrimination between VAD and DAT. A consensus about which qEEG techniques should be recommended for clinical use is needed. Dementias with predominantly frontal pathology show much less EEG abnormality, and in these conditions the EEG is often normal despite obvious clinical dementia. At an early stage of clinical evaluation EEG may be useful in the discrimination of organic dementia from pseudodementia, because EEG is usually normal in depression, confusion, agitation and other psychiatric conditions. Repeated EEG recordings over time would add significantly to the diagnostic information. New techniques such as analysis of the EEG during REM sleep, coherence analysis of the EEG activity, non-linear EEG analysis and the combination of quantified EEG techniques with functional neuroimaging of blood flow and/or metabolism will presumably add to the sensitivity as well as the specificity of the electrophysiological methods in the diagnosis of dementia.

References

1. Steriade M, Gloor P, Llinás R et al, Basic mechanisms of cerebral rhythmic activities. *Electroencephalogr Clin Neurophysiol* (1990) **76**:481–508.
2. Binnie C, Prior P, Electroencephalography. *J Neurol Neurosurg Psychiatry* (1994) **57**: 1308–19.
3. Lopes Da Silva F, Neural mechanisms underlying brain waves: from neural membranes to networks. *Electroencephalogr Clin Neurophysiol* (1991) **79**:81–3.
4. Detari L, Vanderwolf C, Activity of cortically projecting and other basal forebrain neurons during large slow waves and cortical activation in anesthetized cat. *Brain Res* (1987) **437**:1–8.
5. Buzsaki G, Bickford R, Ponomareff G et al, Nucleus basalis and thalamic control of neocortical activity in the freely moving rat. *Neuroscience* (1988) **8**: 4007–26.
6. Riekkinen P Jr, Sirviö J, Riekkinen P, Relationship between cortical choline acetyltransferase content and EEG

delta-power. *Neuroscience Res* (1990) **8**:12–30.

7. Ingvar D, Baldy-Moulinier M, Sulg I, Horman S, Regional cerebral blood flow related to EEG. *Acta Neurol Scand* (1965) Suppl 14:179–82.

8. Ingvar D, Sjölund B, Ardö A, Correlation between EEG frequency, cerebral oxygen uptake and blood flow. *Electroencephalogr Clin Neurophysiol* (1976) **41**:268–76.

9. Saunders M, Westmoreland B, The EEG in evaluation of disorders affecting the brain diffusely. In: Klass D, Daly D, eds. *Current Practice of Clinical Electroencephalography* (Raven Press: New York, 1979) 343–79.

10. Klass D, Brenner P, Electroencephalography of the elderly. *J Clin Neurophysiol* (1995) **12**:116–31.

11. Walter D, Digital processing of bioelectric phenomena. In: Rémond A, ed, *Handbook of Electroencephalography and Clinical Neurophysiology,* Vol 4B (Elsevier: Amsterdam, 1972).

12. Anderer P, Saletu B, Klöppel B et al, Discrimination between demented patients and normals based on topographic EEG slow wave activity: comparison between z statistics, discriminant analysis and artificial neural network classifiers. *Electroencephalogr Clin Neurophysiol* (1994) **91**:108–17.

13. Besthorn C, Zerfass R, Geiger-Kabish C et al, Discrimination of Alzheimer´s disease and normal aging by EEG data. *Electroencephalogr Clin Neurophysiol* (1997) **103**:241–8.

14. Duffy F, Albert M, McAnulty G, Brain electrical activity in patients with presenile and senile dementia of the Alzheimer type. *Ann Neurol* (1984) **16**:439–48.

15. Breslau J, Starr A, Sicotte N et al, Topographic EEG changes with normal aging and SDAT. *Electroencephalogr Clin Neurophysiol* (1989) **72**:281–9.

16. Saletu B, Anderer P, Paulus E et al, EEG brain mapping in diagnostic and therapeutic assessment of dementia. *Alzheimer Dis Assoc Disord* (1991) **5**:57–75.

17. Nuwer M, Quantitative EEG I: techniques and problems of frequency analysis and topographic mapping. *J Clin Neurophysiol* (1988) **5**:89–92.

18. Nuwer M, Quantitative EEG II: frequency analysis and topographic mapping in clinical settings. *J Clin Neurophysiol* (1988) **5**:45–85.

19. Nuwer M, Lehmann D, Lopes da Silva F et al, IFCN guidelines for topographic and frequency analysis of EEGs and EPs. Report of an IFCN committee. *Electroencephalogr Clin Neurophysiol* (1994) **91**:1–5

20. Nuwer M. Assessing digital and quantitative EEG in clinical settings. *J Clin Neurophysiol* (1998) **15**:458–63.

21. Dierks T, Ihl R, Frölich L, Maurer K, Dementia of the Alzheimer type. Effects on the spontaneous EEG described by dipole sources. *Psychiatr Res Neuroimag* (1993) **50**:151–62.

22. Jelic V, Dierks T, Amberla K et al, Longitudinal changes in quantitative EEG during long term tacrine treatment of patients with Alzheimer´s disease. *Neurosci Lett* (1998) **254**:85–8.

23. Nunez P, Srinivasan R, Westdorp A et al, EEG coherency I: statistics, reference electrode, volume conduction, Laplacians, cortical imaging, and interpretation at multiple scales. *Electro-

encephalogr *Clin Neurophysiol* (1997) **103**:499–515.

24. Leuchter A, Newton T, Cook I et al, Changes in brain functional connectivity in Alzheimer-type and multiinfarct dementia. *Brain* (1992) **115**:1543–61.

25. Besthorn C, Förstl H, Geiger-Kabish C et al, EEG coherence in Alzheimer disease. *Electroencephalogr Clin Neurophysiol* (1994) **90**:243–5.

26. Jelic V, Shigeta M, Julin P et al, Quantitative electroencephalography power and coherence in Alzheimer´s disease and mild cognitive impairment. *Dementia* (1996) **7**:314–23.

27. Locatelli T, Cursi M, Liberati D et al, EEG coherence in Alzheimer´s disease. *Electroencephalogr Clin Neurophysiol* (1998) **106**:229–37.

28. Pritchard W, Duke D, Coburn K et al, EEG-based, neural-net predictive classification of Alzheimer's disease versus control subjects is augmented by non-linear EEG measures. *Electroencephalogr Clin Neurophysiol* (1994) **91**:118–30.

29. Jeong J, Kim S, Han S-H, Non-linear dynamic analysis of the EEG in Alzheimer´s disease with optimal embedding dimension. *Electroencephalogr Clin Neurophysiol* (1998) **106**:220–8.

30. Jelles B, van Birgelen J, Slaets J et al, Decrease of non-linear structure in the EEG of Alzheimer patients compared to healthy controls. *Clin Neurophysiol* (1999) **110**:1159–67.

31. Hooijer C, Jonker C, Posthuma J, Visser S, Reliability, validity and follow-up of the EEG in senile dementia: sequelae of sequential measurement. *Electroencephalogr Clin Neurophysiol* (1990) **76**:400–12.

32. Jelic V, *Early diagnosis of Alzheimer´s disease. Focus on quantitative EEG in relation to genetic, biochemical and neuroimaging markers* (Thesis, Stockholm 1999).

33. Prinz P, Peskind R, Vitalino P et al, Changes in the sleep and waking EEGs of nondemented and demented elderly subjects. *J Am Geriat Soc* (1982) **30**:86–93.

34. Günther W, Giunta R, Klages U et al, Findings of electroencephalographic brain mapping in mild to moderate dementia of the Alzheimer type during resting, motor, and music perception conditions. *Psychiatry Res Neuroimag* (1993) **50**:163–76.

35. Wszolek Z, Herkes G, Lagerlund T, Kokmen E, Comparison of EEG background frequency analysis, psychologic test scores, short test of mental status, and quantitative SPECT in dementia. *J Geriatr Psychiatry Neurol* (1992) **5**:22–30.

36. Petit D, Montplasir J, Lorrain D, Gauthier S, Spectral analysis of the rapid eye movement sleep electroencephalogram in right and left temporal regions: a biological marker of Alzheimer's disease. *Ann Neurol* (1992) **32**:172–6.

37. Prinz P, Larsen L, Moe K, Vitiello M, EEG markers of early Alzheimer's disease in computer selected REM sleep. *Electroencephalogr Clin Neurophysiol* (1992) **83**:36–43.

38. Partanen J, Soininen H, Helkala E et al, Relationship between EEG reactivity and neuropsychological tests in vascular dementia. *J Neural Transm* (1997) **104**:905–12.

39. Obrist W, Problems of aging. In: Rémond A, ed, *Handbook of*

Electroencephalography and Clinical Neurophysiology. Vol 6A (Elsevier Amsterdam, 1976) 275–92.

40. Hubbard O, Sunde D, Goldensohn E, The EEG in centenarians. *Electroencephalogr Clin Neurophysiol* (1976) **40**:407–17.

41. Katz R, Horowitz G, Electroencephalogram in the septuagenarian. Studies in a normal geriatric population. *J Am Geriatr Soc* (1982) **30**:273–5.

42. Torres F, Faoro A, Loewenson R, Johnson E, The electroencephalogram of elderly subjects revisited. *Electroencephalogr Clin Neurophysiol* (1983) **56**:391–8.

43. Silverman A, Busse E, Barnes R, Studies in the processes of aging: electroencephalographic findings in 400 elderly subjects. *Electroencephalogr Clin Neurophysiol* (1955) **7**:67–74.

44. Busse E, Barnes R, Friedman E, Kelty E, Psychological functioning of aged individuals with normal and abnormal electroencephalograms. *J Nerv Ment Dis* (1956) **124**:135–41.

45. Visser S, Hooijer C, Jonker C et al, Anterior temporal focal abnormalities in EEG in normal aged subjects; correlations with psychopathological and CT brain scan findings. *Electroencephalogr Clin Neurophysiol* (1987) **66**:1–7.

46. Elmståhl S, Rosén I, Gullberg B, Quantitative EEG in elderly patients with Alzheimer´s disease and healthy controls. *Dementia* (1994) **5**:119–24.

47. Hartikainen P, Soininen H, Partanen J et al, Aging and spectral analysis of EEG in normal subjects, a link to memory and CSF ache. *Acta Neurol Scand* (1992) **86**:148–55.

48. Busse E, Electroencephalography. In: Reisberg B, ed, *Alzheimer's Disease* (The Free Press: New York, 1983) 231–6.

49. Williamson P, Merskey H, Morrison S et al, Quantitative electroencephalographic correlates of cognitive decline in normal elderly subjects. *Arch Neurol* (1990) **47**:1185–8.

50. Elmståhl S, Rosén I, Postural hypotension and EEG variables predict cognitive decline: results from a 5-year follow-up of healthy elderly women. *Dement Geriatr Cogn Disord* (1997) **8**:180–7.

51. Dustman R, Lamarche J, Cohn N et al, Power spectral analysis and cortical coupling of EEG for young and old normal adults. *Neurobiol of Aging* (1985) **6**:193–8.

52. Berger H, Über das Elektrenkephalogramm des Menschen. Dritte Mitteilung. *Arch Psychiat Nervenkr* (1931) **94**:16–60.

53. Berger H, Dritte Mitteilung. Über das Elektrenkephalogramm des Menschen. Fünfte Mitteilung. *Arch Psychiat Nervenkr* (1932) **98**:231–54.

54. Obrist W, Busse E, Eisdorfer R, Kleemeier R, Relation of the electroencephalogram to intellectual function in senescence. *J Geront* (1962) **17**:192–206.

55. Gordon E, Sim M, The EEG in presenile dementia. *J Neurol Neurosurg Psychiatry* (1967) **30**:285–91.

56. Jóhannesson G, Brun A, Gustafson L, Ingvar D, EEG in presenile dementia related to cerebral blood flow and autopsy findings. *Acta Neurol Scand* (1977) **56**:89–103.

57. Soininen H, Partanen V, Helkala E-L, Riekkinen P, EEG findings in senile dementia and normal aging. *Acta Neurol Scand* (1982) **65**:59–70.

58. Schreiter-Gasser U, Gasser T, Ziegler P, Quantitative EEG analysis in early onset Alzheimer's disease: correlations with severity, clinical characteristics, visual EEG and CCT. *Electroencephalogr Clin Neurophysiol* (1994) **90**:267–72.

59. Robinson D, Merskey H, Blume W et al, Electroencephalography as an aid in the exclusion of Alzheimer's disease. *Arch Neurol* (1994) **51**:280–4.

60. Brenner R, Reynolds C, Ulrich R, EEG findings in depressive pseudodementia and dementia with secondary depression. *Electroencephalogr Clin Neurophysiol* (1989) **72**:298–304.

61. Jordan S, Nowacki R, Nuwer M, Computerized electroencephalography in the evaluation of early dementia. *Brain Topogr* (1989) **1**:271–82.

62. Prinz P, Vitiello M, Dominant occipital alpha frequency in early stage Alzheimer's disease and depression. *Electroencephalogr Clin Neurophysiol* (1989) **73**:427–32.

63. Moe K, Larsen L, Prinz P, Vitiello M, Major unipolar depression and mild Alzheimer's disease. *Electroencephalogr Clin Neurophysiol* (1993) **86**:238–46.

64. Coben L, Danziger W, Berg L, Frequency analysis of the resting awake EEG in mild senile dementia of Alzheimer type. *Electroencephalogr Clin Neurophysiol* (1983) **55**:372–80.

65. Penttilä M, Partanen J, Soininen H, Riekkinen P, Quantitative analysis of occipital EEG in different stages of Alzheimer's disease. *Electroencephalogr Clin Neurophysiol* (1985) **60**:1–6.

66. Coben L, Danziger W, Storandt M, A longitudinal EEG study of mild senile dementia of Alzheimer type: changes at 1 year and at 2.5 years. *Electroencephalogr Clin Neurophysiol* (1985) **61**:101–12.

67. Rae-Grant A, Blume W, Lau C et al, The electroencephalogram in Alzheimer-type dementia: a sequential study correlating the electroencephalogram with psychometric and quantitative pathological data. *Arch Neurol* (1987) **44**:50–4.

68. Sloan E, Fenton G, EEG power spectra and cognitive change in geriatric psychiatry: a longitudinal study. *Electroencephalogr Clin Neurophysiol* (1993) **86**:361–7.

69. Soininen H, Partanen J, Laulumaa V et al, Longitudinal EEG spectral analysis in early stage of Alzheimer's Disease. *Electroencephalogr Clin Neurophysiol* (1989) **72**:290–7.

70. Soininen H, Partanen J, Laulumaa V et al, Serial EEG in Alzheimer's disease: 3 year follow up and clinical outcome. *Electroencephalogr Clin Neurophysiol* (1991) **79**:342–8.

71. Helkala E-L, Laulumaa V, Soininen H et al, Different patterns of cognitive decline related to normal or deteriorating EEG in a 3-year follow-up study of patients with Alzheimer's disease. *Neurology* (1991) **41**:528–32.

72. Rodriguez G, Nobili F, Arrigo A et al, Prognostic significance of quantitative electroencephalography in Alzheimer patients: preliminary observations. *Electroencephalogr Clin Neurophysiol* (1996) **99**:123–8.

73. Lopez O, Brenner R, Becker J et al, EEG spectral abnormalities and psychosis as predictors of cognitive and functional decline in probable Alzheimer's disease. *Neurology* (1997) **48**:1521–5.

74. Soininen H, Reinikainen K, Partanen J et al, Slowing of the dominant occipital rhythm in electroencephalogram is associated with low concentration of noradrenalin in the thalamus in patients with Alzheimer's disease. *Neurosci Letts* (1992) **137**: 5–8.

75. Soininen H, Reinikainen K, Partanen J et al, Slowing of electroencephalogram and choline acetyltransferase activity in definitive Alzheimer's disease. *Neuroscience* (1992) **49**: 529–35.

76. Albert M, Duffy F, McAnulty G, Electrophysiological comparisons between two groups of patients with Alzheimer's disease. *Arch Neurol* (1990) **47**: 857–63.

77. Sheridan P, Sato S, Foster N et al, Relation of EEG alpha background to parietal lobe function in Alzheimer's disease as measured by positron emission tomography and psychometry. *Neurology* (1988) **38**:747–50.

78. Edman Å, Matousek M, Wallin A, EEG findings in dementia are related to parietal lobe syndrome. *Dementia* (1995) **6**: 323–9.

79. Rodriguez G, Nobili F, Copello F et al, 99m-Tc-HMPAO regional cerebral blood flow and quantitative electroencephalography in Alzheimer's disease: a correlative study. *J Nucl Med* (1999) **40**:522–9.

80. Pucci E, Belardinelli N, Cacchiò G et al, EEG power spectrum differences in early and late onset forms of Alzheimer's disease. *Clin Neurophysiol* (1999) **110**:621–31.

81. Kuhl D, Minoshima S, Fessler J et al, In vivo mapping of cholinergic terminals in normal aging, Alzheimer's disease, and Parkinson's disease. *Ann Neurol* (1996) **40**:399–410.

82. DeCarli C, Grady C, Clark C et al, Comparison of positron emission tomography, cognition, and brain volume in Alzheimer's disease with and without severe abnormalities of white matter. *J Neurol Neurosurg Psychiatry* (1996) **60**:158–67.

83. Siennicki-Lantz A, Lilja B, Rosén I, Elmståhl S, Cerebral blood flow in white matter is correlated with systolic blood pressure and EEG in senile dementia of the Alzheimer type. *Dement Geriatr Cogn Disord* (1998) **9**:29–38.

84. Jóhannesson G, Hagberg B, Gustafson L, Ingvar D, EEG and cognitive impairment in presenile dementia. *Acta Neurol Scand* (1979) **59**:225–40.

85. Rosén I, Gustafson L, Risberg J, Multichannel EEG frequency analysis and somatosenory evoked potentials in patients with different types of organic dementia. *Dementia* (1993) **4**: 43–9.

86. Neufeldt M, Inzelberg R, Korczyn A, EEG in demented and nondemented Parkinsonian patients. *Acta Neurol Scand* (1988) **78**:1–5.

87. Neufeldt M, Blumen S, Aitkin I et al, EEG frequency analysis in demented and nondemented Parkinsonian patients. *Dementia* (1994) **5**:23–8.

88. Soikkeli R, Partanen J, Soininen H et al, Slowing of EEG in Parkinson's disease. *Electroencephalogr Clin Neurophysiol* (1991) **79**:159–65.

89. Aguglia U, Farnarier G, Tinuper P et al, Subacute spongiform encephalopathy with periodic paroxysmal activities: clinical evolution and serial EEG findings in 20 cases. *Clin Electroencephalogr* (1987) **18**:147–58.

90. Levy S, Chiappa K, Burke C, Young R, Early evolution and incidence of elecroencephalographic abnormalities in Creutzfeldt–Jakob disease. *J Clin Neurophysiol* (1986) **3**: 1–21.
91. Brown P, Cathala F, Castaigne P, Gadjusek D, Creutzfeldt–Jakob disease: clinical analysis of a consecutive series of 230 neuropathologically verified cases. *Ann Neurol* (1986) **20**: 597–602.
92. Takahashi M, Kubota F, Nishi Y, Miyanaga K, Persistent synchronous periodic discharges caused by anoxic encephalopathy due to cardiopulmonary arrest. *Clin Electroencephalogr* (1993) **24**:166–72.
93. Thomas P, Borg M, Reversible myoclonic encephalopathy revealing the AIDS-dementia complex. *Electroencephalogr Clin Neurophysiol* (1994) **90**: 166–9.
94. Gereby G, Elektroenzephalographische Befunde bei nekrotiserender Herpesenzephalitis. *EEG EMG Z Elekroenzephalogr Verwandte Geb* (1981) **12**: 205–11.
95. Smith S, Kocen R, A Creutzfeldt–Jakob like syndrome due to lithium toxicity. *J Neurol Neurosurg Psychiatry* (1988) **51**:120–3.
96. Finelli P, Drug-induced Creutzfeldt–Jakob like syndrome. *J Psychiatry Neurosci* (1992) **17**:103–5.
97. Kuroda Y, Ikeda A, Kurohara K et al, Occurrence of paroxysmal synchronous EEG discharges in subcortical arteriosclerotic encephalopathy (Binswanger's disease). *Intern Med* (1993) **32**:243–6.
98. Yamamoto T, Imai T, A case of Lewi body and Alzheimer's disease with periodic synchronous discharges. *J Neuropathol Exp Neurol* (1988) **47**:536–48.
99. Hachinski V, Iliff L, Zilhka E et al, Cerebral blood flow in dementia. *Arch Neurol* (1975) **32**:632–7.
100. Román G, Tatemichi T, Erkinjuntti T et al, Vascular dementia: diagnostic criteria for research studies. Report of the NINDS-AIREN international workshop. *Neurology* (1993) **43**:250–60.
101. Roberts M, McGeorge A, Caird F, Electroencephalography and computerised tomography in vascular and non-vascular dementia in old age. *J Neurol Neurosurg Psychiatry* (1978) **41**:903–6.
102. Logar C, Enge S, Ladurner G et al, Das EEG bei Multiinfarkten mit und ohne intellektuellen Abbau. *Z EEG-EMG* (1983) **14**: 204–8.
103. Erkinjuntti T, Larsen T, Sulkava R et al, EEG in differential diagnosis between Alzheimer's disease and vascular dementia. *Acta Neurol Scand* (1988) **77**:36–43.
104. Ettlin T, Staehelin H, Kischka U et al, Computed tomography, electroencephalography and clinical features in the differential diagnosis of senile dementia. *Arch Neurol* (1989) **46**:1217–20.
105. Leuchter A, Cook I, Newton T et al, Regional differences in brain electrical activity in dementia: use of spectral power and spectral ratio measures. *Electroencephalogr Clin Neurophysiol* (1993) **87**:385–93.
106. Signorino M, Pucci E, Belardinelli N et al, EEG spectral analysis in vascular and Alzheimer dementia. *Electroencephalogr Clin Neurophysiol* (1995) **94**:313–25.
107. D'Onofrio F, Salvia S, Petretta V et al, Quantified-EEG in normal aging and dementias. *Acta Neurol Scand* (1996) **93**:336–45.

108. Sloan E, Fenton G, Kennedy N, MacLennan J, Neurophysiology and SPECT cerebral blood flow patterns in dementia. *Electroencephalogr Clin Neurophysiol* (1994) **91**:163–70.

109. Szelies B, Mielke R, Herholz K, Heiss W, Quantitative topographical EEG compared to FDG PET for classification of vascular and degenerative dementia. *Electroencephalogr Clin Neurophysiol* (1994) **91**: 131–9.

110. Szelies B, Mielke R, Kessler J, Heiss W, EEG power changes related to regional cerebral glucose metabolism in vascular dementia. *Clin Neurophysiol* (1999)**110**:615–20.

111. Holschneider D, Leuchter A, Uijtdehaage S et al, Loss of high frequency brain electrical response to thiopental administration in Alzheimer´s-type dementia. *Neuropsychopharmacology* (1997) **16**:269–75.

16
Medical management

Leon Flicker

The most important aspect of medical treatment for people with dementia and cerebrovascular disease is to remember that these patients are at much greater risk for having medical illnesses of all types which may go unrecognized because of coexistent cognitive impairment. Forstl et al[1] reviewed the prevalence of medical disorders found in people with Alzheimer's disease (AD) and vascular dementia (VAD) who came to post mortem. People in both categories had a high prevalence of coronary artery disease, peripheral artery disease, evidence of heart failure, renal disease, gastrointestinal tract abnormalities and thyroid abnormalities. This underscores the importance of the diagnosis of unrecognized medical illness in this group of patients.

Unfortunately there is scant information about the specific medical treatment for dementia associated with cerebrovascular disease. At this stage, most of the following recommendations are based on the treatment of patients who have sustained an ischaemic stroke. This information may not specifically apply to patients with dementia associated with cerebrovascular disease, and in particular dementia associated with cerebral haemorrhage.

Specific medical management focuses on prevention of further cerebral damage. This largely focuses on the treatment and prevention of risk factors for cerebrovascular disease. Recognized risk factors associated with dementia include hypertension, diabetes mellitus, advanced age, male sex, smoking and cardiac diseases.[2]

Rogers et al[3] studied a sample of normal elderly volunteers, mean age 70, and demonstrated that the incidence of multi-infarct dementia increased from 7.8 per thousand person-years in the group without risk factors to 16.8 per thousand person-years in subjects with risk factors which included hypertension, heavy cigarette smoking, heart disease and diabetes mellitus. Aronson and colleagues[4] found that a previous history of myocardial infarct was a strong predictor of subsequent dementia in very old women. Other studies have shown that the prognosis of people with stroke who have coexistent dementia is worse than for those without. Loeb et al[5] found that 23% of patients who had sustained a lacunar stroke were affected by dementia by the end of 4 years after their first lacunar stroke. It was also demonstrated that patients with dementia were more likely to have a higher rate of stroke recurrence than those without, emphasizing the importance of secondary prevention in this group of patients. This was confirmed in a study by Tatemichi et al,[6] which showed that the mortality rate was 19 deaths per hundred person-years for people who had a stroke which was complicated by dementia, compared to 6.9 deaths per hundred person years for those who had a stroke which was uncomplicated by dementia. The relative risk for death associated with dementia was 3.9 [95% confidence interval (CI): 1.8, 5.4]. As well as mortality, dementia after stroke increases the risk of long-term stroke recurrence.[7] That study found a relative risk of 2.7 (95% CI: 1.4, 5.4) for recurrent stroke in those individuals who had dementia following their initial stroke.

This evidence would suggest that patients who have cerebrovascular disease and dementia are at heightened risk for further stroke and thus should be targeted for secondary prevention of stroke. The options for this include control of hypertension, antiplatelet therapy, anticoagulant therapy, control of diabetes mellitus, stopping smoking, reducing hypercholesterolaemia and perhaps other therapies designed to affect rheological properties or vasodilatation of the cerebral vasculature.

Control of hypertension

There have been numerous studies looking at the use of antihypertensives in elderly people. Unfortunately very few of these studies specifically address the endpoint of the appearance or worsening of VAD. Many of these studies have now been systematically reviewed. For example, Mulrow et al[8] reviewed 15 trials which included 21 908 elderly subjects. They found that treatment of hypertension in older people, 60–80 years of age, reduced cardiovascular morbidity and mortality from 177 to 126 (95% CI of the difference 31–73) events per thousand participants over 5 years. Cardiovascular mortality was reduced from 69 to 50 deaths, total mortality was reduced from 129 to 111 deaths. They reviewed, separately, three trials which addressed the question of isolated systolic hypertension and found that cardiovascular morbidity and mortality was reduced over a 5-year period from 157 to 104 events per thousand participants (95% CI of the difference 12–89). One of the studies included in this systematic review[9] found a mean systolic blood pressure difference between active and placebo groups of 10.1 mmHg and a diastolic difference of 4.5 mmHg. The stroke rate was reduced from 13.7 to 7.9 per thousand patient-years which represented a highly significant 42% reduction. The first line medication used in this study was nitrendipine although another study of systolic hypertension in the elderly found chlorthalidone to be efficacious.[10]

At this stage there appears to be clear evidence for treating healthy older people with either diastolic hypertension or isolated systolic hypertension. However, the evidence for the aggressive treatment of hypertension in individuals who have already had VAD is scant. A study performed by Starr et al[11] suggested that there may be benefits for aggressively treating hypertension in those individuals with some cognitive impairment. Because of disturbance in autoregulation it has been argued that excessive lowering of blood pressure may precipitate vascular damage. However, there seems to be little randomized trial evidence to confirm this impression.[12]

Anticoagulation

Again, the evidence for anticoagulation following the onset of dementia associated with cerebrovascular disease is scant but there has been more substantial evidence available to address the question of treatment of non-embolic ischaemic stroke or transient ischaemic attack with anticoagulation, and this evidence has been systematically reviewed.[13] Nine trials were available for inclusion in a meta-analysis. The reviewers concluded that there was no evidence that anticoagulation significantly reduced the odds of death or dependency, with an odds ratio of 0.83 (95% CI 0.52, 1.34) and it did not reduce the risk of ischaemic or recurrent stroke, odds ratio 0.79 (95% CI 0.56, 1.13). However, anticoagulation did increase the odds of major bleeding with the risk for fatal intracranial haemorrhage increasing, odds ratio 2.54 (95% CI 1.19, 5.45) and for major extracranial haemorrhage, odds ratio 4.87 (95% CI 2.50, 9.49). The reviewers concluded there was no clear evidence of benefit from long-term anticoagulation therapy in patients with non-embolic stroke who were not in atrial fibrillation.

However, this is clearly not the case with those patients who have atrial fibrillation from either rheumatic or non-rheumatic causes. A meta-analysis by Koudstaal[14] showed that the risk for recurrent stroke was reduced by two thirds, odds ratio 0.36 (95% CI 0.22–0.58) and the risk was halved for all vascular events for patients with pre-existing stroke or transient ischaemic attack. The clear recommendation following this analysis was that anticoagulants should be given to patients with non-rheumatic atrial fibrillation and recent cerebral ischaemia if at all possible and this recommendation should probably be echoed for those patients with dementia associated with cerebrovascular disease, although, of course, issues of compliance and monitoring may be much more problematic in patients with dementia.

Antithrombotic treatment

The evidence for aspirin as an effective secondary prevention for all patients with either pre-existing cardiovascular or cerebrovascular disease has been extensively reviewed.[15] Jonas[16] reviewed the evidence for the effect of aspirin on the risk of stroke or death in those who had suffered cerebral ischaemia and found that the odds ratio for both women and men was 0.83 (95% CI 0.73, 0.95); it was found that the odds ratio for men only and women only was not substantially different. Clearly aspirin should be given to all patients with dementia associated with cerebrovascular disease where there are no contraindications. Aspirin has also been used in a small pilot study as therapy for patients with multi-infarct dementia[17] and significant improvements were found in cognitive performance. Unfortunately, larger studies of this type are not available. However, further questions regarding antiplatelet therapy remain.

First, does dipyridamole add to the effect of aspirin? A meta-analysis by Lowanthal and Buyse[18] found a trend for reduction in vascular events following a combination of dipyridamole and aspirin vs aspirin alone, but it was not conclusive. A recent study, The European Stroke Prevention Study, found benefits with a combination of dipyridamole and aspirin compared to aspirin alone.[19] The stroke risk was reduced by 18% in patients with aspirin alone, by 16% with dipyridamole alone and by 37% with the combination. It should be noted that, in this study, aspirin was used in a dose of 50 mg daily and the dipyridamole was used in a modified release form at a dose of 200 mg twice daily.

Another question is whether ticlopidine is more efficacious than aspirin and whether it should be a first-line treatment. Ticlopidine at a dose of 250 mg twice daily has been found to have benefits over aspirin at a dose of 1300 mg daily for prevention of recurrent cerebrovascular events.[20] Significant side effects were found with ticlopidine, including diarrhoea, rash and neutropenia. In general the greater cost and the need to monitor for side-effects has resulted in the use of ticlopidine as second line treatment for recurrent cerebrovascular events.

The use of antiplatelet vs anticoagulation therapy for the secondary prevention of recurrent stroke in patients with atrial fibrillation from non-rheumatic causes has been compared within a systematic review, but it is essentially based on one trial.[21] Anticoagulants in general reduce the risk of recurrent stroke by about half compared to aspirin, odds ratio 0.55 (95%CI 0.36, 0.83), whereas, unfortunately, major bleeding complications occurred nearly five-fold more often, odds ratio 4.65 (95% CI 1.66, 12.99). The absolute difference in risk of these bleeding consequences was small. On the basis of these data, the clear recommendation is that anticoagulation is preferred to antiplatelet treatment in the secondary prevention of further cerebral damage in those people with atrial fibrillation unless there are clear contraindications.

Control of diabetes mellitus

Diabetes mellitus is a known risk factor for vascular diseases. Recent evidence would suggest that it is a potent risk factor for dementia. Ott and colleagues[22] from the Rotterdam Study have reported a positive association between diabetes and dementia with an odds ratio of 1.3 (95% CI 1.0, 1.9), even after adjusting for age and sex. More impressively, the risk of VAD was increased 5.4-fold (95% CI 1.2, 23.8) for those people with diabetes treated with insulin, and 3.2-fold (95% CI 1.4, 7.4) for those patients treated with oral medications. The overall risk for VAD associated with the presence of diabetes mellitus was 2.1 (95% CI 1.1, 4.0), but the risk of VAD was not increased for patients who had no drug treatment for diabetes.

These results may reflect evidence for increased severity of diabetes associated with VAD, that is, if patients have severe and long-standing diabetes they are more likely to develop VAD. However, it does raise the issue of whether high endogenous or exogenous insulin levels may be complicated by VAD. This has implications in the treatment of people with diabetes mellitus and VAD, although evidence from the UK Prospective Diabetes Study[23] found benefits from intensive treatment of type 2 diabetes mellitus. The risk of any diabetes-related endpoint which included death, myocardial infarction, stroke or amputation, blindness or cataract was reduced by 12% with more intensive treatment. Using stroke as a single endpoint, there was no significant reduction in risk for either fatal or non-fatal stroke in the more intensively treated group. In this study, just as important as control of type 2 diabetes was the control of hypertension, with tight blood pressure control associated with a 44% reduction in strokes (95% CI 11–65%).[24] Blood pressure treatments were found to be cost effective.[25]

Control of elevated cholesterol

The association between hypercholesterolaemia and stroke has been relatively controversial. However, intervention studies seem to be less contentious. Initially systematic reviews, for example, that of Atkins et al,[26] failed to reveal a reduction in risk for fatal and non-fatal stroke. This may have been related to the earlier types of treatment, such as clofibrate or cholestyramine. A more recent meta-analysis by Herbert et al[27] examined whether the use of HMG-CoA reductase inhibitors (statin drugs) reduces the risk of total mortality. A total of 16 individual trials with 29 000 subjects was analysed. The average reduction in total cholesterol was 22%. The authors found a reduction in the risk of stroke of 29% (95% CI 14–41%) and an overall reduction in total mortality of 22% (95%CI 12–31%), which was attributable to a significant reduction in cardiovascular disease. This suggests that patients with dementia and cerebrovascular disease may benefit from a review of serum cholesterol and appropriate treatment with the statin drugs if hypercholesterolaemia is found and not amenable to treatment with lifestyle modification.

Other measures

Clearly the cessation of smoking is efficacious, not only for the prevention of subsequent strokes, but also for its association with a reduction in coronary vascular disease and lung cancer. Of other treatments, one that perhaps has had the most investigation is pentoxifylline. A study reported in 1992[28] found a reduction in the deterioration of the AD assessment scale which was not statistically significant ($P = 0.06$). Another recent study, reported by the European Pentoxifylline Multi-infarct Dementia Study Group (EPMID)[29] found some benefits of pentoxifylline 400 mg tds over a 9-month period for the outcome measure of the Gottfries, Brane, Steen scale, but this was not confirmed by a conventional intention-to-treat analysis. A recent meta-analysis of pentoxifylline[30] for acute ischaemic stroke failed to reveal sufficient evidence to recommend its use, but also concluded that insufficient patients had been studied to date, with an odds ratio of 0.49 (95% CI 0.20, 1.20) for the combined outcome of death or deterioration. A meta-analysis of nimodipine in the treatment of primary degenerative, mixed and VAD[31] failed to find convincing evidence of treatment effects; few trials were available for meta-analysis. The odds ratio of 0.53 (95% CI 0.25, 1.13) for the outcome of overall clinical efficacy revealed a trend for benefit. Another treatment that is currently undergoing investigation is hormone replacement therapy,[32] but at present no evidence is available for the endpoints of VAD or stroke.

Other treatments that have been studied include buflomidil,[33] nicergoline[34] and memantine,[35] but although some suggestive evidence of beneficial effects has been found, the studies are small and non-convincing. Bromocriptine was found to be ineffective.[36]

Conclusions

At this stage the best evidence of the benefits of medical management for the prevention of further cerebrovascular damage is for the control of hypertension. In those patients with diabetes mellitus, antihypertensive treatment may even be more important than aggressive control of hyperglycaemia, although modest benefits may be obtained from this intervention as well. The use of antiplatelet agents, and in particular aspirin, is efficacious, and is preferred in patients without contraindications and who are not in atrial fibrillation. In those patients with atrial fibrillation consideration should be given to the use of anticoagulation therapy. In selected patients with hypercholesterolaemia, the statin medications may have a definite role.

References

1. Forstl H, Cairns N, Burns A et al, Medical disorders in Alzheimer's disease and vascular dementia, *Postgrad Med J* (1991) **670**: 742–4.

2. Skoog I, Risk factors for vascular dementia: a review, *Dementia* (1994) **5**:137–44.

3. Rogers RL, Mayer JS, Mortel KF, Decreased cerebral blood flow precedes multi-infarct dementia but follows senile dementia of Alzheimer's type, *Neurology* (1986) **36**:1–6.

4. Aronson MK, Ooi WL, Morgenstern H et al, Women, myocardial infarction, and dementia in the very old, *Neurology* (1990) **40**:1102–6.

5. Loeb C, Gandolfo C, Croce R, Conti M, Dementia associated with lacunar infarction, *Stroke* (1992) **23**:1225–9.

6. Tatemichi TK, Paik M, Bagiella E et al, Risk of dementia after stroke in a hospitalised cohort: results of a longitudinal study, *Neurology* (1994) **44**:1885–91.

7. Moroney JT, Bagiella E, Tatemichi TK et al, Dementia after stroke increases the risk of long-term stroke recurrence, *Neurolgy* (1997) **5**:1317–25.

8. Mulrow C, Lau J, Cornell J et al, Antihypertensive drug therapy in the elderly (Cochrane Review). In: *The Cochrane Library*, Issue 4 (Update Software: Oxford, 1998).

9. Staessen JA, Fagard R, Thijs L et al, Randomised double-blind comparison of placebo and active treatment for older patients with isolated systolic hypertension. The Systolic Hypertension in Europe (Syst-Eur) Trial investigators, *Lancet* (1997) **350**:757–64.

10. Probstfield JL, Prevention of stroke by antihypertensive drug treatment in older persons with isolated systolic hypertension: final results of the Systolic Hypertension in the Elderly Program (SHEP), *JAMA* (1991) **265**:3255-64

11. Starr JM, Whalley LJ, Deary IJ. The effects of antihypertensive treatment on cognitive function: results from the HOPE study, *J Am Geriatr Soc* (1996) **44**:411–15.

12. Konno S, Meyer JS, Terayama Y et al, Classification, diagnosis and treatment of vascular dementia, *Drugs Aging* (1997) **11**:361–73.

13. Liu M, Counsell C, Sandercock P, Anticoagulation versus no anticoagulation following non-embolic ischaemic stroke or transient ischaemic attack (Cochrane Review). In: *The Cochrane Library*, Issue 4 (Update Software: Oxford 1998).

14. Koudstaal P, Secondary prevention following stroke or transient ischemic attack in patients with nonrheumatic atrial fibrillation: anticoagulant versus antiplatelet therapy (Cochrane Review). In: *The Cochrane Library*, Issue 4 (Update Software: Oxford, 1998).

15. Antiplatelet Trialists' Collaboration, Collaborative overview of randomised trials of antiplatelet ther-

apy in various categories of patients, *Br Med J* (1994) **308**: 81–106.

16. Jonas S, Effect of aspirin on risk of stroke or death in women who have previously suffered cerebral ischaemia, *Cerebrovasc Dis* (1994) **4**:157–62.

17. Meyer JS, Rogers RL, McClintic K et al, Randomised clinical trial of daily aspirin therapy in multi-infarct dementia. A pilot study, *J Am Geriatr Soc* (1989) **37**:549–55.

18. Lowenthal A, Buyse M. Secondary prevention of stroke: does dipyridamole add to aspirin? *Acta Neurol Belg* (1994) **94**:24–34.

19. Diener HC, Cunha L, Forbes C et al, European stroke prevention study. 2. Dipyridamole and acetylsalicylic acid in the secondary prevention of stroke, *J Neurol Sc* (1996) **143**:1–13.

20. Hass WK, Easton JD, Adams HP Jr et al, A randomised trial comparing ticlopidine hydrocholoride with aspirin for the prevention of stroke in high-risk patients, *N Engl J Med* (1989) **321**:501–7.

21. Koudstaal P, Secondary prevention following stroke or transient ischemic attack in patients with nonrheumatic atrial fibrillation: anticoagulant therapy versus control (Cochrane Review). In: *The Cochrane Library*, Issue 4 (Update Software: Oxford, 1998).

22. Ott A, Stolk RP, Hofman A et al, Association of diabetes mellitus and dementia: the Rotterdam Study, *Diabetologia* (1996) **39**: 1392–7.

23. UK Prospective Diabetes Study (UKPDS) Group. Intensive blood-glucose control with sulphonylureas or insulin compared with conventional treatment and risk of complications in patients with type 2 diabetes (UKPDS 33), *Lancet* (1998) **352**:837–53.

24. UK Prospective Diabetes Study Group, Tight blood pressure control and risk of macrovascular and microvascular complications in type 2 diabetes: UKPDS 38, *Br Med J* (1998) **317**:703–13.

25. UK Prospective Diabetes Study Group, Cost effectiveness analysis of improved blood pressure control in hypertensive patients with type 2 diabetes: UKPDS 40, *Br Med J* (1998) **317**:720–6

26. Atkins D, Psaty BM, Koepsell TD et al, Cholesterol reduction and the risk of stroke in men: a meta-analysis of randomised, controlled trials, *Ann Intern Med* (1993) **119**:136–45.

27. Herbert PR, Gaziano JM, Chan KS et al, Cholesterol lowering with statin drugs, risk of stroke and total mortality. An overview of randomized trials, *JAMA* (1997) **278**:313–21.

28. Black RS, Barclay LL, Nolan KA et al, Pentoxifylline in cerebrovascular dementia, *J Am Geriatr Soc* (1992) **40**:237–44.

29. European Pentoxifylline Multi-infarct Dementia Study Group (EPMID), European pentoxifylline Multi-infract Study, *Eur Neurol* (1996) **36**:315–21.

30. Bath PMW, Bath FJ, Asplund K, Pentoxifylline, propentofylline and pentifylline in acute ischaemic stroke (Cochrane Review). In: *The Cochrane Library*, Issue 4 (Update Software: Oxford, 1998).

31. Qizilbash N, Lopez Arrieta J, Birks J, Nimodipine in the treatment of primary degenerative, mixed and vascular dementia (Cochrane Review). In: *The Cochrane Library*, Issue 4 (Update Software: Oxford, 1998).

32. McBee WL, Dailey ME, Dugan E et al, Hormone replacement therapy and other potential treatments for dementias, *Endocrinol Metab Clin N Am* (1997) **26**:329–45.

33. Cucinotta D, Aveni Casucci MA,

Pedrazzi F et al, Multicentre clinical placebo-controlled study with buflomedil in the treatment of mild dementia of vascular origin, *J Int Med Res* (1992) **20**:136–49.

34. Saletu B, Paulus E, Linzmayer L et al, Nicergoline in senile dementia of Alzheimer type and multi-infarct dementia: a double blind, placebo controlled, clinical and EEG/ERP mapping study, *Psychoparmacology* (1995) **117**:385–95.

35. Ditzler K, Efficacy and tolerability of memantine in patients with dementia syndrome. A double blind, placebo controlled trial, *Arzneim Forsch Drugs Res* (1991) **41**:773–80.

36. Nadeau SE, Malloy PF, Andrew ME, A crossover trial of bromocriptine in the treatment of vascular dementia, *Ann Neurol* (1998) **24**:270–72.

17
Management of psychiatric disorders

David Ames

Introduction

As House and colleagues[1] have shown, the range of psychiatric disorders which occur after stroke is protean. Patients may manifest delirium, frontal disinhibition, behavioural disturbances, schizophrenia-like and delusional states, mania, depressive disorders, emotional lability and a range of conditions in which anxiety is the predominant symptom. These syndromes may occur alone or in association with a dementia. This chapter will draw on published evidence where available, to advise practical management strategies for specific psychiatric syndromes occurring in the context of cerebrovascular disease in general and dementia associated with cerebrovascular disease in particular. However, as management of generalised behavioural disturbances is addressed in the next chapter and family interventions in the one after that, these topics will not be covered in any detail here.

Dementia

Information and support

Unlike pure Alzheimer's disease (AD), dementia associated with cerebrovascular disease may have an abrupt onset. This may make adjustment for carers even harder than in the more insidious forms of dementia. As with AD, providing clear information to patient and family about the diagnosis, prognosis and community services will be vital.[2] Early education and support for carers have the potential to ameliorate distress and retard the need for institutional care of those with dementia, while delivering such information late may be less effective.[3] In countries with an Alzheimer Association or Alzheimer Society, carers of those with VAD should be advised to join, obtain written information about dementia and attend at least one support group session to see whether they find such involvement helpful.

Cognitive enhancers and related drug therapies

It is possible that cholinergic deficits similar to those found in AD may sometimes underlie at least some of the cognitive deficits found in individuals with VAD.[4] In addition, a significant number of people with dementia occurring in the context of cerebrovascular disease will have coexistent Alzheimer pathology.[4] Thus trials of the cholinesterase inhibitor donepezil hydrochloride, which has proven (if mild) efficacy in the relief of cognitive impairment associated with AD,[5] are now underway. Results of this research should become available during 2000. If efficacy in ameliorating cognitive deficits is shown, one would expect other cholinesterase inhibitors such as rivastigmine also to show utility in similar clinical situations. In the meantime there is insufficient evidence to recommend the routine use of a cholinesterase inhibitor in patients with apparent VAD, though their referral to evaluative trials is to be encouraged. However, when dementia presents with insidious gradual onset in a patient whose stroke predated the cognitive decline by months or years, if assessment and investigations are not suggestive of new strokes, there may be grounds for a trial of therapy with a cholinesterase inhibitor on the assumption that the pathology producing cognitive decline is likely to be AD.

The US trial of *Ginkgo biloba* extract EGb 761 in the treatment of dementia[6] had some methodological flaws and a high drop-out rate. Patients receiving EGb 761 showed slight but statistically significant improvement in cognitive function at 1 year (1.4 ADAS-Cog points better than the placebo group) and their relatives rated them as very slightly improved. However, the clinician global impression of change measure failed to show evidence of efficacy. The study included 73 patients with multi-infarct dementia in addition to 236 with AD, but did not analyse treatment outcomes for these two diagnostic groups separately.

There was no higher rate of adverse events in the group receiving EGb 761 than among those who took placebo. Although the evidence in favour of the usefulness of EGb 761 in VAD is weak, where patients and their families are keen that it be tried it seems unlikely to do harm. The results of future, better designed evaluative studies would be of some interest.

Frontal disinhibition

Personality change after stroke is a major cause of relationship strain and where frontal damage leads to disinhibition, most of the patient's family members will struggle to adjust to the alteration. Education, altered expectations and firm but kind supervision (for example to prevent driving, to control inappropriate spending) should be the mainstay of management. Sometimes it will be necessary for the patient to cede power of attorney or to be placed under an administration order to prevent financial disaster. There is little evidence that psychotropic drugs are helpful when frontal disinhibition is prominent, but the lack of properly conducted studies means that it is impossible to make dogmatic statements on this topic. Where some calming or control is felt to be of paramount necessity a trial of antipsychotic medication in low dose, increasing according to tolerance and/or response, would not seem to be unreasonable. Because of the high levels of morbidity associated with older antipsychotic drugs it would be prudent to use newer agents such as olanzapine, risperidone or ziprisadone. If the therapy seems not to be helpful it should be withdrawn. If it is continued, regular review is essential.

Occasionally patients with frontal disinhibition make repeated and unwanted sexual advances. Most but not all of these patients are male. Such behaviour can present a significant risk to frail, demented co-residents in long-term care facilities. The author has occasionally seen the antiandrogen cyproterone acetate prescribed for these patients followed in some cases by amelioration of intrusive sexual behaviour. However, the medicolegal and ethical implications of such use present something of a minefield. Where such prescribing is contemplated it would be wise to obtain a second expert opinion, discuss the situation with the patient's relatives and, depending on the legislative environment, seriously consider whether the opinion of a mental health review board or guardianship court should be sought.

Delirium

Delirium will sometimes follow stroke[7] and may be due to cerebral oedema or a range of associated conditions including infection, drug intoxication/withdrawal and metabolic abnormalities.[7] If reversible causes are detected and appropriately managed, most cases will recover from the delirium or die without needing specific psychiatric treatment. Where delusions, hallucinations or grossly disturbed behaviour are of a severity which necessitates temporary suppression, the empirical use of an antipsychotic in low dose may be considered. Drugs with strong anticholinergic properties should be avoided in delirium, doses should be kept low (for example 0.5 mg haloperidol bd, 0.5 mg risperidone nocte) and the drug tapered rapidly once the delirium starts to subside. A significant number of people who have strokes have been heavy consumers of alcohol and it is important to evaluate the possibility that post-stroke delirium may be associated with alcohol withdrawal. Thiamine replacement and a reducing benzodiazepine regime may be life-saving in such occasional cases.

Schizophrenia-like states, hallucinations and delusions

No stroke patient in the large longitudinal cohorts of Robinson and colleagues was found to develop a schizophrenia-like syndrome,[8] which suggests that such sequelae are relatively uncommon. Nevertheless, both Robinson's group and others have described patients presenting with delusions and hallucinations which developed after a definite stroke event and the author of this chapter recently managed a patient who developed a florid psychosis with numerous first-rank symptoms after a series of well-documented small strokes. Where the symptoms are distressing or disruptive, an antipsychotic drug should be used and there is anecdotal evidence that symptomatic improvement will often, but not always, ensue.[8] Now that novel antipsychotics are widely available, low-dose therapy with olanzapine, risperidone or ziprisadone should be seriously considered. The elderly, especially those with cerebrovascular disease, are very vulnerable to parkinsonism and other extrapyramidal syndromes which are commonly induced by conventional dopamine-blocking agents which should be avoided. Where cerebrovascular disease is associated with convulsive activity, comorbid psychotic phenomena may improve after the institution of anticonvulsant drugs.[9]

Mania

There is a scanty literature on the treatment of post-stroke mania and bipolar disorder. Only Starkstein, Robinson and colleagues[8,10] have reported a case series as opposed to individual cases. In their experience 10/27 patients with secondary mania after stroke (as opposed to those patients with a prior affective history who had strokes and subsequently became manic) showed clear improvement on lithium carbonate and only three showed no benefit at all. Thus it seems sensible to consider the use of lithium both for initial and subsequent prophylactic treatment in post-stroke mania. Antipsychotics may assist with control of mania in this population, but because of the high likelihood of adverse effects from typical agents it would seem prudent to use novel agents with sedative properties in cautious initial doses (for example olanzapine 2.5–5 mg per day at first), and for short duration.

Depression

Up to 22% of stroke patients may develop major and up to 17% non-major depression.[8] There is evidence of efficacy for antidepressant therapy from three double-blind placebo-controlled studies which utilised nortriptyline, trazodone and citalopram. All studies found active treatment superior to placebo, but the total number of patients randomised was only 99 in all three studies combined.[8]

In two retrospective uncontrolled case series of stroke patients receiving electroconvulsive therapy (ECT) covering a total of 34 patients, only three failed to show significant improvement and no patient in either study had a further stroke or worsening of their neurological impairment.[8]

There have been no formal trials of psychological treatment in those with post-stroke depression, but individual case reports and accounts of therapies modified to accommodate the cognitive and linguistic deficits of stroke patients do exist.[11]

There is compelling evidence to indicate that the presence of cerebrovascular disease retards recovery and increases the risk of depressive relapse, death and dementia in elderly people with major depression.[12]

When considering how and whether to treat a depressed patient who has had a stroke, practitioners must consider not only the possible adverse effects of the treatments they plan to use, but also the fact that untreated post-stroke depression is associated with worse rehabilitative outcome and reduced post-stroke survival.[8] The poor outcome of older depressed people with cerebrovascular disease[12] is an argument for energetic early treatment, not therapeutic nihilism. Where the syndrome meets criteria for major depression and is not improving over a 2-week period and also where milder depressive syndromes are persisting and interfering with rehabilitation it seems reasonable to commence therapy with a short-acting selective serotonin reuptake inhibitor (SSRI). Tricyclics should be reserved for resistant cases in view of the propensity of the older patient to experience anticholinergic effects and the risk of postural hypotension in an individual with established vascular disease. ECT will be indicated where depression is severe, especially if delusions are present, if life-threatening behaviours (suicide attempts, failure to eat or drink) are present, or if the patient has a past history of ECT-responsive depression. Despite the reassuring findings from research,[8] it seems prudent to delay ECT if possible to at least 3 months post-stroke, but clinical considerations will sometimes occasion earlier intervention. The fact that there is no specific evidence base in favour of psychological therapy should not deter practitioners from providing supportive therapy at least, and occasional cases may warrant an empirical trial of cognitive behavioural therapy or grief counselling.

From an examination of the research literature in this field it is clear that despite the relatively high prevalence of post-stroke depression, there is a lack of quality treatment studies of large numbers of patients. Further studies of all modes of therapy are urgently needed. Indeed any services which see a high number of stroke patients have a duty to promote and execute treatment research in this field so that management strategies may be informed by quality evidence.

Emotional lability

Around one-fifth of all patients who have a stroke will experience pathological laughing and/or crying within the first year of the stroke event.[8] Although the condition may occur in association with a depressive disorder, many patients are seen in whom emotional lability appears to occur independent of depression.[8] The condition seems to respond to antidepressants. There is some evidence that nortriptyline, citalopram and fluoxetine produce improvement more often than placebo in such patients, although no study has randomised more than 28 patients.[8] Where emotional lability is persistent and distressing a trial with short half-life SSRI should be attempted.

Anxiety

Sharpe and colleagues[13] found 12 of 60 stroke patients to suffer from anxiety disorders 3 to 5 years after their index stroke, yet far less research has been done on the management of post-stroke anxiety and related disorders than on the management of post-stroke depression.

The widespread use of benzodiazepines for post-stroke anxiety should be discouraged in view of the potential of this class of agents to cause tolerance and dependence as well as the association of the longer-acting agents with hip fractures.[14] There also is a possibility of accentuating disinhibition in those whose strokes have a frontal focus. Where a benzodiazepine is needed for control of anxiety or severe sleep disturbance in the post-stroke period it is wise to employ shorter-acting agents such as oxazepam and to limit therapy to a maximum of 4 weeks or to use therapy intermittently (for example temazepam 10 mg nocte no more than thrice weekly).

There are no useful data on the use of buspirone in post-stroke anxiety. This drug affects serotonergic transmission and its onset of action is over a 2-week period. It does not cause drowsiness or addiction but it is quite expensive.

Where phobic disorder or panic is prominent, one could take note of findings in patients with functional disorders of similar phenomenology and undertake a trial of therapy with an SSRI (for example sertraline 25 mg mane increasing to 50–100 mg according to tolerance or response) or in extreme cases a tricyclic antidepressant.

Cognitive behavioural therapy (CBT) is now seen as the psychological treatment of choice for functional anxiety disorders, but little systematic research has been conducted on those who experience such symptoms after stroke. In many health systems there is a gross shortage of available trained practitioners funded to provide such treatment. Nevertheless, where cognition is sufficiently preserved for the patient to engage in CBT and a therapist is available to undertake the treatment it should be the first intervention attempted. CBT may be used in combination with drugs as well as without them.

Conclusion

In reviewing the literature on psychiatric treatment of those with cerebrovascular disease one is struck by the fact that despite the work of a few indefatigable researchers, what we do not know and need to find out far exceeds what we do know and can utilise in the care of our patients who have strokes and/or VAD. The interested reader will find more detailed expositions of the field in very good recent books by Robinson[8] and Birkett.[11] It is to be hoped that, after reading them, some young researchers will dedicate themselves to this fascinating, important, but still under-researched area.

References

1. House A, Dennis M, Mogridge L et al, Mood disorders in the year after stroke, *Br J Psychiatry* (1991) **158**:83–92.

2. Brodaty H, *Managing Alzheimer's Disease in Primary Care* (Science Press: London, 1998).

3. Brodaty H, Gresham M, Luscombe G, The Prince Henry Hospital dementia caregivers' training programme, *Int J Geriatr Psychiatry* (1997) **12**:183–92.

4. Bowler JV, Hachinski V, Vascular cognitive impairment: a new approach to vascular dementia, *Baillières Clin Neurol* (1995) **4**:357–67.

5. Burns A, Rossor M, Hecker J et al, The effects of donepezil in Alzheimer's disease—results from a multinational trial, *Dementia Geriatr Cog Disord* (1999) **10**:237–44.

6. Le Bars PL, Katz MM, Berman N et al, A placebo controlled, double-blind, randomized trial of an extract of Ginkgo biloba for dementia, *JAMA* (1997) **278**: 1327–32.

7. Lindesay J, Macdonald AJD, Starke I, *Delirium and the Elderly* (Oxford University Press: Oxford, 1990).

8. Robinson RG, *The Clinical Neuropsychiatry of Stroke* (Cambridge University Press: Cambridge, 1998).

9. Levine DN, Finkelstein S, Delayed psychosis after right temporoparietal stroke or trauma: relation to epilepsy, *Neurology* (1982) **32**: 267–73.

10. Starkstein SE, Fedoroff JP, Berthier ML, Robinson RG, Manic depressive and pure manic states after brain lesions, *Biol Psychiatry* (1991) **29**:149–58.

11. Birkett DP, *The Psychiatry of Stroke* (American Psychiatric Press: Washington DC, 1996).

12. O'Brien J, Ames D, Chiu E et al, Severe deep white matter lesions and outcome in elderly patients with major depressive disorder: follow up study, *Br Med J* (1998) **317**:982–4.

13. Sharpe M, Hawton K, House A et al, Mood disorders in long-term survivors of stroke: associations with brain lesion location and volume, *Psychol Med* (1990) **20**:815–28.

14. Ray WA, Griffin MR, Downey W, Benzodiazepines of long and short elimination half-life and the risk of hip fracture, *JAMA* (1989) **62**:3303–7.

18
Vascular dementia: consequences for family carers and implications for management

Henry Brodaty and Alisa Green

There is an aphorism in geriatric medicine that when a person is diagnosed with dementia there is usually a second patient, the family carer. Such recognition has resulted in a vast literature on carers and dementia. However, much less has been written about carers and vascular dementia (VAD) or on carers and stroke. This chapter attempts to redress this.

The impact of dementia on the family carer

Living with a person with a mental disability is an unremitting burden.[1] The decline in cognitive abilities, the loss of functional capacity, the dwindling companionship and the increasing demands of physical care impose escalating stresses on family carers.[2]

Such stresses manifest themselves psychologically, physically, socially, financially, and by increased use of health services.[2] Research indicates that carers have high levels and rates of psychological distress and depression[2-5] and a corresponding decline in physical health,[6] exacerbation of pre-existing medical conditions, such as hypertension,[7] and compromised immune function.[8]

The provision of care to a spouse or parent with dementia often requires the carer to leave or reduce paid employment,[9] as what may initially be part-time assistance can often become an all-encompassing role.[10] This is reflected in the findings of one study that (primary) family carers spent an average of 60 hours per week on their caring responsibilities.[11] Carers must cope with restrictions on social and leisure activities, disruption of household and work routines, conflicting multiple role demands, disruption of family relationships, and lack of support and assistance from other family members and from health and agency professionals.[12]

Effects of stroke on the family carer

Stroke, which is often the harbinger of VAD, may have distinct effects on carers, who are likely to be particularly stressed at several points on the post-stroke trajectory:[13]

- immediately after the stroke when the carer has to come to terms with an event that is usually dramatically sudden and potentially life-threatening;
- during the treatment phase and in-patient care;
- at the time of discharge from hospital when the carer realises that she (or he) is suddenly to be given responsibility for the patient; and
- in the weeks and months following hospital discharge when professional support dwindles and the carer may become exhausted.

Carers may already have feelings of guilt about the stroke, for example did they give the patient the wrong diet, or could they have called for help earlier. Subsequently they may fear leaving the patient alone or become overprotective.[14]

Predictors of stress in carers of persons with stroke

Factors associated with carer stress up to 6 months after a stroke include the (objective) severity of the stroke,[15–17] behavioural or mood disturbances in the stroke patient[16] and concerns by the carer over the future care of the stroke patient.[17] From 6 months after a stroke, additional factors associated with stress in carers include dissatisfaction with their social life,[17–19] poor physical health,[17] less family support[20] and demographic variables such as income and occupation. Increased levels of depression and psychological distress in carers have been found to persist for up to 3 years after the stroke.[17–19]

Comparison of the effects of vascular dementia and Alzheimer's disease

Research into carers' needs has mainly focused on dementia in general, or Alzheimer's disease (AD) in particular.[2,10,21] However, there is a growing recognition that the demands of caring and the needs of the care recipient differ according to the type of dementia.[22,23]

Alzheimer's disease and VAD together account for approximately 80% of dementia cases in the elderly.[24] Though similar in many ways, there are clinical reasons why their impacts may differ. These disorders vary in their antecedent risk factors, onset, nature of disease progression, neuropsychological profile, neurological features and associated physical ill health.[25] Additionally, risk factors for VAD such as hypertension, cardiovascular disease, cerebrovascular disease (CVD) and diabetes mellitus have their own morbidity and may have independent effects on family members prior to the onset of stroke or VAD.

Differences in onset and progression

The sudden onset of VAD can have an immediate and marked impact on the family, leaving them devoid of time to prepare for the changes.[23] By contrast, the usual progression of AD is gradual and allows more time for carers to adapt to their role.[21] By contrast, carers of persons with VAD, especially of those with multi-infarct dementia (MID), must repeatedly adapt to unexpected sudden deteriorations inherent in that dementia's 'step-wise' decline. Further, the patient's fluctuating mental state, more typical of VAD, may be confusing to carers.

Differences in patients' psychological and physical disability

VAD is more likely than AD to leave the individual's personality superficially intact, so that persons with VAD may not seem to other family members and friends to have changed much.[23] This may lessen carer burden or paradoxically make it more difficult for family carers coping with cognitive decline in a person perceived by others to be functioning normally. Similarly, physical disability, which is more likely to complicate the picture in VAD, may increase the burden on family carers but may also legitimise the carer role. Finally, depression is a more common feature of VAD than AD.[26,27] Depression in such cases is directly associated with psychological morbidity in carers.[28,29]

Differences in psychological effects on carers

Despite clinical differences, empirical evidence that there are differential effects on carers of VAD, stroke and AD is equivocal. In a comparison of stroke and dementia carers, Draper et al[19] found that subjective burden and psychological morbidity in carers was independent of the patient's diagnosis. A subsequent study by the same group reported that the risk factors identified for carer stress in stroke and dementia care were similar.[30] However, Reese et al[31] found that AD carers reported significantly greater feelings of burden than stroke carers or a control group of noncarers. Other studies have found AD carers may be less satisfied with the assistance they receive from family and friends than carers of stroke patients,[19] have less social support[32] and have fewer social resources even after controlling for age and socio-economic status.[31] This may result in part from the common perception that AD is a mental illness [33] while stroke is clearly identified as a physical disorder.

The disparate findings of these studies could reflect amalgamation of different subtypes of dementia and disability—physical, cognitive and behavioural. Thus, Draper et al[19] compared patients with dementia (including MID) and those who had had a stroke but without dementia, and Reese et al[31] compared AD and stroke patients. We could not locate any studies comparing AD and VAD directly; most compare the effects of AD or unspecified dementia and stroke.

Ethnic and cultural influences on the management of VAD

Ethnic and cultural factors must be considered in the management of dementia, as the prevalences of AD and VAD differ, as do the ways in which these diseases present themselves, and the ways in which families respond. Whereas AD is more common in Western countries, VAD tends to be the more prevalent subtype of dementia in Asian countries.[34-36] These findings may reflect methodological, genetic, social, cultural or environmental differences[34,37,38] and the difficulties with diagnosis resulting from language differences and cultural bias inherent in many diagnostic instruments.

Family attitudes vary with ethnicity and strongly influence care and management. For instance, minority family carers in the USA, particularly African-American carers, are more likely to maintain their elderly at home, rather than admit them to nursing homes.[39] Even within ethnic groups, minor nuances of cultural variations in family custom can become important: in some groups, such as Italian Americans, the family eats together at set times. This practice can cause tension if a patient is unable to eat in a socially acceptable way.[40]

Carers from different cultures appear to experience the stresses of caregiving independent of dementia subtype. For instance, in the USA African-American carers experience lower rates of depression and subjective burden than Caucasian carers.[41] They also appear to find caring tasks less stressful and consider themselves effective, in contrast to Caucasian carers.[6] Such differences may reflect cultural variation in factors such as expectations about caring and previous experiences with adversity[6] as well as socio-economic status.[39]

Cultural variance also appears to affect the way that family members approach and view their caring role and responsibilities. In some cultures, traditional gender role expectations may mean that the older son or his wife, rather than a daughter, may take on the major burden of caring, or that sons may be the ones responsible for making decisions, while daughters provide day-to-day care.[42,43] Different cultures vary in the extent to which families will place relatives in nursing homes.[39,42] Placing an elderly relative in a nursing home may be considered abandonment and therefore unthinkable, even in cases of extreme stress and burden to the carer.[42]

Thus, diverse minority and ethnic groups often require special services to meet their unique needs, which may easily be overlooked or poorly understood. Awareness of the needs of different cultural groups can assist in the establishment of more culturally appropriate services that are also more valued by the individuals in need of such services.[44]

However, multiple barriers impede access to needed services: language, dependence upon others for translation, lack of cultural relevance of services and misconceptions that mean that behaviours related to dementia evoke little concern until symptoms are quite advanced.[45] For example, many cultures view confusion, disorientation and memory loss as normal parts of aging, while others regard these as signs of 'craziness'.[42] The most frequent obstacle to diagnosis and management of dementia is lack of a common language. For instance, ethnic carers may be unable to understand medical instructions, which can lead to incorrect medication administration or non-compliance.[46]

In English-speaking countries, non-English-speaking elders depend on their English-speaking relatives to learn about and make use of services.[45] Access to services for ethnic populations can be facilitated by locating programmes within the ethnic community, using personnel who are culturally compatible with the target group and providing social and health services alongside with existing services in the community. Close working relationships with community agencies already serving minority populations (for example within a neighbourhood health facility where the residents are accustomed to receiving primary medical care) help strengthen and encourage referrals, and provide training and education for staff members.[47]

Management of VAD together with the family

Until dementia can be reversed or 'cured', management aims to maximise the quality of life of the patient and, where there is a family, that of the carer. Management planning requires a long-term view and the establishment of partnerships between the principal protagonists—patients, families and clinicians. The family is critical to both diagnosis and management.

A knowledge of the likely trajectory of the dementia assists in planning. The greater variability and unpredictability of VAD forces variation from the 'staged management' model.[48] For example, the shock of the sudden development of dementia following a stroke, the uncertainty of how much improvement will occur in the long term and the fact that sometimes the patient has a more severe dementia right from the start without ever evolving through the stages of early dementia may exacerbate the carer's distress and make care more difficult. Even so, it is useful to conceptualise the course of VAD as progressing through early, middle and late stages. New challenges arise for the family in each stage and management can be formulated accordingly.[48]

Early stage of dementia

The first concern after making a diagnosis is how to inform the patient and the family. This is a sensitive and delicate process which requires the clinician to determine the extent to which each wishes to be informed of the diagnosis and its implications, and thus to 'titrate' the amount of information provided against the patient's and carer's reactions. Patients have a right to know their diagnosis but, equally, not to have this forced on them if they do not wish to know. Family members may express strong views about withholding the diagnosis from the patient, though, paradoxically, wishing to be informed were they in the same situation.[49] This may run counter to the clinician's duty to the patient. Usually it is possible to resolve this impasse by alleviating the family's fears through discussion and/or by allowing the family time to consider the matter further. Well-judged disclosures rarely distress patients and may even afford relief, as they can then understand why they have been experiencing difficulties.

Assessment is more than mere diagnosis; it requires an evaluation of the patient's particular capabilities and deficits. This will guide management, which should build on strengths and compensate for deficits, for example by the use of memory aids such as a notebook by the phone for messages and the establishment of a daily routine.

In the early stage of dementia family members may undergo a reaction similar to grieving or bereavement—for the loss of the person they knew, or in anticipation of such a loss. It is important to allow family members the opportunity to voice their concerns; referral to a local support group may be of assistance. The patient and family members may differ in the extent to which they wish to learn about dementia; questions are often best answered by organisations such as the Alzheimer's Association or the Stroke Society, which can recommend books and other information kits and offer local support group meetings.

Prognosis is commonly raised. Many patients and families are (mistakenly) relieved to learn that the dementia is vascular in aetiology and not of the Alzheimer's type. This is a misconception as evidence suggests that VAD has poorer prognosis, with earlier residential care placement and death.[50–52]

Other issues prominent in the management of early dementia include safety with driving and work, especially for younger people with dementia (more likely with VAD than with AD); financial and legal management; planning for the future; enduring power of attorney; wills; and the use of anti-dementia medication. The absence of specific treatments for VAD akin to those available for AD such as the acetylcholinesterase inhibitors is a source of disappointment for some carers. However control of risk factors for stroke such as hypertension, smoking, obesity, diabetes mellitus and hyperlipidaemia, promotion of regular exercise and use of aspirin may reassure carers (and patients) that something active is being done. Unfortunately data are not yet available to answer the frequently posed question of heritability of VAD.

Middle stage dementia

In the middle stage of dementia, patients will become increasingly dependent upon others as they are unable to compensate for deficits. Concerns include the loss of the ability to manage more complex household tasks and transport independently, and increasing ineptitude in other day-to-day activities. An occupational therapist can recommend strategies to maximise the patient's capacity for self-care within the home.

Personality changes and behavioural disturbances are also likely to become more apparent, and these are a potent source of burden and distress for the carer. A useful technique for carers is to make a note of the instances of the troublesome behaviours, what preceded them and what caused them to subside. This allows patterns to be identified and management strategies can be formulated that may prevent or reduce problem behaviours.[53] Comprehensive training programmes and counselling for carers can reduce their distress, increase their coping skills and knowledge, enhance the quality of life for them and their dependants and, importantly, delay institutionalisation.[3,54]

During this middle stage of dementia, patients are also more likely to suffer from depression, delusions, hallucinations and behavioural disturbances. If these follow a cerebrovascular event such phenomena may be transient or part of a delirium. If they persist and are troublesome to patients, carers or other people, behavioural management techniques[55] and/or medication, such as antidepressants or neuroleptics,[56] may be indicated.

Late stage dementia

The late stage of dementia brings new challenges for carers as the patient continues to deteriorate, requiring increasing help with basic self-care activities such as dressing, bathing, feeding and going to the toilet. Carers may need to enlist more practical assistance, respite care and community nursing. In some cases increasing cognitive decline and apathy may mean that previous problem behaviours diminish.

At this time, carers are most likely to consider placing the patient in a hostel or nursing home. Carers often experience intense anguish or guilt when making this decision. It is sometimes helpful to point out that admission to a residential facility may actually improve the quality of life of both patient and carer, by enabling them to spend more time together that is enjoyable. The decision for placement is usually made when caring duties exceed the carer's capacities: the patient becomes incontinent, problem behaviours become unmanageable, there is a breakdown in the family carer's health or the patient no longer recognises the family carer.

In the terminal stages, family carers may be forced to make complex ethical end-of-life decisions: should tube feeding be instituted for the patient who loses the ability to swallow or should antibiotic treatment be commenced for an infection when there is no discernible quality of life?

Finally, the death of the patient, although often anticipated, is a time of distress and grief for the carer, as they suddenly find themselves relieved of the full-time duty of caring for the patient. At this time, grief counselling for the carer may be appropriate.

Prognosis of VAD

Institutionalization

In order to make decisions about management and care, families wish to know about the prognosis—how long before before the patient will need to be admitted to a nursing home, how long is the patient likely to live?[57] The extent to which a patient can be cared for at home usually relies on the continued availability of a carer, which in itself depends on the extent to which the carer can continue to cope with the patient's condition.[48] Characteristics of the carer are better predictors of institutional placement than characteristics of the care-recipient.[58] Care-recipients are significantly more likely to be institutionalised when carers experience burden, employ confrontational or immature problem-solving strategies, rely on social support or are unwilling to accept responsibility for caring. Increased carer strain and feelings of carer stress are related both to the desire to institutionalise and to actual institutionalisation.[50]

Patient characteristics predicting institutionalisation include the severity of the dementia, the rate of progression, the presence of behavioural complications, the patient's age[59,60] and possibly the type of dementia—a higher rate of nursing home placement has been found for patients with VAD compared to those with AD.[50,52,61]

Mortality

A higher incidence of mortality has been reported for patients with VAD (30.4–63.6%) than patients with AD (22.6–33.8%).[50,51] The average survival time in AD has been found to be 8–10 years, although the range can be quite variable.[62] By comparison, the mean survival time for VAD has been found to be around 5 years.[63]

For individuals with VAD, a longer life expectancy is linked with female gender,[64] higher educational level and better performance on measures of cognitive ability. Surprisingly, coexisting diabetes, hypertension and heart disease were not significant predictors of survival in patients with VAD.[65] van Dijk et al[64] found that nursing home patients with dementia appeared to have a less favourable prognosis compared with dementia sufferers who resided in the community, and that 50% of patients in nursing homes survive an average of 2 years after admission.

Conclusion

Although management of VAD follows the management model of dementia in general, there are differences between VAD and AD in their effects on carers and for framing strategies. Variations in aetiology, onset and course of the illness, comorbidity, drug treatments and prognosis are noteworthy and can have clinical implications.

References

1. Anderson R, The unremitting burden on carers, *Br Med J* (1987) **204**:73.
2. Brodaty H, Hadzi-Pavlovic D, Psychosocial effects on carers of living with persons with dementia, *Aust NZ J Psychiatry* (1990) **24**:351–61.
3. Mittelman MS, Ferris SH, Shulman E et al, A comprehensive support program: effect on depression in spouse-caregivers of AD patients, *Gerontologist* (1995) **35**:792–802.
4. Morris RG, Morris LW, Britton PG, Factors affecting the emotional wellbeing of the caregivers of dementia sufferers, *Br J Psychiatry* (1988) **53**:147–56.
5. Poulshock SW, Deimling GT, Families caring for elders in residence: issues in the measurement of burden, *J Gerontol* (1984) **39**:230–9.
6. Haley WE, The family caregiver's role in Alzheimer's disease, *Neurology* (1997) **48**(S6):S25–S29.
7. Schulz R, Visintainer P, Williamson G, Psychiatric and physical morbidity effects of caregiving, *J Gerontol* (1990) **45**:181–91.
8. Kiecolt-Glaser JK, Glaser R, Shuttleworth EC et al, Chronic stress and immunity in family caregivers of Alzheimer's disease victims, *Psychosom Med* (1987) **49**:523–35.
9. Stone R, Cafferata GL, Sangel J, Caregivers of the frail elderly: a national profile, *Gerontologist* (1987) **27**:616–25.
10. Aneshensel CS, Pearly LI, Mullan JT et al, *Profiles in Caregiving: The Unexpected Career* (Academic Press: San Diego, 1995).
11. Max W, Webber P, Fox P, Alzheimer's disease: the unpaid burden of caring *J Aging Health* (1995) **7**:179–99.

12. Biegel DE, Sales E, Schulz R, *Family Caregiving in Chronic Illness. Alzheimer's Disease, Cancer, Heart Disease, Mental Illness, and Stroke* (Sage Publications: California, 1991).
13. Holbrook M, Stroke: social and emotional outcome, *J R Coll Physicians Lond* (1982) **116**:100–4.
14. Warlow CP, Dennis MS, van Gijn J et al, *Stroke. A Practical Guide to Management* (Blackwell Science: Oxford, 1996) 534–6.
15. Wade DT, Legh-Smith J, Hewer RL, Effects of living with and looking after survivors of a stroke, *Br Med J* (1986) **293**:418–20.
16. Brocklehurst JC, Morris P, Andrews K et al, Social effects of stroke, *Soc Sci Med* (1981) **15A**:35–9.
17. Schulz R, Tompkins CA, Rau MT, A longitudinal study of the psychosocial impact of stroke on primary support persons, *Psychology Aging* (1988) **3**:131–41.
18. Carnwath TC, Johnson DA, Psychiatric morbidity among spouses of patients with stroke, *Br Med J* (1987) **294**:409–11.
19. Draper B, Poulos CJ, Cole AMD et al, A comparison of caregivers for elderly stroke and dementia victims, *J Am Geriatr Soc* (1992) **40**:896–901.
20. Silliman RA, Fletcher RH, Earp JL, Wagner EH, Families of elderly stroke patients. Effects of home care, *J Am Geriatr Soc* (1986) **34**:643–8.
21. Nolan M, Grant G, Keady J, *Understanding Family Care* (Open University Press: Buckingham, 1996).
22. Vitaliano PP, Russo J, Young HM et al, The screen for caregiver burden, *Gerontologist* (1991) **31**: 76–83.
23. Hoffman SB, Platt CA, *Comforting the Confused: Strategies for Managing Dementia* (Springer: New York, 1991).
24. Evans DA, Funkenstein HH, Albert MS et al, Prevalence of Alzheimer's disease in a community of older persons: higher than previously reported, *JAMA* (1989) **262**:2551–6.
25. Nolan BH, Swihart AA, Pirozzolo FJ, The neuropsychology of normal aging and dementia: an introduction. In: Wedding D, Horton AM, Webster J, eds, *The Neuropsychology Handbook: Behavioral and Clinical Perspectives* (Springer: New York, 1986) 410–40.
26. Mega MS, Cummings JL, Fiorello T, Gornbein J, The spectrum of behavioural changes in Alzheimer's disease, *Neurology* (1996) **46**:130–5.
27. Donaldson C, Tarrier N, Burns A, Determinants of carer stress in Alzheimer's disease, *Int J Geriatr Psychiatry* (1998) **13**:248–56.
28. Brodaty H, Luscombe G, Depression in persons with dementia, *Int Psychogeriatr* (1996) **8**: 609–22.
29. Brodaty H, Luscombe G, Psychological morbidity in caregivers is associated with depression in patients with dementia, *Alzheimer Dis Assoc Disord* (1998) **12**: 62–70.
30. Draper B, Poulos R, Poulos CJ et al, Risk factors for stress in elderly caregivers, *Int J Geriatr Psychiatry* (1996) **11**:227–31.
31. Reese D, Gross AM, Smalley DL, Meeser SC, Caregivers of Alzheimer's disease and stroke patients: immunological and psychological considerations, *Gerontologist* (1994) **34**:534–40.
32. Franks MM, Stephens MAP, Social support in the context of caregiving: husbands' provision of support to wives involved in parent care, *J Gerontol* (1996) **51**:P43–P52.

33. Aronson MK, *Understanding Alzheimer's Disease: What It Is, How To Cope With It, Future Directions*, (Charles Scribner's Sons: New York, 1988).

34. White L, Petrovich H, Ross WG et al, Prevalence of dementia in older Japanese-American men in Hawaii: the Honolulu-Asia aging study, *JAMA* (1996) **276**:955–60.

35. Ueda D, Kawano H, Hasuo Y, Fujishima M, Prevalence and etiology of dementia in a Japanese community, *Stroke* (1992) **23**: 798–803.

36. Yoshiitake T, Kiyohar Y, Kato I et al, Incidence and risk factors of vascular dementia and Alzheimer's disease in a defined elderly Japanese population: the Hisayama Study, *Neurology* (1995) **45**:1161–8.

37. Mayreux R, Stern Y, Ottman R et al, The apolipoprotein epsilon 4 allele in patients with Alzheimer's disease, *Ann Neurol* (1993) **34**: 752–4.

38. Hendrie HC, Osuntokun BO, Hall KS et al, Prevalence of Alzheimer's disease and dementia in two communities: Nigerian Africans and African Americans, *Am J Psychiatry* (1995) **152**: 1485–92.

39. Wallsten SM, Elderly caregivers and care receivers. Facts and gaps in the literature. In: Nussbaum PD, ed, *Handbook of Neuropsychology and Aging* (Plenum Press: New York, 1997) 467–82.

40. Birkett DP, The family. In: Birkett DP, ed, *The Psychiatry of Stroke* (American Psychiatric Press: Washington, 1996) 311–19.

41. Lawton MP, Rajagopal D, Brody E et al, The dynamics of caregiving for demented elderly among black and white families, *J Gerontol* (1992) **47**:S156–S164.

42. Yeo G, Background. In: Yeo G, Gallagher-Thompson D, eds, *Ethnicity and the Dementias* (Taylor & Francis: Bristol, 1996) 3–7.

43. Johnson TW, Utilising culture in work with aging families. In: Smith GC, Tobin SS, Robertson-Tchabo EA, Power PW, eds, *Strengthening Aging Families* (Sage Publications: Thousand Oaks, 1995) 175–95.

44. Larson EB, Imai Y, An overview of dementia and ethnicity with special emphasis on the epidemiology of dementia. In: Yeo G, Gallagher-Thompson D, eds, *Ethnicity and the Dementias* (Taylor & Francis: Bristol, 1996) 9–20.

45. Valle R, Cultural and ethnic issues in Alzheimer's disease family research. In: Light E, Leibowitz BD (eds) *Alzheimer's Disease and Family Stress: Directions for Research*, Rockville, MD: National Institute of Mental Health (1989) **89–1569**:122–54.

46. Espino DV, Lewis R, Dementia in older minority populations, *Am J Geriatr Psychiatry* (1998) **6**: S19–S25.

47. Hart VR, Gallagher-Thompson D, Davies HD et al, Strategies for increasing participation of ethnic minorities in Alzheimer's disease diagnostic centers: a multifaceted approach in California, *Gerontologist* (1996) **36**:259–62.

48. Brodaty H, *Managing Alzheimer's Disease in Primary Care* (Science Press: London, 1998).

49. Maguire CP, Kirby M, Cohen R et al, Family members' attitudes toward telling the patient with Alzheimer's disease their diagnosis, *Br Med J* (1996) **313**:529–30.

50. Brodaty H, McGilchrist CA, Harris L et al, Time until institutionalisation and death in patients with dementia, *Arch Neurol* (1993) **50**:643–50.

51. Barclay LL, Zemcov A, Blass JP et al, Survival in Alzheimer's disease and vascular dementias, *Neurology* (1985) **35**:834–40.

52. Fragtiglioni L, Forsell Y, Aguero TH et al, Severity of dementia and institutionalisation in the elderly: prevalence data from an urban area in Sweden, *Neuroepidemiology* (1994) **13**:79–88.

53. Carrier L, Brodaty H, Mood and behavior management. In: Gauthier S, ed, *Clinical Diagnosis and Management of Alzheimer's Disease*, 2nd edn (Martin Dunitz: London, 1999).

54. Brodaty H, Gresham M, Luscombe G, The Prince Henry Hospital dementia caregivers-training programme, *Int J Geriatr Psychiatry* (1997) **12**:183–92.

55. Teri L, Logsdon R, Uomoto J et al, Treatment of depression in dementia patients: a controlled clinical trial, *J Gerontol B Psychol Sci Soc Sci* (1997) **52**:159–66.

56. Peisah C, Brodaty H, Practical guidelines for the treatment of behavioural complications of dementia, *Med J Aust* (1994) **161**:558–63.

57. Brodaty H, Griffin D, Hadzi-Pavlovic D, A survey of dementia carers: doctor's communications, problem behaviours, and institutional care, *Aust NZ J Psychiatry* (1990) **24**:362–70.

58. Wells Y, Over R, Institutional placement of a dementing spouse: the influence of appraisal, coping strategies, and social support, *Aust J Psychol* (1998) **50**:100–5.

59. Hope T, Keene J, Gedling K et al, Predictors of institutionalization for people with dementia living at home with a carer, *Int J Geriatr Psychiatry* (1998) **13**:682–90.

60. Haupt M, Kurz A, Predictors of nursing home placement in patients with Alzheimer's disease, *Int J Geriatr Psychiatry* (1993) **8**:741–6.

61. Drachman DA, O'Donnell BF, Lew RA, Swearer JM, The prognosis in Alzheimer's disease: 'How far' rather than 'how fast' best predicts the course, *Arch Neurol* (1990) **47**:851–6.

62. Geldmacher DS, Whitehouse PJ, Current concepts: evaluation of dementia, *N Engl J Med* (1996) **335**:330–6.

63. Herbert R, Brayne C, Epidemiology of vascular dementia, *Neuroepidemiology* (1995) **14**:240–57.

64. van Dijk PTM, Dippel DWJ, Habbema JDF, Survival of patients with dementia, *J Am Geriatr Soc* (1991) **39**:603–10.

65. Hier DB, Warach JD, Gorelick PB et al, Predictors of survival in clinically diagnosed Alzheimer's disease and multi-infarct dementia, *Arch Neurol* (1989) **46**:1213–16.

19
The provision of long-term care and the management of behavioural disorders in cerebrovascular disease and dementia

Edmond Chiu

'The provision of care for people suffering from dementia represents a considerable challenge to the research and clinical community. Examples of good practice abound but there is a dearth of empirical research to support what should properly be regarded as good practice and which improves the quality of care and the quality of life of patients and their carers.'
      Alistair Burns, Editorial Introduction. *International Journal of Geriatric Psychiatry* (1999) **14**:83.

Introduction

Number 2, Volume 14 of the *International Journal of Geriatric Psychiatry* (1999) was mostly devoted to a collection of papers and critical commentaries presented at a symposium entitled 'What works in dementia care' held at the Centre for Social Research in Dementia at the University of Stirling, Scotland, in June 1998. The compelling need to be clear about what works in dementia care was ably demonstrated,[1] as was the very unsatisfactory state of the evidence-based research in dementia care. However, it was argued that evidence-based practice, while laudable, is at present immature and would limit us to drug interventions which, while having a tradition of data collection through randomized controlled trials (RCTs), would not necessarily totally satisfy the objective of providing the best quality of life for people with dementia.

In the relative absence of hard evidence, the discussion of principles and consensus in the long-term care of people with dementia should proceed in order to provide a framework for debate and research. In this context, the discussion of the management of behavioural disorders in cerebral vascular disease and dementia is relevant as the two areas frequently co-exist. Indeed, behavioural disorder is a major risk factor that leads to early or premature institutionalization into long-term care,[2,3] is present in up to 90% of patients in nursing homes,[4] and has a negative impact on the quality of life of patients and families.[5]

Principles of long-term care

The principles of long-term care of persons with dementia do not necessarily differentiate between subtypes of dementia and may be applied equally in dementia related to cerebral vascular disease as well as in other forms of dementia. The pathways of many types of dementia as progressive, deteriorating brain disease converge to a common final pathway when the long-term management is conceptualized, planned and implemented.

A study of official policy documents from each country of the European Union by the European Trans-national Alzheimer's Study of the University of Glenmorgan was summarized by Marshall,[6] who identified five key principles emphasized by all member states. These are:

1. People with dementia should be enabled to remain at home for as long as possible.
2. Carers should receive as much help as possible in order to facilitate the above.
3. Sufferers should retain maximum control over the support they receive.
4. All relevant services should be coordinated at the local level.
5. Sufferers in institutional care should live in surroundings which are as 'homely' as possible.

Four key principles were emphasized by most member states:

1. There should be a systematic attempt to equate the provision of services with need.
2. Categorical care should be replaced by care which addresses the general need of sufferers.
3. Early diagnosis of dementia should be encouraged
4. The needs of people with dementia are not addressed separately from the needs of older people in general at the national level.

To these key principles of policy may be added, although currently without supporting research evidence, the following:

1. Long-term care in dementia is care throughout the whole pathway of dementia, not just at the high dependency end of the disease process.
2. The style of long-term care emphasizes care throughout the whole life (continuity) and all of life (holistic).

3. Ability enhancement should have higher priority than disability minimization.
4. Care should be underpinned by a sense of optimistic humanity which embraces the person with dementia, despite the multiple negative impacts of the dementia processes on the individual.
5. The ultimate criterion of care outcome is best quality of life, and is translated to a decision-making approach valuing all activities that adds to quality of life and eschews decisions which will detract from quality of life for the person with dementia.

What determines entry into long-term care?

Multidisciplinary assessment of the elderly is a well-established strategy to prevent inappropriate nursing home admissions.[7–9] Behavioural disorders,[2,3] carer burden,[10] dementia, stroke, hip and other fractures,[11] and cognitive impairment in combination with functional decline (or higher level of dependence in activities of daily living)[12] are factors related to admission to long-term residential care.

In answer to the question of whether early intervention can reduce the number of elderly people with dementia admitted to institutions of long-term care, O'Connor et al[13] offered a wide range of help, including financial benefits, physical aids, home helps, respite admissions, practical advice, and psychiatric assessment. Their conclusion was that 64% of intervention subjects were admitted at the end of 2 years compared with 8% of the non-intervention (control) group. This study is at variance with the findings of Challis et al,[14,15] which indicated that the provision of specially tailored help reduced admission rates. However, the mentally frail elderly in these studies had higher admission rates to long-term care institutions compared with the physically frail elderly. O'Connor et al[13] concluded that special assistance to the mentally frail elderly with dementia might actually increase rather than decrease the number admitted to institutions, particularly for those living alone.

Quality of life and quality of care in long-term facilities

It is an accepted axiom that quality of life is the ultimate test of any health care programme. It is assumed that quality of life can only be achieved through quality of care in a long-term care environment. In 1987 Kane[16] proposed a framework to merge the health care and social side of institutional care into a system that uses quality of life as its major outcome. She suggested a tripartite scheme which integrates the *health care component* (medical care, nursing, rehabilitation and various specialized therapies), *personal care* (assistance with routines of living such as bathing, toileting, grooming, mobility and feeding) and the *social milieu* in which such care takes place (the physical/built environment, activities, rules and expectations).

The measure of achievement of such quality of care is in the outcome of functional capacity, emotional and social well-being, autonomy, freedom and choice; these should be well balanced and integrated with an acceptance of the progressive nature of the disease process that leads the patient into long-term care. Quality of life is a multidimensional concept and reflects a patient's retained abilities, preferences, interests and perceived satisfaction.

McCurdy,[17] after reading Kitwood's vignettes of nursing home experience in the USA,[18] was moved to propose the centrality of 'personhood' in dementia care to counter 'depersonalization'—a failure to treat the resident with dementia 'fully as a person'. The widespread belief that there is 'no cure, no help, no hope' for people with dementia shapes attitudes and behavioural responses to them, and must be countered. It was argued that, despite underlying despair in both patients and carers, the need and capacity for spirituality are no less because of increasing dependence, declining verbal communication and cognitive impairment. A more expansive view of spirituality could recognize that 'connectedness' with others[19] and the presence of supportive community-based care will help to maintain the dementia sufferer's sense of spirituality. The dignity of an individual as a spiritual being is grounded in 'the belief that others held us in high regard, should rest on the fundamental knowledge that intimates, care givers and even strangers think well of me and recognizes . . . me to be as fully human as they are'.[20] The critique of Kitwood[18] is that the minimalist interpretation of 'palliation' in dementia care, that led to the sense of hopelessness as reflected in such terms as 'the death that leaves the body behind', 'keeping the patient comfortable', is not worthy of the true principles of palliative care. An essential task of providing quality care for quality of life is the cultivation of attitudes that are hopeful, open and receptive of spirituality and humanity in both the patient and the carer.

Quality environment for people with dementia

Mary Marshall[6,21] described design principles for people with dementia living in long-stay establishments. Buildings for people with dementia should:

1. make sense
2. help them to find their way
3. provide a therapeutic environment
4. provide a safe environment
5. provide good facilities for staff.

Marshall argued that good design is integral to good care, and technological development should provide new opportunity for increasing dependence, dignity and privacy. There exists a remarkable international consensus on design for people with dementia, as summarized in Table 19.1.[6] The application of such sound design principles can lead to further research into the efficacy in outcome for people with dementia who live in such environments. The application of these principles in other cultures may require the identification of different characteristics to those for developed or economically advantaged Western societies. The increasing emphasis on people with dementia living in their own homes will call for the development of modifications of these design characteristics for homes and domestic dwellings.

The role of the primary care physician in long-term care

The primary care physician is increasingly taking a more important part in the long-term care of people with dementia. This has arisen from a combination of social policy imperatives to keep people at home as long as

Table 19.1 The consensus on principles and key design features.

The consensus on principles of design includes:
- design should compensate for disability
- design should maximize independence
- design should enhance self-esteem and confidence
- design should demonstrate care for staff
- design should be orientating and understandable
- design should reflect a balance of safety and autonomy
- design should reinforce personal identity
- design should welcome relatives and the local community
- design should allow control of stimuli

The consensus on design features includes:
- small
- familiar, domestic, homely in style
- plenty of scope for ordinary activities (unit kitchens, washing lines, garden sheds)
- unobtrusive concern for safety
- different rooms for different functions
- age-appropriate furniture and fittings
- safe outside space
- single rooms big enough for lots of personal belongings
- good signage and multiple cues where possible, e.g. sight, smell, sound
- use of objects rather than colour for orientation
- enhanced visual access
- controlled stimuli, especially noise

Reproduced with permission from the *International Journal of Geriatric Psychiatry*.

possible and the allocation of primary care physicians to nursing homes as the responsible physicians. In response to this, Jarvik and Wiseman[22] offered a very practical approach using the mnemonic FICS'M (Family, Intellectual Status, Continence, Sleep and Mobility) to help physicians to address treatable problems associated with people with dementing illnesses. They also advocated that both the patient and the carer-giver(s) should be evaluated at regular intervals.

Support and education for the patient's family includes the provision of accurate and understandable answers to their questions, referral to appropriate services and resources, treatment of disturbing behaviours, assistance in the negotiation of long-term placement and support through post mortem investigations. It is important that the patient's intellectual status be observed through identification and treatment of delirium, depression and iatrogenc effects and that information be supplied regarding drug trials for cognitive impairments. Any continence issues should be discussed thoroughly, to be followed by investigation and retraining regimes. Sleep problems pose a considerable burden for both patients and carers, therefore counselling on sleep hygiene and the treatment of insomnia is very useful. Mobility impairment, which frequently accompanies ageing, orthopaedic disorders or stroke should be energetically investigated and treated. Prevention of mobility decline by early intervention through physiotherapy should be anticipated. Reduction of mobility side effects of medication (akathisia, rigidity, falls, ataxia) by close surveillance of both prescribed and over-the-counter medication is necessary. Removal of hazards in the home and modifications to the built environment to prevent falls will require the services of an occupational therapist through referral by the primary care physician. This reinforces the idea that the primary care physician is in the best position to undertake case management to ensure that the total health, well-being and social circumstances be provided for in an integrated and comprehensive manner.

Such interventions should take into account the physical, psychological and social problems associated with dementia and will substantially increase mobility and improve the quality of life of both patient and carers.

Behavioural and psychological symptoms of dementia

In the spring of 1996 the International Psychogeriatric Association (IPA) convened a Consensus Conference on the Behavioural Disturbance of Dementia to:

1. review current knowledge on behavioural disturbances of dementia, and

2. to reach some consensus in the four critical areas of nosology, aetiology, clinical symptoms and research direction.

This consensus group of some 60 experts in the field from 16 countries produced a statement on the definition of BPSD: 'Symptoms of disturbed perception, thought content, mood and behaviour that frequently occur in patients with dementia.[23]

Non-cognitive behavioural changes in dementia have been a major management issue in long-term care and have been a subject for research efforts over many years. However, very few studies differentiated between the behavioural and psychological symptoms of dementia in subtypes of dementia, as they were mainly directed at dementia in Alzheimer's disease (AD). Where vascular dementia (VAD) subjects have been included, no separate analysis has been undertaken.[24] The longitudinal study by Hope et al[24] identified 75 patients with AD, seven with VAD and 15 with mixed dementia in a sample of subjects living at home, but did not attempt to analyse the VAD data separately due to the small number of VAD subjects in this study.

Eight of the most common behavioural changes were reported by Hope et al using the present behaviour examination (PBE) schedule.[25] These were:

- moving and mislaying objects
- verbal aggression
- walking or other activities at night
- eating less
- apparent sadness
- hyperphagia
- changed food choice and
- repeated request or demands.

This study of home dwelling subjects complements the study of Burns et al[26] in clinic and hospital subjects with lower cognitive function. By statistical analysis, Hope[27] classified such behaviour into three behavioural syndromes:

- *overactivity* (walking more, aimless walking, trailing and checking)
- *aggressive behaviour* (aggressive resistance in the context of intimate care, physical aggression, verbal aggression
- *psychosis* (hallucinations, persecutory ideas, anxiety).

In addition, depressive mood was noted as an entity in its own right and not closely related to the described behavioural syndromes.

The management of BPSD can be readily divided into pharmacological and non-pharmacological strategies. Pharmacological treatment targets symptoms which may respond to a particular drug treatment and should be time limited. Antipsychotics, both conventional and newer agents, can be useful in the treatment of psychotic symptoms of hallucinations, delusions, hostility, aggression, agitation, violent behaviour and sleep–wake cycle disturbances. Benzodiazepines help to reduce anxiety, agitation, tension and sleep disturbance. For depressive symptoms the whole range of antidepressants is available, although the traditional tricyclic antidepressants do have significant unwanted side effects which are to be avoided in the elderly. The elderly tolerate better the newer products such as selective serotonin reuptake inhibitors (SSRI), serotonin and norepinephrine reuptake inhibitors (SNRI) and other novel agents. Anticonvulsants such as carbamazepine and valproic acid are increasingly being used for BPSD,[28,29] particularly in patients with cerebral vascular disease and dementia.

Non-pharmacological modalities of treatment, especially those of psychosocial methodology, have been reported to be effective but lack the vigour of randomized controlled trials. However, the reported efficacy in environmental interventions,[30] recreational, adjunctive and social strategies[31,32] and psychological interventions[33] do point to possibilities in improving the quality of life of patients in long-term care through a variety of non-drug interventions.

Conclusion

In the area of long-term care for patients with dementia of all types there remains many unanswered research questions. Any evidence that may be available is derived from the study of patients with AD and not specifically VAD subjects. Whether studies in AD patients can be generalized to patients with non-Alzheimer's type dementia is a major issue awaiting clarification.

Another essential question requiring vigorous research is whether patients with cerebrovascular disease and dementia will respond to interventions (either pharmacological or non-pharmacological) in the same way as AD patients.

Grouping together all patients with dementia cannot clarify these questions. However, separating subjects with non-Alzheimer's subtypes from the AD group places the researchers in the invidious position of having small sample sizes and lacking statistical power in quantitative studies. While multi-centre studies may address the problem, this raises considerable logistical difficulties which will need to be overcome if we are to have a better understanding of the outcomes of interventions that target patients with cerebral vascular disease and dementia.

Qualitative methodology in combination with quantitative methodology may go some way towards resolving this dilemma. Woods[34] suggested that while, methodologically, RCTs are not able to provide the answers to all the complex issues, the evaluation of consecutive single case studies in terms of treatment failure and success will continue to be valuable. In clinical practice single case methodology frequently provides the initial basis for the development of a hypothesis which can then be tested and evaluated using group study methodology including RCTs.

With the improvements in the number of people surviving stroke (see Chapter 20), it is possible that some of these may proceed to develop VAD and thereby add to the pool of patients requiring long-term care. Therefore, more targeted research is needed into long-term care for patients of this group in order to provide the best quality of life for them through their pathway of dementia.

References.

1. Downs MG, Zarit SH, What works in dementia care? Research evidence for policy and practice, Part I, *Int J Geriat Psychiatry* (1999) **14**:83–5.
2. Colerick EJ, George LK, Predictors of institutionalisation amongst care-givers of patients with Alzheimer's disease, *J Am Geriatr Soc* (1986) **7**:493–8.
3. O'Donnell BF, Drachman DA, Barnes HJ et al, Incontinence and troublesome behaviour predict institutionalisation in dementia, *J Geriatr Psychiatry Neurol* (1992) **5**:45–52.
4. Finkel SI, The signs of the behavioural and psychological symptoms of dementia, *Clinician* (1998) **16**:33–42.
5. Finkel SI, Costa e Silva J, Cohen G et al, Behavioural and psychological signs and symptoms of dementia: a consensus statement on the current knowledge and implications for research and treatment, *Int Psychogeriatr* (1996) **8**(Suppl 3):497–500.
6. Marshall M, What do service planners and policy makers need from research? *Int J Geriatr Psychiatry* (1999) **14**:86–96.
7. Kane RI, Rubenstein LZ, Brook RH et al, Utilization review in nursing homes: making implicit level-of-care judgments explicit, *Med Care* (1981) **19**:3–13.
8. Quartararo M, O'Neill TJ, Tang G et al, Assessing the residential care needs of nursing home applicants, *Aus J Pub Health* (1991) **15**:222–7.
9. George S, Measures of dependency: the use in assessing the need for residential care for the elderly, *J Pub Health Med* (1991) **13**:178–81.
10. Rabins PV, Mace NL, Lucas MJ, The impact of dementia on the family, *JAMA* (1982) **248**:333–5.
11. Temkin-Greener H, Meiners MR, Transitions in long term care, *Gerontol* (1995) **15**:196–206.
12. Quartararo M, Glasziou P, Kerr CB, Classification trees for decision-making in long term care, *J Geronto* (1995) **50A**:M298–302.
13. O'Connor DW, Pollitt PA, Brook CPB et al, Does early intervention reduce the number of elderly people with dementia admitted to institutions for long term care? *Br Med J* (1991) **302**:871–5.
14. Challis D, Davies B, *Case Management in Community Care: An Evaluated Experiment in the Home Care of the Elderly* (Gower: Aldershot, 1986).

15. Challis D, Chessum R, Chesterman J et al, *Case Management in Social and Health Care* (University of Kent Personal Social Science Research Unit: Canterbury, 1990).
16. Kane RA, Quality of life in long term institutions—is a regulatory strategy feasible? *Dan Med Bull* (1987) Special Suppl Series No **5**:73–81.
17. McCurdy DB, Personhood, spirituality and hope in the care of human beings with dementia, *J Clin Ethics* (1998) **9**:81–92.
18. Kitwood T, *Dementia Reconsidered: The Person Comes First* (Open University Press: Philadelphia, 1997).
19. Richards M, Seicol S, The challenge of maintaining spiritual connectedness for persons institutionalised with dementia, *J Relig Gerontol* (1991) **7**:38.
20. Holstein M, Reflections on death and dying, *Acad Med* (1997) **72**:850.
21. Marshall M, Better quality environment for people with dementia. In: Jacoby R, Oppenheimer K eds, *Psychiatry of the Elderly* (Oxford University Press: Oxford, 1998).
22. Jarvik LF, Wiseman EJ, A checklist for managing the dementia patient, *Geriatrics* (1991) **46**:31–40.
23. International Psychogeriatric Association, *BPSD Educational Pack* (Gardiner-Calwall: Macclesfield, 1998).
24. Hope T, Keene J, Gedling K et al, Behavioural changes in dementia: 1. Point of entry data of a prospective study, *Int J Geriatr Psychiatry* (1997) **12**:1062–73.
25. Hope T, Fairburn C, The present behavioural examination (PBE): the development of an interview to measure current behavioural abnormalities, *Psychol Med* (1992) **22**:223–30.
26. Burns A, Jacoby R, Levy R, Psychiatric phenomena in Alzheimer's disease I, II, III, IV, *Br J Psychiatry* (1990) **157**:72–94.
27. Hope T, Keene J, Fairburn C et al, Behaviour changes in dementia: 2. Are there behavioural syndromes, *Int J Geriatr Psychiatry* (1997) **12**:1074–8.
28. Tariot PN, Erb R, Podgorski CA et al, Efficacy and tolerability of carbamazepine for agitation and aggression in dementia, *Am J Psychiatry* (1998) **155**:54–61.
29. Lott AD, McElroy SC, Keys MA, Sodim valporate in the treatment of behavioural agitation in elderly patients with dementia. *J Neuropsychiatry Clin Neurosci* (1995) **7**:314–9.
30. Burgio L, Interventions for the behavioural complications of Alzheimer's disease, *Int Psychogeriatr* (1996) **8**(Suppl 1):45–52.
31. Rovner B, Steele CD, Shmuely Y et al, A randomized control trial of dementia care in nursing homes, *J Am Geriatr Soc* (1996) **44**:7–13.
32. Hanser SB, Music therapy to reduce anxiety, agitation and depression, *Nursing Home Med* (1996) **4**:286–91.
33. Miller MD, Opportunity for psychotherapy for patients with dementia, *J Geriatr Psychiatry Neurol* (1989) **2**:11–17.
34. Woods B, Promoting wellbeing and independence for people with dementia, *In J Geriatr Psychiatry* (1999) **14**:97–109.

20
Prevention

Stephen M Davis

Introduction

Despite the varied pathologies causing vascular dementia (VAD), it is generally presumed to be the only preventable form of dementia.[1,2] Post-stroke dementia is common. One study found an incidence, 1 year after stroke, of 5% in patients over 60 and 10% over 90 years.[3] It is more common than Alzheimer's disease (AD) in Asia and other developing regions and may therefore be the commonest form of dementia worldwide.[4]

As discussed in earlier chapters of this book, VAD encompasses a range of pathologies, some of which overlap with AD.[5] This interface first includes the mixed dementias, where there are pathological features suggesting a direct contribution of both aetiologies,[6] and second the concept that some types of vascular disease, notably amyloid angiopathy, are directly implicated in the pathology of AD.

Cognitive impairments related to strokes can also be due to a variety of pathological types and locations of the underlying cerebral lesions. Earlier studies linked the development of dementia to multiple cortical infarcts producing cumulative brain volume loss. Dementia can also be produced by small yet strategically placed infarcts in the thalamus, caudate head or angular gyrus (Figure 20.1). The association of dementia with multiple subcortical lacunar infarcts was recognized early in the French literature (*etat lacunaire*). Lacunar infarcts and other manifestations of deep white matter ischaemia were historically recognized by Binswanger as a cause of VAD.[7] The concept of leukoaraiosis was introduced by Hachinski in the 1980s to describe manifestations of subcortical white matter ischaemia demonstrated on neuroimaging techniques such as computed tomography (CT) and magnetic resonance imaging (MRI).[8] The magnitude of white matter changes on MRI has been correlated with cognitive impairments.[9] The recent delineation of CADASIL (cerebral autosomal dominant arteriopathy with subcortical infarcts and leukoencephalopathy), a genetically determined cause of white matter pathology and dementia, provided further insights into a genetically-determined cause of VAD (Figure 20.2).[10]

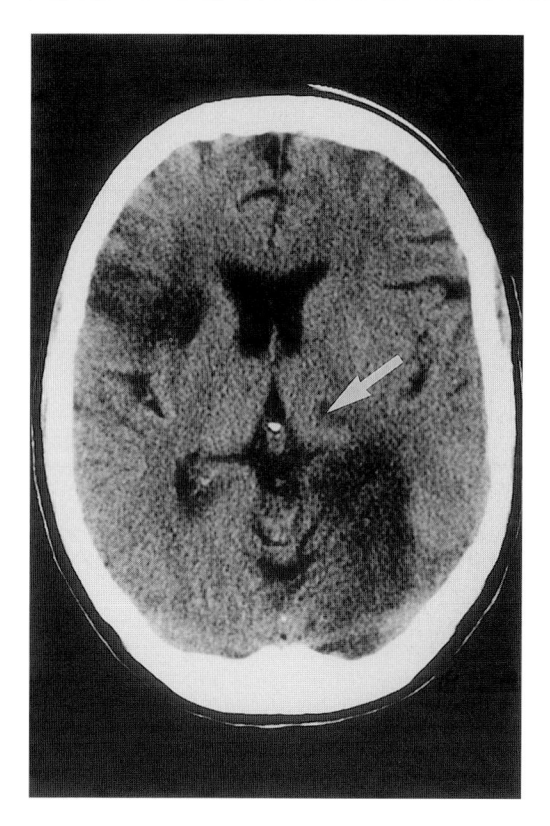

Figure 20.1

An example of multiple cerbral infarcts shown on CT scan. Regions of cerebral infarction include infarction in the right middle cerbral and left posterior cerebral artery (PCA) territory. The left PCA infarct includes infarction of the thalamus, a common cause of memory abnormalities (arrow).

In most Western countries, there has been an impressive fall in population-based stroke mortality over the past few decades.[11] However, with the ageing of the population and lack of decline in the incidence of stroke, a marked increase in stroke prevalence has been predicted.[12] Furthermore, age is the strongest independent risk factor for the development of VAD.[13] In the individual patient, the impressive advances in stroke prevention via a range of proven strategies should translate to a lowered risk of the development of VAD. There have been few studies to test this hypothesis specifically. Hence, this chapter will involve a brief review of the major modifiable risk factors for stroke and the effects of primary and secondary stroke prevention, based on the evidence from randomized, controlled clinical trials.

Prevention of VAD: an overall approach

Stroke prevention involves primary and secondary strategies. Primary prevention includes treatment of risk factors and cerebrovascular lesions,

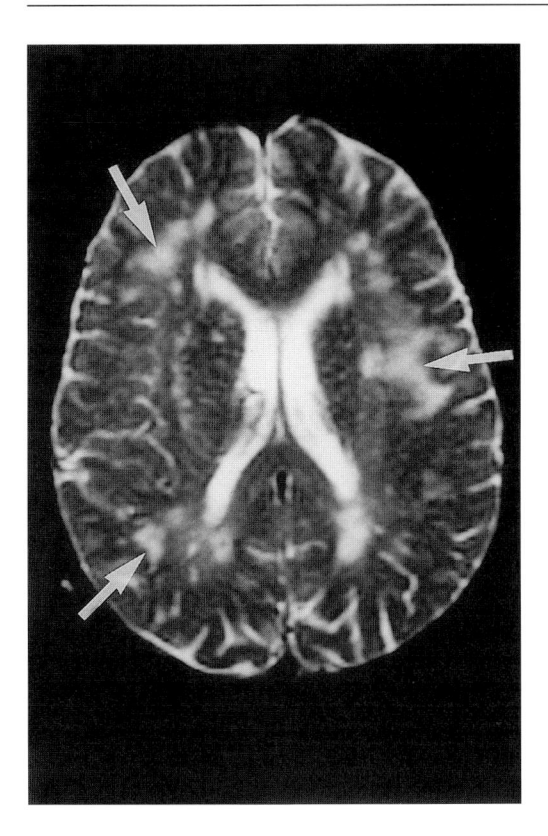

Figure 20.2
MR scan showing multifocal white matter abnormalities (arrow) in a 46-year-old man presenting with cerebral infarction. He had no conventional risk factors for stroke and a brother in his 40s had a stroke with very similar MR abnormalities, suggestive of CADASIL (cerebral autosomal dominant arteriopathy with subcortical infarcts and leukoencephalopathy).

in individuals who have not experienced cerebrovascular symptoms. Secondary prevention involves strategies used after a stroke or transient ischaemic attack (TIA), which should be tailored to the specific type of cerebrovascular pathology. Stroke is the third most common cause of death in most Western countries and the commonest cause of chronic adult disability. While most stroke prevention studies have focused on a reduction in the incidence of stroke and neurological disability, prevention of VAD should be a crucial endpoint. This is now being addressed in some stroke prevention trials such as the PROGRESS study (perindopril protection against recurrent stroke study).[14]

Primary prevention

Primary prevention strategies target the major risk factors for stroke (Table 20.1). In the consideration of risk factors and stroke, the population attributable risk is a useful concept to evaluate the overall importance of a risk factor, combining the relative risk of the individual factor and its prevalence.[15]

Table 20.1 Risk factors for ischaemic stroke (adapted from Srikanth and Donnan[16]).

Risk factor	Relative risk of stroke	Modifiable	Benefits proven
Age and gender	Increasing age, male gender	No	
Smoking	1.0–4.0	Yes	Yes
Previous stroke, TIA	5.0-10.0	Yes	Yes
Hypertension	2.0–4.0	Yes	Yes
Diabetes	2.0–8.0	Yes	Yes
Heart disease (particularly atrial fibrillation)	6.0–8.0	Yes	Yes
Hypercholesterolaemia	1.0–2.0	Yes	Yes
Miscellaneous (obesity, lack of exercise, snoring, high haematocrit, elevated fibrinogen)	Variable	Yes	Some (e.g. exercise)

Age and gender
In general, the frequency of stroke increases with advancing age, although there are important differences between stroke subtypes. For example, patients with subarachnoid haemorrhage are usually aged 30–60 years; it often affects young and middle-aged adults in their productive years. Conversely, cerebral infarcts due to extracranial vascular disease occur in older individuals. Overall, male gender is associated with increased stroke risk. Among older patients there is a slightly higher rate of stroke in females, but this may simply reflect the greater longevity of women.

Hypertension
Hypertension is the most important risk factor for both cerebral infarction and haemorrhage.[15,17] The population attributable risk from hypertension has been estimated as 26%.[15] Numerous population studies have demonstrated an increased frequency of stroke with both systolic and diastolic hypertension.[14] Hypertension can be correlated with common pathogenetic stroke mechanisms. These include cardiac disease with the increased risk of cerebral embolism, intracerebral small vessel disease producing lacunar infarction, extracranial atherosclerosis producing thromboembolism, development of cerebral aneurysms and rupture of deep perforating vessels producing intracerebral haemorrhage.

A meta-analysis of 14 randomized trials of antihypertensive therapy showed that modest blood pressure reduction of 5–6 mmHg reduces stroke risk by about 40%.[18] This benefit also extends to those with mild hypertension. Most of these trials of antihypertensive agents involved beta blockers and diuretics, rather than the newer agents such as the angiotensin converting enzyme inhibitors, angiotensin II blockers and calcium channel antagonists. Effective antihypertensive therapy should translate to a lower risk of VAD.[19]

Cardiac disease

Valvular heart disease, from a congenital or rheumatic cause, has long been recognized as a cause of cerebral embolism. The decline in the incidence of rheumatic heart disease, associated with a 17-fold increase in stroke risk in those with atrial fibrillation, has probably contributed to the reduction in population-based stroke mortality.[20] Attention has more recently been focused on other forms of cardiac disease, particularly non-valvular atrial fibrillation, the most common cause of cardiogenic cerebral infarction in Western countries. It is associated with a six to eight times increase in stroke risk.[20] Atrial fibrillation represents an extraordinarily important opportunity for stroke prevention.[21] An Australian study indicated that approximately 1.7% of the population aged 60 years had atrial fibrillation, rising to 11% in those older than 75 years.[22]

Recent clinical trials have demonstrated a substantial relative risk reduction of about 70% in the stroke rate in patients with non-valvular atrial fibrillation but without cerebrovascular symptoms, treated with warfarin.[21] In compliant patients, there are quite low risks of major haemorrhagic complications with careful monitoring, maintaining the international normalized ratio (INR) in the 2–3 range. There is also a modest therapeutic benefit with aspirin, although it is only about half as effective as warfarin.[21] Aspirin should be used when patients are not candidates for anticoagulation, and in those under the age of 60 years with atrial fibrillation, but without risk factors or echocardiographic features of structural heart disease ('lone atrial fibrillation').

In patients with valvular heart disease and atrial fibrillation, the risk of stroke is far higher than in those with non-valvular atrial fibrillation.[20] Warfarin is effective and is combined with aspirin to convey additional benefit in patients with prosthetic heart valves and atrial fibrillation or prior thrombo-embolism.[23]

Diabetes

Diabetes mellitus is associated with a two- to five-fold increase in the rate of stroke.[24] This is due to both accelerated atherogenesis in the extracranial arteries (macrovascular disease) and also to the development of small vessel, lacunar infarcts (microvascular disease). Diabetes is also associated with intravascular factors that potentiate stroke, such as increased blood viscosity. The prognosis of acute stroke in diabetic and other hyperglycaemic patients is worse than in those with normal blood sugar levels, probably due to the production of excessive lactate and increased tissue damage.[25] Optimal control of blood glucose is likely to reduce the vascular complications of diabetes.

Smoking
Smoking is an important specific risk factor for stroke, particularly ischaemic stroke and subarachnoid haemorrhage.[26,27] It at least doubles stroke risk in both men and women.[28] Like diabetes, smoking accelerates atherogenesis and has intravascular effects on platelet adhesion and viscosity. The intravascular effects appear to be particularly important, in that there is a substantial reduction of stroke risk within 2–4 years of smoking cessation.[28,29] Chronic smoking also lowers cerebral blood flow. For these reasons, reduction in population-based smoking rates is an important public health strategy for stroke prevention.[30]

Hypercholesterolaemia
Hyperlipidaemia, and in particular hypercholesterolaemia, has been thought to be a somewhat weaker risk factor for stroke than ischaemic heart disease in epidemiological studies.[31] However, elevation of the low density lipoprotein (LDL) cholesterol fraction is significantly related to increased cerebrovascular atherosclerosis. Recent trials of the HMG-CoA reductase inhibitors (the 'statin' drugs), which produce potent cholesterol reduction, have shown in patients with ischaemic heart disease and cholesterol ranging from normal to high levels a marked reduction in the risk of stroke.[32,33] The efficacy of these drugs is likely to reflect other pharmacological actions also, including antiplatelet effects and actions on atherosclerotic plaque.

Heavy alcohol use
Heavy alcohol usage is associated with an increased risk of both ischaemic and haemorrhagic stroke, particularly subarachnoid haemorrhage. In contrast, some studies have suggested that low to moderate alcohol intake may actually be stroke-protective.[30]

Miscellaneous factors
Polycythaemia is an important and treatable risk factor for cerebral infarction. An elevated haematocrit, even in the upper 'physiological' range, is associated with increased stroke risk and stroke severity. Leisure-time physical activity has been linked with reduced risk of ischaemic stroke.[34]

Asymptomatic carotid disease
Carotid bruits occur in at least 4% of asymptomatic adults over the age of 40 years, of which only a proportion are due to severe internal carotid

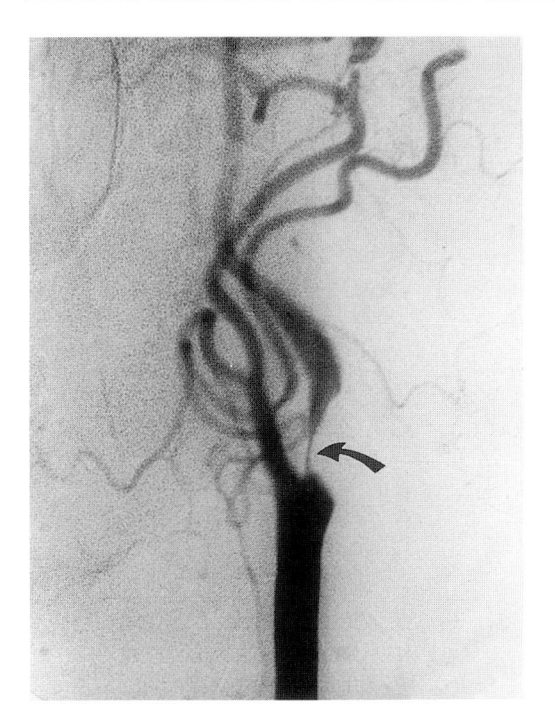

Figure 20.3
Angiogram showing severe left internal carotid stenosis (arrow).

stenosis (Figure 20.3). They are associated with a mild increase in stroke risk, and are a stronger predictor of myocardial infarction. There have been a number of randomized controlled trials to determine whether carotid endarterectomy (CEA) is indicated in patients with severe but asymptomatic carotid stenosis (Figure 20.3). The most definitive of these indicated that there was an 11% stroke rate in the hemisphere ipsilateral to a 60% or greater carotid stenosis, reduced significantly to 5% by CEA in good surgical hands.[35] However, this study also confirmed that the natural history of asymptomatic carotid stenosis was relatively benign. Therefore, a large number of operations would be required to prevent one stroke. The place of CEA for asymptomatic carotid stenosis therefore remains controversial.[36]

Secondary prevention

Secondary prevention strategies after stroke, unlike the primary prevention techniques, are tailored to the underlying stroke pathology. The range of secondary prevention strategies continues to expand (Table 20.2).[37] The last decade has seen the development of a number of new antiplatelet strategies, proof of the efficacy of warfarin in patients with

Table 20.2 Therapeutic opportunities in secondary prevention.

Strategy	Indication	Level of evidence
Antiplatelet and anticoagulant strategies		
· Combination antiplatelet strategies		II (Combined aspirin/dipyridamole)
· Aspirin		I
· Ticlopidine		II
· Clopidogrel		II
· Dipyridamole		II
· Glycoprotein IIb/IIIa inhibitors		Not yet available
· Warfarin	Non-valvular atrial fibrillation, valvular heart disease	I
Surgical and interventional strategies		
· Carotid endarterectomy	Symptomatic carotid stenosis	I
· Angioplasty/stenting	Not yet proven, possibly patients with extracranial, intracranial symptomatic atherosclerotic stenosis	III No randomized, controlled trials yet confirming benefits

Quality of Evidence Ratings (NHMRC Guidelines, December 1996)

Level I: Evidence is obtained from a systematic review of all relevant randomised controlled trials.
Level II: Evidence is obtained from at least one properly designed randomised controlled trial.
Level III: Evidence is obtained from well designed controlled trials without randomisation; from well designed cohort or case-control analytic studies, preferably from more than one centre or research group; from multiple time series with or without the intervention; or from dramatic results in uncontrolled experiments.
Level IV: Opinions of respected authorities, based on clinical experience, descriptive studies, or reports of expert committees.

non-valvular atrial fibrillation (both primary and secondary prevention), better delineation of the indications for carotid endarterectomy for symptomatic and asymptomatic disease, and the introduction of cerebrovascular angioplasty.

Antiplatelet strategies

The benefits of aspirin were first established by pivotal studies two decades ago, with a relative risk reduction of about 22% for the composite outcomes of stroke, death or myocardial infarction.[38] Over this period, there was heated controversy about the most effective and safe dose of aspirin in secondary prevention. Recent meta-analysis of the 10 secondary prevention trials where aspirin was tested against placebo showed no discernible difference between high, medium and low doses of aspirin.[39] The general consensus amongst stroke investigators today is that doses in the 'low' 50–325 mg range are preferred.

The effectiveness of aspirin depends on the inhibition of platelet cyclooxygenase, but other antiplatelet strategies with differing actions have also been proven to be effective in stroke prevention. Ticlopidine was shown to have a significant protective effect after thrombo-embolic stroke and to be more effective than aspirin in a trial which involved direct comparison of the agents.[40] Ticlopidine, however, is associated with a 1–2% risk of severe although reversible neutropenia and a 5–10% rate of troublesome diarrhoea. Clopidogrel, like Ticlopidine, inhibits platelet ADP. It was shown in the CAPRIE (Clopidogrel vs aspirin in patients at risk of ischaemic events) trial to be more effective than aspirin in stroke prevention, without the risk of neutropenia.[41] The CAPRIE trial showed a relative risk reduction of 8.7% for Clopidogrel over aspirin. By inference, if one assumes about a one-quarter reduction of vascular events in 'at risk' patients using aspirin, this can be improved to approximately one-third with Clopidogrel. However, because of the small absolute risk reduction (approximately 0.5% per year) and the cost of the drug, it is likely that Clopidogrel will be mainly used as second line therapy in patients who are either intolerant of aspirin or are aspirin failures. Clopidogrel and aspirin are likely to have an additive or synergistic effect because of their different actions. This is currently being tested in cardiac trials and probably will be evaluated in patients with prior TIA or stroke.

Dipyridamole reduces platelet aggregation by raising the antiaggregating effects of cyclic AMP and cyclic GMP. A synergistic effect between aspirin and dipyridamole was demonstrated in the European Stroke Prevention Study (ESPS) 2 trial.[42] In this factorial design, the relative stroke risk was reduced by 18% with aspirin, 16% with dipyridamole, and an apparently additive 37% with the combination of these two therapies.

The platelet glycoprotein IIb/IIIa receptor is the final common pathway of platelet aggregation. Oral platelet GPIIb/IIIa antagonists prevent the binding of fibrinogen to platelets and are currently being investigated as a potentially potent strategy in the prevention of major vascular events after stroke and acute myocardial infarction.[43,44]

Warfarin
Most of the recent trials evaluating warfarin with non-valvular atrial fibrillation have evaluated warfarin as a primary prevention strategy, as patients with prior stroke or transient ischaemic attack were excluded. The European Atrial Fibrillation trial[45] compared warfarin, aspirin and placebo in secondary stroke prevention after recent TIA or ischaemic stroke. While both warfarin and aspirin were significantly effective in reducing stroke risk, warfarin was substantially more effective than aspirin and is the recommended strategy in appropriate anticoagulation candidates.

Carotid endarterectomy
Two large trials (the North American Symptomatic Carotid Endarterectomy Trial, NASCET, and the European Carotid Surgery Trial, ECST) showed major benefits for carotid endarterectomy over optimal medical therapy in patients with greater than 70% carotid stenosis and either TIA or non-disabling stroke (Figure 20.3).[46,47] In the NASCET study, an absolute risk reduction of 17% over 18 months was achieved, indicating that one stroke could be prevented for every six patients treated over this period.[46]

Cerebrovascular angioplasty
Percutaneous transluminal angioplasty, of established value for coronary artery disease, has been more recently used for symptomatic carotid stenosis, usually combined with endovascular stenting.[48] A large number of uncontrolled studies have demonstrated that the risks of the procedure are approximately equivalent to those of carotid endarterectomy. The technique is appealing in that a good radiological result can be demonstrated with reduced inpatient length of stay. However, the long-term benefits remain unclear. Large trials are being conducted to compare the safety and efficacy of carotid angioplasty/stenting with carotid endarterectomy, in patients with symptomatic carotid stenosis. The technique has also been used in small numbers of patients with surgically inaccessible, intracranial stenoses. It may have a role in patients with asymptomatic carotid stenosis.

Conclusions

In summary, despite the heterogeneity of pathologies underlying VAD, most share common risk factors which can be modified by primary prevention strategies. Secondary prevention strategies should impact on relevant pathologies, such as cardioembolic cerebral infarction, lacunar infarction, and large vessel disease with thrombo-embolism. As indicated above, most of these studies have recorded composite outcomes of death, stroke, myocardial infarction and stroke related disability, but have not evaluated the development of dementia. Hence, more information is needed to gauge the efficacy of prevention strategies for VAD. Scientific validation is required with careful trial design and longer outcome studies. In the interim, promotion of primary and secondary vascular prevention strategies should emphasize the prevention of VAD, as well as stroke, myocardial infarction and vascular death.

References

1. Hachinski V, Preventable senility: a call for action against the vascular dementias, *Lancet* (1992) **340**: 645–8.
2. Butler RN, Ahronheim J, Fillit H et al, Vascular dementia: stroke prevention takes on new urgency, *Geriatrics* (1993) **48**:32–42.
3. Tatemichi TK, Foulkes MA, Mohr JP et al, Dementia in stroke survivors in the stroke data bank cohort. Prevalence, incidence, risk factors, and computed tomographic finds, *Stroke* (1990) **21**:858–66.
4. Gorelick PB, Roman GC, Vascular dementia: a time to 'seize the moment', *Neuroepidemiology* (1993) **12**:139–40.
5. Pasquier F, Leys D, Why are stroke patients prone to develop dementia? *J Neurol* (1997) **244**: 135–42.
6. Bowler JV, Eliasziew M, Steenhuis R et al, Comparative evolution of Alzheimer disease, vascular dementia and mixed dementia, *Arch Neurol* (1997) **54**:697–703.
7. Hachinski VC, Binswanger's disease: neither Binswanger's nor a disease (editorial), *J Neurol Sci* (1991) **103**:1.
8. Hachinski VC, Potter P, Merskey H, Leuko-araiosis, *Arch Neurol* (1987) **44**:42.
9. Breteler MMB, van Swieten JC, Bots M L et al, Cerebral white matter lesions, vascular risk factors, and cognitive function in a population-based study: The Rotterdam Study, *Neurology* (1994) **44**: 1246–52.
10. Dichgans M, Mayer M, Uttner I et al, The phenotypic spectrum of CADASIL: clinical findings in 102 cases, *Ann Neurol* (1998) **44**: 731–9.
11. Bennett S, Cardiovascular risk factors in Australia: trends in socioeconomic inequalities, *J Epidemiol Community Health* (1995) **49**: 363–72.
12. Jamrozik K, Stroke: a looming epidemic? *Aust Fam Physician* (1997) **26**:1137–43.
13. Gorelick PB, Status of risk factors for dementia associated with stroke, *Stroke* (1997) **28**:459–63.
14. MacMahon S, Rodgers A, Antihypertensive agents and stroke prevention, *Cerebrovasc Dis* (1994) **4**:11–15.
15. Whisnant JP, Modeling of risk factors for ischemic stroke: the Wills Lecture, *Stroke* (1997) **28**:1840–4.
16. Srikanth V, Donnan DA, Stroke: a current perspective, *Curr Therap* (1998) **39**:39–45.
17. Rodgers A, MacMahon S, Gamble

G et al for the UK Transient Ischaemic Attack Collaborative Group, Blood pressure and risk of stroke in patients with cerebrovascular disease, *Br Med J* (1996) **313**:147.
18. Collins R, Peto R, MacMahon S et al, Epidemiology, *Lancet* (1990) **335**:827–38.
19. Whitlock G, MacMahon S, Anderson C et al, Blood pressure lowering for the prevention of cognitive decline in patients with cerebrovascular disease, *Clin Exper Hypertension* (1997) **19**:843–55.
20. Atrial Fibrillation Investigators, Risk factors for stroke and efficacy of antithrombotic therapy in atrial fibrillation. Analysis of pooled data from five randomized controlled trials, *Arch Intern Med* (1994) **154**:1449–57.
21. Lake FR, Cullen KJ, de Klerk NH et al, Atrial fibrillation and mortality in an elderly population, *Aust NZ J Med* (1989) **19**:321–6.
22. Wolf PA, Dawber TR, Emerson TH, Kannel WB, Epidemiologic assessment of chronic atrial fibrillation and risk of stroke: the Framingham Study, *Neurology* (1978) **28**:973–7.
23. Turpie AGG, Gent M, Laupacis A et al, A comparison of aspirin with placebo in patients treated with warfarin after heart-valve replacement, *N Engl J Med* (1993) **329**:524–9.
24. Zimmet PZ, Alberti KGMM, The changing face of macrovascular disease in non-insulin-dependent diabetes mellitus: an epidemic in progress, *Lancet* (1997) **350**:1–4.
25. Kiers L, Davis SM, Larkins R et al, Stroke topography and outcome in relation to hyperglycaemia and diabetes, *J Neurol Neurosurg Psychiatry* (1992) **55**:263–70.
26. Shinton R, Beevers G, Meta-analysis of relation between cigarette smoking and stroke, *Br Med J* (1989) **298**:789–94.
27. Donnan GA, You R, Thrift A, McNeil JJ, Smoking as a risk factor for stroke, *Cerebrovasc Dis* (1993) **3**:129–38.
28. Robbins AS, Manson JE, Lee IM et al, Cigarette smoking and stroke in a cohort of US male physicians, *Ann Intern Med* (1994) **120**:458–62.
29. Kawachi I, Colditz GA, Stampfer MJ et al, Smoking cessation and decreased risk of stroke in women, *JAMA* (1993) **269**:232–6.
30. Jamrozik K, Broadhurst RJ, Anderson CS, Stewart-Wynne ED, The role of lifestyle factors in the etiology of stroke: a population-based case-control study in Perth, Western Australia, *Stroke* (1994) **25**:51–9.
31. Atkins D, Pstay BM, Koepsell TD et al, Cholesterol reduction and the risk for stroke in men. A meta-analysis of randomized, controlled trials, *Ann Intern Med* (1993) **119**:136–45.
32. Blauw GJ, Lagaay AM, Smelt AHM, Westendorp RGJ, Stroke, statins and cholesterol. A meta-analysis of randomized, placebo-controlled, double-blind trials with HMG-CoA reductase inhibitors, *Stroke* (1997) **28**:946–50.
33. Bucher HC, Griffith LE, Guyatt GH, Effect of HMG-CoA reductase inhibitors on stroke. A meta-analysis of randomized controlled trials, *Ann Intern Med* (1998) **128**:89–95.
34. Sacco RL, Gan R, Boden-Albala B et al, Leisure-time physical activity and ischemic stroke risk. The Northern Manhattan Stroke Study, *Stroke* (1998) **29**:380–7.
35. Executive Committee for the Asymptomatic Carotid Atherosclerosis Study, Endarterectomy for asymptomatic carotid artery stenosis, *JAMA* (1995) **273**:1421–8.
36. National Health and Medical Research Council (NHMRC), *Clini-*

cal Practice Guidelines: Prevention of Stroke (December 1996).
37. Davis SM, Donnan GA, Secondary prevention for stroke after CAPRIE and ESPS 2, Cerebrovasc Dis (1998) **8**:73–7.
38. Antiplatelet Trialists Collaboration, Collaborative overview of randomised trials of antiplatelet treatment, Part 1. Prevention of death, myocardial infarction, and stroke by prolonged antiplatelet therapy in various categories of patients, Br Med J (1994) **343**:139–42.
39. Algra A, van Gijn J, Aspirin at any dose above 30mg offers only modest protection after cerebral ischaemia, J Neurol Neurosurg Psychiatry (1996) **60**:197–9.
40. Hass WK, Easton JD, Adams HP Jr et al, A randomised trial comparing ticlopidine hydrochloride with aspirin for the prevention of stroke in high-risk patients, N Engl J Med (1989) **321**:501–7.
41. CAPRIE Steering Committee, A randomised, blinded, trial of clopidogrel versus aspirin in patients at risk of ischaemic events (CAPRIE), Lancet (1996) **348**:1329–39.
42. Diener H, Cunha L, Forbes C et al, European Stroke Prevention Study 2, Dipyridamole and acetylsalicylic acid in the secondary prevention of stroke, J Neurol Sci (1996) **143**:1–13.
43. Lefkovits J, Plow EF, Topol EJ, Platelet glycoprotein IIb/IIIa receptors in cardiovascular medicine, N Engl J Med (1995) **332**:1553–9.
44. Mousa SA, Mu DX, Lucchesi BR, Prevention of carotid artery thrombosis by oral platelet GPIIb/IIIa antagonist in dogs, Stroke (1997) **28**:830–6.
45. EAFT (European Atrial Fibrillation Trial) Study Group, Secondary prevention in non-rheumatic atrial fibrillation after transient ischaemic attack or minor stroke, Lancet (1993) **342**:1255–62.
46. North American Symptomatic Carotid Endarterectomy Trial Collaborators, Beneficial effect of carotid endarterectomy in symptomatic patients with high grade carotid stenosis, N Engl J Med (1991) **325**:445–53.
47. European Carotid Surgery Trialists' Collaborative (ECST) Group, MRC European Carotid Surgery Trial: interim results for symptomatic patients with severe (70–99%) or with mild (0–20%) carotid stenosis, Lancet (1991) **337**:1235–43.
48. Bladin CF, Davis SM, Burton K et al, Recommendations on the use of percutaneous transluminal angioplasty (PTA) for the treatment of extracranial atherosclerotic vascular disease—The Australian Association of Neurologists, Aust NZ J Med (1998) **28**:654–6.

Index

Note: Page numbers in *italic* refer to tables or figures in the text

activities of daily living (ADL) training **139**
ADDTC criteria **8–9**
   diagnosis of probable VAD **106**
   neuroimaging requirements **153, 154,** *155*
   subtypes of VAD **102**
administration orders **193**
affective disorders **7–8, 89–91**
   treatment **194**
   see also depression
African-American populations
   family carers **202–3**
   stroke risk **30**
ageing, normal
   confounding VAD **69–70**
   EEG changes **167–8**
   ischaemic stroke risk **224**
   white matter changes **80–1, 153**
aggressiveness **126–7**
AIDS dementia complex **170**
akinesia **120–1**
alcohol use
   ischaemic stroke risk **226**
   withdrawal **193**
Alzheimer's Association **191, 204**
Alzheimer's Disease (AD)
   confusional episodes **88**
   differentiation from VAD
     cognitive deficits **137–8**
     imaging **147–8**
   EEG changes **168–9**
   impacts on family carers **200–2**
   institutional placement **206**
   mortality **206–7**
   regional prevalence **40–2, 60, 65–6**
   research **1**
   SPET scanning changes **157–9**
   vascular risk factors **22**
   white matter changes **80**
amnestic syndromes **89, 135**
amyloid angiopathy **70, 74, 92**
angiotensin-converting enzyme (ACE) inhibitors **225**
angiotensin II blockers **225**
angular gyrus lesions **87, 134**
anosognosia **125**
antiandrogens **193**
anticoagulation **183, 184, 225, 230**
anticonvulsants **194, 218**

antidepressants **194–5, 196**
antihypertensive agents **182–3, 225**
antiplatelet agents **139, 184, 229–30**
antipsychotic agents **217–18**
   frontal disinhibition **193**
   post-stroke mania **194**
   schizophrenia-like states **194**
Anton's syndrome **126**
anxiety disorders **123–4**
   management **196**
apallic syndromes **70–1**
apathy **120–1**
aphasia **133**
apolipoprotein E genotypes **29, 136**
apoplexy **3–4**
apraxia **133**
aprosodia **133**
aspirin **139, 184, 186–7, 225**
aspontaneity **120–1**
atrial fibrillation
   anticoagulation **183, 184, 225, 230**
   antiplatelet therapy **184**
   stroke risk **225**
   warfarin therapy **230**
auditory perception disorders **122**

barbiturate-induced EEG changes **166, 171**
BD, *see* Binswanger's disease
behavioural changes in dementia **216–17**
   and the family carer **205**
   non-pharmacological management **218**
   pharmacological management of **217–18**
behavioural psychiatric symptoms of VAD *124*
behavioural therapy, *see* cognitive behavioural therapy
benzodiazepines **166, 193, 196, 218**
beta blockers **225**
Binswanger's disease (BD) **72–3**
   cognitive impairments **136**
   depression **91**
   EEG changes **170**
   primary symptoms **120**
bipolar disorder **90–1**
   management **194**
body image disturbances **122**
border zone infarcts **74, 81**

brain reserve capacity **69–70**
brainstem lesions **89**
bromocriptine **186**
buflomidil **186**
building design features **139, 214–15**
Bürgers disease **8**
buspirone **196**

CADASIL, *see* cerebral autosomal dominant arteriopathy with subcortical infarcts and leukoencephalopathy
calcium channel antagonists **225**
California criteria, *see* ADDTC criteria
Canada, cerebrovascular disease **30**
Capgras syndrome *122*
CAPRIE trial **229**
carbamazepine **218**
cardiac disease **7, 71–2, 225**
care, *see* family carer; long-term care
carotid angioplasty, percutaneous transluminal **230**
carotid bruits **226–7**
carotid endarterectomy **227, 230**
carotid stenosis **226–7**
CASI, *see* Cognitive Abilities Screening Instrument
caudate infarcts **86–7, 135**
cerebral arteriosclerosis, increases in **25**
cerebral autosomal dominant arteriopathy with subcortical infarcts and leukoencephalopathy (CADASIL) **6, 73, 221, 223**
  symptoms **120, 136**
cerebral blood flow (CBF) **5**
  SPET scanning **157–9**
  and white matter infarction **81–2**
Cerebral Embolism Task Force **71**
cerebral metabolism **157, 169, 171**
China, epidemiology studies
  ageing population **47,** *48*
  attitudes to the elderly **48**
  care-givers study **51**
  dementia study review **49**
  family structure **47–8**
  health facilities for the elderly **48–9**
  heterogeneity of population **53**
  incidence of VAD **50**
  mortality of VAD **53**
  prevalence of VAD **50–1,** *52*
Chinese-American populations **30**
chlorthalidone **182**
cholestyramine **185**
cholinesterase inhibitors **192**
choreoatheloic movements **87**
cigarette smoking **59, 186, 226**
citalopram **194–5, 196**
classification of VAD
  approaches to **99–100**
  by clinical syndrome *100*

  historical perspective **3–4**
  by location of lesion *100*
  subtypes **102–3,** *105*
  by type of lesion *100*
  by vascular aetiology **70–1,** *100*
  see also clinical criteria for VAD
clinical criteria for VAD **8–9, 26–7, 104–8**
  comparison of systems **109,** *110*
  need for international agreement **109**
  neuroimaging requirements in **26–7, 108–9, 153–6**
  subtypes **102–3,** *105*
  see also individual clinical criteria
clofibrate **185**
clopridogrel **229**
Cognitive Abilities Screening Instrument (CASI) **35–6**
  feasibility study in Japan **36–8**
cognitive assessment **131–2**
cognitive behavioural therapy (CBT) **139**
  anxiety disorders **196–7**
  depression **195**
cognitive enhancing agents **192**
cognitive impairments in VAD **116–17**
  Binswanger's disease **136**
  differentiation from other dementias **137–8**
  inherited arteriolopathies **136**
  medical treatment **138–9, 192**
  mixed dementias **137**
  multi-infarct dementia **133**
  strategic infarct dementia **133–5**
  white matter infarcts **135–6**
collagen vascular disease **74**
computed tomography (CT) **26–7, 145–6**
  differentiation of VAD/AD **148**
  white matter changes **150–1,** *152*
confusional episodes **88, 126**
consciousness, clouding of **88–9**
Consortium of Canadian Centers for Clinical Cognitive Research Consensus Statement **25–6**
cortical and subcortical infarct dementia *71,* **73–4**
cortical synapse loss **70**
cortico-bulbar tract lesions **89**
Creutzfeldt-Jakob disease (CJD) **138, 170**
cribiform state **80–1, 153**
crying **121**
CT, *see* computed tomography
cyproterone acetate **193**

death of patient **206**
De Clerambault syndrome *122*
delirium **126**
  aetiology **88**
  management **193**
delusions **126**
  management of **194**
dementia of the senium **70**

dementia support groups **191**
denial of illness **126**
depersonalization in care **214**
depression
  assessment of **125**
  and cognitive deficits **90, 125**
  and left hemisphere lesions **7–8, 89–90, 125, 133**
  Binswanger's disease **91**
  in family carer **202**
  multi-infarct dementia **91**
  symptoms **124–5**
  treatment **194–5**
  white matter lesions **91**
depressive pseudodementia **168**
design features of institutions **214–15**
diabetes mellitus
  control **185, 186–7**
  stroke risk **225–6**
  VAD risk **185**
diaschisis **157, 158**
dipyridamole **184, 229**
disinhibition **121**
  management of **192–3**
diuretics **225**
donepezil hydrochloride **192**
dopamine-blocking agents **194**
drop attacks **88**
DSM-III-R criteria **8, 50–1**
DSM-IV criteria **8, 104**
  neuroimaging requirements **153,** *155*
dysarthria-clumsy hand syndrome **119**
dyscalculia **87**
dysgrafia **87**

EAFT, *see* European Atrial Fibrillation Trial
East Boston Study **20**
eating problems **125, 202**
ECST, *see* European Carotid Surgery Trial
electroconvulsive therapy (ECT) **195**
electroencephalogram (EEG) **165–72**
  basic features **165–6**
  brain mapping **157, 166–7**
  coherence analysis **167, 171**
  eyes closed/eyes open ratio **167, 171**
  and functional neuroimaging **169, 171**
  non-linear analysis **167**
  in non-vascular dementias **168–70**
  in normal ageing **167–8**
  periodic sharp wave complexes **170**
  quantitative techniques **166**
  rapid eye movement sleep recording **167**
  reproducibility **167**
  serial studies **169**
  in VAD **170–1**
emotional blunting **119, 121**
emotional lability **121**
  management **196**
environment of dementia patient **139, 214–15**

epidemiology of VAD
  age **56, 57–8, 65**
  ageing of populations **66–7**
  diagnostic criteria **63**
  diagnostic methods **55, 63–4**
  gender **58–9, 60, 64, 65**
  historical trends **66**
  incidence **57–60, 65**
  institutionalized subjects **19–20, 64**
  limitations of data **55–6**
  methodological variation **63–4**
  mixed dementias **55–6**
  prevalence **56–7, 64**
  regional differences **59–60, 65–6**
  see also individual countries and regions
EPMID, *see* European Pantoxifylline Multi-infarct Dementia Study Group
ESPS, *see* European Stroke Prevention Study
etat crible **80–1, 153**
EURODEM project **57**
European Atrial Fibrillation Trial (EAFT) **230**
European Carotid Surgery Trial (ECST) **230**
European Pantoxifylline Multi-infarct Dementia Study Group (EPMID) **186**
European Stroke Prevention Study (ESPS) **184, 229**
European Trans-National Alzheimer's Study **212**
Europe, epidemiology
  auxiliary examinations **18–19**
  diagnostic criteria application **20–1**
  differential diagnosis of VAD **21**
  differential mortality **19**
  incidence **17–18**
  inclusion of institutionalized subjects **19–20**
  inclusion of stroke subjects **21–2**
  prevalence **15–16**
exercise **226**
extrapyramidal syndromes **194**

familial vascular encephalopathies **6, 120, 136**
family carer
  comparative effects of VAD and AD **200–2**
  depression **202**
  early stages of dementia **204–5**
  education and support for **191**
  ethnic and cultural factors **202–3**
  financial and legal management **193, 204**
  impacts of dementia **199**
  impacts of stroke **200**
  institutional placement of patient **206**
  language difficulties **203**
  late and terminal stages of dementia **205–6**

family carer – *cont.*
  middle stages of dementia **205**
  predictors of stress **200**
  and primary care physician **215–16**
  traditional gender roles **202**
FICS'M mnemonic **216**
finger dysgnosia **87**
fluctuating course of VAD **87–9**
fluoxetine **196**
Fregoli syndrome *122*
frontal disinhibition **121**
  management **192–3**
frontal lobe symptoms **86–7**, *118*, **121**
frontotemporal dementia (FTD) **6**
  cognitive impairments **138**
  EEG changes **169**
  white matter changes **80**

gait problems **87**
gender
  and ischaemic stroke risk **224**
  and VAD risk **58–9, 64, 65**
genetics of dementia **6, 29, 136**
Gerstmann syndrome **87, 134**
Ginkgo biloba extract **192**
global brain syndrome *118*
globus pallidus infarcts **135**
glycosaminoglycan angiopathy **74**
Gothenburg study **20**

Hachinski Ischemic Scale (HIS) **26, 87, 153**, *154*
  clinical features *131*
  development **5**
  differentiation of VAD/AD **137**
haematocrit, elevated **226**
haemorrhagic dementia **71, 74, 224, 226**
hallucinations **88, 126**
  management **194**
haloperidol **193**
herpes encephalitis **170**
hippocampus
  atrophy **148, 159**
  infarcts **89, 119**
Hispanic-American populations **30**
HMG-CoA reductase inhibitors **185–6, 226**
hormone replacement therapy **186**
Huntington's disease **87, 138**
hydrocephalic dementia **87**
hypercholesterolaemia **185–6, 226**
hyperglycaemia **226**
hypertension **5, 22, 224–5**
  control **182–3**
  diabetes mellitus **185, 186**
hypomania **90**
hypoperfusion **5**
  white matter infarction **81–2**
hypotension **5, 81–2**
  episodic postural, case study **91–2**

hypoxic-hypoperfusive dementia **5, 70–1, 74, 81–2**

ICD–10 criteria
  definition of VAD **8, 104–5**
  neuroimaging requirements **153**, *154*
  VAD subtypes **102**, *105*
inflammatory vascular disease **8**
information and support services **191, 204**
  primary care physician **216**
inheritance, patterns of **6**
insight **121, 125**
institutional building design **214–15**
institutional placement **206**
  delaying **213**
  cultural/ethnic factors **202–3**
  and prognosis **206–7**
  see also long-term care
intermetamorphosis syndrome *122*
internal capsule, genu, infarcts **134**
International Psychogeriatric Association (IPA) **216–17**
ischaemic penumbra **72, 88**
Italian Americans families **202**

Japan, epidemiology studies
  ageing population **33**
  awareness of mental health **34**
  CASI feasibility study **35–8**
  change in AD/VAD prevalence **40–2**
    procedural factors **42–4**
    socio-demographic factors **43–4**
  diagnostic interviews **34–5**
  incidence studies **44**
  screening methods **34**, *35*
  survey response rates **34**
Japanese-American populations **40, 44, 66**

KAME project **40, 44, 66**
Kungsholmen Project **18**

lacunar state, *see* subcortical vascular dementia
language impairment **137–8**
large vessel dementia **70, 71–2**
  see also multi-infarct dementia; strategic infarct dementia
left cerebral hemisphere lesions **7–8, 89–90, 125, 133**
leukoaraiosis **26, 150–3, 221**
Lewy body dementia **88, 138, 151**
lithium carbonate **194**
lithium toxic encephalopathy **170**
long-term care **211–219**
  principles **212–13**
  quality of the environment **214–15**
  quality of life **213–14**
  research **211, 218–19**
low density lipoprotein (LDL) **226**

Index

magnetic resonance imaging (MRI) **26–7, 146**
   white matter changes **151,** *152*
   differentiation of VAD and AD **148**
magnetic resonance spectroscopy **157**
mamillary body infarct **89**
management, medical **138–9, 181–7**
   anticoagulation **183, 184, 225, 230**
   antithrombosis **139, 184, 229–30**
   diabetes mellitus **185, 225–6**
   hypercholesterolaemia **185–6, 226**
   hypertension **182–3, 224–5**
management, psychiatric disorders **191–7**
   anxiety states **196–7**
   cognitive impairment **138–9, 192**
   delirium **193–4**
   depression **194–5**
   emotional lability **196**
   frontal disinhibition **192–3**
   information/support **191**
   mania **194**
   schizophrenia-like states **194**
mania **90–1**
   management **194**
memantine **186**
memory failure **89, 134–5**
microvascular disease, *see* small vessel dementia
middle temporal gyrus lesions **88**
migraine with aura **120**
Mini-Mental State (MMS) examination **38, 125, 132**
misidentification syndromes **122**
mixed dementias
   cognitive impairments **137**
   in epidemiology studies **55**
   neuroimaging **159**
   white matter changes **79–80**
mobility of patient **216**
mood disorders, *see* affective disorders
mortality of VAD **206–7**
motor agitation **125**
MRI, *see* magnetic resonance imaging
multi-infarct dementia (MID) **5, 26, 71–2**
   cognitive impairments **133**
   and depression **91**
   primary symptoms **117–19**
myocardial infarction **181**
myoinositol **157**

N-acetyl aspartate (NAA) levels **157**
narcosis **70**
NASCET trial **230**
native Americans **30**
neurochemical imaging **159–60**
neurofibrillary tangles **70**
neuroimaging **6–7**
   clinical criteria requirements **26–7, 108–9, 153–6**
   functional imaging **157–9**
   combined with EEG **169, 171**
   in mixed dementias **159**
   role in diagnosis **145**
   structural imaging **145–7**
      changes in dementia **149–50**
      differentiating VAD and AD **147–8, 159**
      extent of change causing dementia **149**
      interpretation of changes **147, 153**
      white matter changes **150–3**
neuropathology of VAD
   ageing process **69–70**
   classification of VAD subtypes **70–1**
   haemorrhagic dementia **74**
   hypoxic-hypoperfusive dementia **74**
   large vessel dementia **71–2**
   small vessel dementia **72–4**
neurotransmitter levels **89**
nicergoline **186**
nimodipine **186**
NINDS-AIREN criteria **9, 20–1, 26–7, 131–2**
   diagnosis of probable VAD **107–8**
   multi-infarct dementia **133**
   neuroimaging requirements **108, 153–6**
   neuropsychological evaluation **132**
   subtypes of VAD **102**
nitrendipine **182**
nocturnal confusion **88**
North America, epidemiology studies
   development of diagnostic criteria **26–7**
   historical studies **26**
   incidence studies **28–30**
   prevalence **28**
   stroke incidence **29–30**
   vascular cognitive impairment **27**
nortriptyline **194–5, 196**
Nun study **29**
nursing homes, *see* institutional placement
nystagmus **88**

occupational therapist **205, 216**
olanzapine **193, 194**
orthostatic hypotension, case study **91–2**
oxazepam **196**

panic **196**
paramedian mesencephalic-diencephalic infarcts (PMDI) **119**
parietal lobe syndrome **87,** *118*
Parkinson's disease **138, 159**
   EEG changes **169–70**
patho-anatomical classification of VAD **70–1**
pentoxifylline **186**
penumbra zone **72, 88**
personality changes **121**
   management of **192–3**
'personhood' **214**
PET, *see* positron emission tomography

phobic disorders **196**
Pick's disease **80, 138**
platelet glycoprotein IIb/IIIa antagonists **229–30**
polyarteritis nodosa **8**
polycythaemia **226**
polymyalgia rheumatica **8**
population ageing **66–7**
    China **47**, *48*
    Japan **33**
posatirelin **139**
positron emission tomography (PET) **157**
    combined with EEG **169, 171**
posterior cerebral artery occlusion **89**
present behaviour examination (PBE) **217**
prevention **138–9, 222–3**
    primary strategies **223–7**
    secondary strategies **181–2, 227–31**
    see also individual risk factors
primary care physician **215–16**
progressive supranuclear palsy **138**
PROGRESS study **223**
propentofylline **138–9**
prognosis of VAD **206–7**
pseudodementia **168**
psychological symptoms of VAD **122–7**, *123*
psychological therapy **139**
    anxiety disorders **196–7**
    depression **195**
psychotropic drugs **193**

quality of environment **214–15**
quality of life **213–14**

recognitions, false **122**
reduplication paramnesia **126**
regional brain syndromes **117**, *118*
rehabilitation, cognitive **139**
rheumatic heart disease **225**
right cerebral hemisphere lesions **89–90**
right-left disorientation **87**
risk factors for stroke **181–2**, *224*, *see also individual risk factors*
risperidone **193, 194**
ritualistic behaviour **122**
rivastigmine **192**
Rotterdam Study **17–18, 185**
Russia, prevalence of VAD **57**

schizophrenia-like states **194**
screaming behaviour **125**
selective incomplete white matter infarction (SIWI) **79**
    in Alzheimer's disease **80**
    in frontotemporal dementias **80**
selective neuronal loss **72**
selective serotonin reuptake inhibitors (SSRIs) **195, 196, 218**
semiapallic syndromes **70–1**
senile plaques **70**

serotonin and norepinephrine reuptake inhibitors (SNRI) **218**
sertraline **196**
sexual advances **193**
silent stroke **86, 150**
single photon emission tomography (SPET) **157–9**
    combined with EEG studies **169, 171**
    compared to structural imaging **159**
sleep disturbance **125, 216**
small vessel dementia **8**, *71*, **72–3**
    cortical and subcortical **73–4**
    subcortical **73**
    see also subcortical vascular dementia
SNRI, *see* serotonin and norepinephrine reuptake inhibitors
spaced retrieval **139**
SPET, *see* single photon emission tomography
spirituality **214**
SSRI, *see* selective serotonin reuptake inhibitors
statin drugs **185–6, 226**
Stepwise Comparative Status Analysis (STEP) **116**
'step-wise' decline **86, 87–9**
    effects on family carer **201**
stereotypical behaviour **122**
steroid-sensitive dementias **8**
strategic infarct dementia **5**, **72**, **103**, *222*
    cognitive impairments **133–5**
    primary symptoms **119**
Stroke Society **204**
subarachnoid haemorrhage *71*, **74, 224**
    and cigarette smoking **226**
subcortical arteriosclerotic encephalopathy, *see* Binswanger's disease
subcortical brain syndrome *118*
subcortical disconnection syndromes **91**
subcortical vascular dementia **73, 103**
    cognitive impairments **135–6**
    primary symptoms **119–20**
summational dementia **70**
symptoms of VAD
    correlation with pathology **85**
        affective symptoms **89–91**
        fluctuations **86, 87–9**
        frontal lobe **86–7**
        onset and progress **86**
        parietal lobe **87**
    general description **115–16**
    history and status examination **116**
    primary **117, 120–2**
        in familial vascular encephalopathies **120**
        regional syndromes **117**, *118*
        in strategic infarct dementia **119**
        in subcortical vascular dementia **119–20**

secondary psychiatric **122–7**
   behavioural *124*
   psychological *123*
   see also individual symptoms
synapse loss, cortical **70**
systemic lupus erythematosus (SLE) **8**
Syst-Eur trial **22**

temazepam **196**
temporal lobe atrophy **148, 159**
terminal care **206**
thalamic infarcts **72, 119,** *222*
   cognitive impairments **134–5**
thiamine replacement **193**
ticlopidine **139, 184, 229**
   side effects **229**
trazodone **194–5**
tricyclic antidepressants **195, 218**

UK Prospective Diabetes Study **185**
urinary incontinence **87, 216**

valproic acid **218**
valvular heart disease **225**
vascular cognitive impairment **27, 116–17**
'vascular depression' **8, 91**
venous occlusions **71, 74**

verbal memory loss **134**
vertebro-basilar insufficiency **88–9**
vertigo, episodic **88**
vitamin deficiency **70, 193**

Wallerian degeneration **81**
wandering behaviour **125**
warfarin **225, 230**
white matter changes **5–6, 77–83**
   in Alzheimer's disease **80**
   clinical detection **82**
   deep **151–3**
   and depression **91**
   diagnosis and differentiation **82–3**
   diffuse **78**
   diffuse pathology alone **79**
   focal **77–8**
   focal and diffuse **78–9**
   in frontotemporal dementia **80**
   histopathological detection **82**
   mood disorders **90–1**
   neuroimaging **150–3**
   in normal ageing **80–1, 153**
   pathogenesis **81–2**
   periventricular **151,** *152*
   volume of lesions **91**

ziprisadone **193, 194**